1999
YEAR BOOK OF
OPHTHALMOLOGY®

Statement of Purpose

The YEAR BOOK Service

The YEAR BOOK series was devised in 1901 by practicing health professionals who observed that the literature of medicine and related disciplines had become so voluminous that no one individual could read and place in perspective every potential advance in a major specialty. In the final decade of the 20th century, this recognition is more acutely true than it was in 1901.

More than merely a series of books, YEAR BOOK volumes are the tangible results of a unique service designed to accomplish the following:

- to *survey* a wide range of journals of proven value
- to *select* from those journals papers representing significant advances and statements of important clinical principles
- to provide *abstracts* of those articles that are readable, convenient summaries of their key points
- to provide *commentary* about those articles to place them in perspective

These publications grow out of a unique process that calls on the talents of outstanding authorities in clinical and fundamental disciplines, trained literature specialists, and professional writers, all supported by the resources of Mosby, the world's preeminent publisher for the health professions.

The Literature Base

Mosby and its editors survey approximately 500 journals published worldwide, covering the full range of the health professions. On an annual basis, the publisher examines usage patterns and polls its expert authorities to add new journals to the literature base and to delete journals that are no longer useful as potential YEAR BOOK sources.

The Literature Survey

The publisher's team of literature specialists, all of whom are trained and experienced health professionals, examines every original, peer-reviewed article in each journal issue. More than 250,000 articles per year are scanned systematically, including title, text, illustrations, tables, and references. Each scan is compared, article by article, to the search strategies that the publisher has developed in consultation with the 270 outside experts who form the pool of YEAR BOOK editors. A given article may be reviewed by any number of editors, from one to a dozen or more, regardless of the discipline for which the paper was originally published. In turn, each editor who receives the article reviews it to determine whether the article should be included in the YEAR BOOK. This decision is based on the article's inherent quality, its probable usefulness to readers of that YEAR BOOK, and the editor's goal to represent a balanced picture of a given field in each volume of the YEAR BOOK. In addition, the editor indicates when to include figures and tables from the article to help the YEAR BOOK reader better understand the information.

Of the quarter million articles scanned each year, only 5% are selected for detailed analysis within the YEAR BOOK series, thereby assuring readers of the high value of every selection.

The Abstract

The publisher's abstracting staff is headed by a seasoned medical professional and includes individuals with training in the life sciences, medicine, and other areas, plus extensive experience in writing for the health professions and related industries. Each selected article is assigned to a specific writer on this abstracting staff. The abstractor, guided in many cases by notations supplied by the expert editor, writes a structured, condensed summary designed so that the reader can rapidly acquire the essential information contained in the article.

The Commentary

The YEAR BOOK editorial boards, sometimes assisted by guest commentators, write comments that place each article in perspective for the reader. This provides the reader with the equivalent of a personal consultation with a leading international authority—an opportunity to better understand the value of the article and to benefit from the authority's thought processes in assessing the article.

Additional Editorial Features

The editorial boards of each YEAR BOOK organize the abstracts and comments to provide a logical and satisfying sequence of information. To enhance the organization, editors also provide introductions to sections or individual chapters, comments linking a number of abstracts, citations to additional literature, and other features.

The published YEAR BOOK contains enhanced bibliographic citations for each selected article, including extended listings of multiple authors and identification of author affiliations. Each YEAR BOOK contains a Table of Contents specific to that year's volume. From year to year, the Table of Contents for a given YEAR BOOK will vary depending on developments within the field.

Every YEAR BOOK contains a list of the journals from which papers have been selected. This list represents a subset of approximately 500 journals surveyed by the publisher and occasionally reflects a particularly pertinent article from a journal that is not surveyed on a routine basis.

Finally, each volume contains a comprehensive subject index and an index to authors of each selected paper.

The 1999 Year Book Series

Year Book of Allergy, Asthma, and Clinical Immunology: Drs. Rosenwasser, Boguniewicz, Borish, Routes, Spahn, and Weber

Year Book of Anesthesiology and Pain Management®: Drs. Tinker, Abram, Chestnut, Roizen, Rothenberg, and Wood

Year Book of Cardiology®: Drs. Schlant, Collins, Gersh, Graham, Kaplan, and Waldo

Year Book of Chiropractic®: Dr. Lawrence

Year Book of Critical Care Medicine®: Drs. Parrillo, Balk, Calvin, Franklin, and Shapiro

Year Book of Dentistry®: Drs. Meskin, Berry, Jeffcoat, Leinfelder, Roser, Summitt, and Zakariasen

Year Book of Dermatology and Dermatologic Surgery™: Drs. Thiers and Lang

Year Book of Diagnostic Radiology®: Drs. Osborn, Birdwell, Dalinka, Groskin, Maynard, Pentecost, Ros, Smirniotopoulos, and Young

Year Book of Emergency Medicine®: Drs. Wagner, Dronen, Davidson, King, Niemann, and Hamilton

Year Book of Endocrinology®: Drs. Bagdade, Braverman, Fitzpatrick, Horton, Kannan, Landsberg, Molitch, Morley, Odell, Poehlman, and Rogol

Year Book of Family Practice®: Drs. Berg, Bowman, Davidson, Dexter, and Scherger

Year Book of Gastroenterology: Drs. Aliperti and Fleshman

Year Book of Hand Surgery®: Drs. Amadio and Hentz

Year Book of Medicine®: Drs. Klahr, Frishman, Malawista, Mandell, Jett, Young, Barkin, and Bagdade

Year Book of Neonatal and Perinatal Medicine®: Drs. Fanaroff, Maisels, and Stevenson

Year Book of Nephrology, Hypertension, and Mineral Metabolism: Drs. Schwab, Bennett, Emmett, Hostetter, and Moe

Year Book of Neurology and Neurosurgery®: Drs. Bradley and Gibbs

Year Book of Nuclear Medicine®: Drs. Gottschalk, Blaufox, Coleman, Strauss, and Zubal

Year Book of Obstetrics, Gynecology, and Women's Health®: Drs. Mishell, Herbst, and Kirschbaum

Year Book of Oncology®: Drs. Ozols, Eisenberg, Glatstein, Loehrer, and Urba

Year Book of Ophthalmology®: Drs. Wilson, Augsburger, Cohen, Eagle, Grossman, Laibson, Maguire, Nelson, Penne, Rapuano, Sergott, Spaeth, Tipperman, Ms. Gosfield, and Ms. Salmon

Year Book of Orthopedics®: Drs. Morrey, Beauchamp, Currier, Tolo, Trigg, and Swiontkowski

Year Book of Otolaryngology–Head and Neck Surgery®: Drs. Paparella, Holt, and Otto

Year Book of Pathology and Laboratory Medicine®: Drs. Raab, Cohen, Dabbs, Olson, and Stanley

Year Book of Pediatrics®: Dr. Stockman

Year Book of Plastic, Reconstructive, and Aesthetic Surgery®: Drs. Miller, Bartlett, Garner, McKinney, Ruberg, Salisbury, and Smith

Year Book of Psychiatry and Applied Mental Health®: Drs. Talbott, Ballenger, Frances, Lydiard, Meltzer, Jensen, and Tasman

Year Book of Pulmonary Disease®: Drs. Jett, Castro, Maurer, Peters, Phillips, and Ryu

Year Book of Rheumatology, Arthritis, and Musculoskeletal Disease™: Drs. Panush, Hadler, Hellmann, LeRoy, Pisetsky, and Simon

Year Book of Sports Medicine®: Drs. Shephard, Drinkwater, Eichner, Torg, Alexander, and Mr. George

Year Book of Surgery®: Drs. Copeland, Bland, Deitch, Eberlein, Howard, Luce, Seeger, Souba, and Sugarbaker

Year Book of Urology®: Drs. Andriole and Coplen

Year Book of Vascular Surgery®: Dr. Porter

1999
The Year Book of OPHTHALMOLOGY®

Editor-in-Chief
Richard P. Wilson, M.D.
Attending Surgeon, Glaucoma Service, Wills Eye Hospital; Professor of Ophthalmology, Jefferson Medical College of Thomas Jefferson University, Philadelphia, Pennsylvania

Wills Eye Hospital®

Mosby

St. Louis Baltimore Boston Carlsbad Naples New York Philadelphia Portland London
Madrid Mexico City Singapore Sydney Tokyo Toronto Wiesbaden

Mosby
Dedicated to Publishing Excellence

Publisher: Cheryl A. Smart
Associate Publisher: Susan Patterson
Developmental Editor: Colleen Cook
Manager, Periodical Editing: Kirk Swearingen
Production Editor: Stephanie M. Geels
Project Supervisor, Production: Joy Moore
Production Assistant: Karie House
Manager, Literature Services: Idelle L. Winer
Illustrations and Permissions Coordinator: Chidi C. Ukabam

1999 EDITION

Printed in the United States of America
Composition by Reed Technology and Information Services, Inc.
Printing/binding by Maple-Vail

Editorial Office:
Mosby, Inc.
11830 Westline Industrial Drive
St. Louis, MO 63146
Customer Service: customer.support@mosby.com
www.mosby.com/Mosby/CustomerSupport/index.html

International Standard Serial Number: 0084-392X
International Standard Book Number: 0-8151-9714-4

Editorial Board

Table of Contents

Journals Represented

Mosby and its editors survey approximately 500 journals for its abstract and commentary publications. From these journals, the editors select the articles to be abstracted. Journals represented in this YEAR BOOK are listed below.

Acta Paediatrica
American Journal of Human Genetics
American Journal of Managed Care
American Journal of Neuroradiology
American Journal of Ophthalmology
American Journal of Pathology
Anaesthesia
Annals of Neurology
Archives of Ophthalmology
British Journal of Ophthalmology
Clinical Pharmacology and Therapeutics
Cornea
Investigative Ophthalmology and Visual Science
Journal of Cataract and Refractive Surgery
Journal of Neurosurgery
Journal of Pediatric Ophthalmology and Strabismus
Journal of Thoracic and Cardiovascular Surgery
Journal of the American Association for Pediatric Ophthalmology and Strabismus
Journal of the American Medical Association
Journal of the American Optometric Association
Laboratory Investigation
Medical Care
Medical Economics
Medical Group Management Journal
Neurology
New England Journal of Medicine
Ophthalmic Plastic and Reconstructive Surgery
Ophthalmic Surgery and Lasers
Ophthalmologica
Ophthalmology
Physician's Advisory
Radiotherapy and Oncology
Stroke
Transactions of the American Ophthalmological Society
World Journal of Surgery

STANDARD ABBREVIATIONS

The following terms are abbreviated in this edition: acquired immunodeficiency syndrome (AIDS), cardiopulmonary resuscitation (CPR), central nervous system (CNS), cerebrospinal fluid (CSF), computed tomography (CT), deoxyribonucleic acid (DNA), diopter (D), electrocardiography (ECG), health maintenance organization (HMO), human immunodeficiency virus (HIV), intensive care unit (ICU), intramuscular (IM), intravenous (IV), magnetic resonance (MR) imaging (MRI), ribonucleic acid (RNA), and ultrasound (US).

NOTE

The YEAR BOOK OF OPHTHALMOLOGY® is a literature survey service providing abstracts of articles published in the professional literature. Every effort is made to assure the accuracy of the information presented in these pages. Neither the editors nor the publisher of the YEAR BOOK OF OPHTHALMOLOGY® can be responsible for errors in the original materials. The editors' comments are their own opinions. Mention of specific products within this publication does not constitute endorsement.

To facilitate the use of the YEAR BOOK OF OPHTHALMOLOGY® as a reference tool, all illustrations and tables included in this publication are now identified as they appear in the original article. This change is meant to help the reader recognize that any illustration or table appearing in the YEAR BOOK OF OPHTHALMOLOGY® may be only one of many in the original article. For this reason, figure and table numbers will often appear to be out of sequence within the YEAR BOOK OF OPHTHALMOLOGY®.

Introduction

Few readers read introductions. Our busy lives force us to concentrate on the essentials. The time required for our professional obligations has expanded dramatically. Physicians are forced to carve out time from patient care or their private lives to accommodate the added burden of night and weekend meetings devoted to facing the challenges of health care reform. Almost as aggravating to the obsessive-compulsive (I freely admit I fall into that category, and I would certainly want any physician taking care of me to also exhibit those traits) is the information explosion. What we thought was turning into a paperless world is now engulfing us in more and more paper. The plethora of ophthalmic throwaways increases daily, along with the glut of advertisements and solicitations. Join one conservation group and you are inundated with heart-wrenching and graphic examples of environmental collapse from 30 other organizations that bought the mailing list from the first group to which you contributed. Each appeal pulls at your conscience, imploring you to contribute money or time, or both. The only way to maintain equilibrium is to slash and burn, to eliminate whole categories of paper crossing your tabletop. But the nagging question is always there: Did I miss something important?

The YEAR BOOK OF OPHTHALMOLOGY shines in this arena. No longer are you forced to scan the reams of paper that land on any horizontal surface in your home or office like silt on the bottom of the Mississippi River, obliterating important memos and articles in masses of everyday matters. With the YEAR BOOK, you have contracted with a recognized group of experts to select the most important happenings in ophthalmology and put them in perspective for you.

Although I clearly think we do an excellent job at this, we are always looking to improve. As we adapt to the changes in health care, our information-gathering systems must also be adjusted. I have tried to meet your needs by adding sections on practice management by Patricia Salmon and health law by Alice Gosfield. These additions may not be enough. I would appreciate any suggestions you have concerning substance, style, or other areas we should be covering. Please contact me by E-mail (wilson@wills-glaucoma.org), fax (215-928-0166), or mail (Glaucoma Service, Wills Eye Hospital, 900 Walnut Street, Philadelphia, PA 19107).

Richard P. Wilson, M.D.

1 Cataract

Cataract Surgery 1998

by Richard Tipperman, M.D.

There were many advances in cataract surgery in 1998. It is exciting to read increasing numbers of articles reporting on the safety and efficacy of phakic intraocular lenses. In addition, for the practicing anterior segment surgeon there were several articles that should help improve the safety and outcomes of cataract surgery.

Pseudoexfoliation, Zonular Weakness, and Capsule Tension Rings

One of the most common problems routinely encountered in cataract surgery is weak zonules in the presence of pseudoexfoliation syndrome. As noted in two articles reviewed in this YEAR BOOK, pseudoexfoliation syndrome is associated with increased complications of capsular rupture and vitreous loss. In addition, the zonular weakness associated with pseudoexfoliation syndrome can lead to late intraocular lens (IOL) dislocation.

Sun and Gimbel (Abstract 1–12) reported an in vitro study of the efficacy of the capsular tension ring in managing zonular dialysis at the time of cataract surgery. The capsular tension ring was also reviewed in the 1997 YEAR BOOK OF OPHTHALMOLOGY. The zonular tension ring can be placed immediately after capsulorhexis is performed to support the capsule during phacoemulsification. The ring is then left in place to help ensure IOL centration. By stabilizing a weak zonular support system, the ring should make cataract removal safer and also improve the long-term centration of IOLs implanted in patients with zonular compromise. Several-sized rings are available, depending on the characteristics of the patients' intraocular anatomy. Capsular tension rings have not yet been approved by the Food and Drug Administration in the United States. Currently a core FDA study is under review, and it is hoped that they may be approved by next year.

Staining of the Lens Capsule With Indocyanine Green

The technique of staining the lens capsule with indocyanine green has "revolutionized" the management of mature cataracts! Performing capsulorhexis for patients with mature cataracts (or any poor red reflex) is extremely technically demanding. Because of the inability to adequately view the capsule, it can be impossible at times to perform a complete curvilinear capsulorhexis. In these instances, cataract removal becomes more difficult because the presence of radial tears makes it dangerous to perform a nuclear "cracking" technique and increases the possibility of posterior extension of a radial tear.

Horiguchi, Miyake, Ohta, et al. (Abstract 1–8) report using indocyanine green to stain the anterior lens capsule of patients with a mature cataract. Since reading this article I have personally used this technique on numerous occasions, and it is unbelievable how the visualization of the anterior lens capsule is dramatically improved. When the indocyanine green is initially injected, it does not stain the capsule an obvious green; however, once capsulorhexis is begun, the white cortical portion of the cataract stands out, brightly contrasted against the capsule, and this makes localizing and controlling the capsulorhexis significantly safer. If you read only one article on cataract surgery in 1998, this should be the one.

Phakic Intraocular Lenses

The implantation of phakic IOLs represents a gray area between refractive surgery and cataract surgery. It may represent one of the most important future areas for the practicing anterior segment surgeon, and I have therefore chosen to highlight it in this section. Two articles in this YEAR BOOK (Abstracts 1–3 and 1–4) describe series of patients with moderate to high myopia and hyperopia who underwent implantation of a phakic IOL. Although the follow-up in both series was brief (3-6 months), the safety and efficacy of these procedures was impressive. Rosen and Gore (Abstract 1–4) did describe one patient who had significant difficulties with postoperative glaucoma; however, this was caused by a lack of patency of the peripheral iridotomies that had been created before the placement of his phakic IOL.

Phakic IOLs may hold particular promise for the treatment of patients with high refractive errors. Although it was initially believed that laser in situ keratomileusis (LASIK) could be used to treat almost any degree of refractive error, experience has shown that there is a maximal degree of corneal flattening that can be produced to still achieve a high-quality visual result. For these patients, phakic IOLs may be especially useful. Obviously, there are many questions yet to be answered regarding phakic IOLs. These include long-term safety issues such as cataract formation or the development of glaucoma. Nonetheless, it is likely that phakic IOLs will be profiled in the 2000 YEAR BOOK as well.

Limbal Relaxing Incisions With Cataract Surgery

Budak K, Friedman NJ, Koch DD (Baylor College of Medicine, Houston)
J Cataract Refract Surg 24:503-508, 1998 1–1

Introduction.—Surgical correction could be used to increase uncorrected visual acuity and decrease distortion from meridional magnification

TABLE 1.—Modified Gills Nomogram for Limbal Relaxing Incisions to Correct Astigmatism With Cataract Surgery

Astigmatism (D)	Incision Type	Length (mm)	Optical Zone
1	One LRI	6.0	At limbus
1-2	Two LRIs	6.0	At limbus
2-3	Two LRIs	8.0	At limbus
>3	Two LRIs + corneal relaxing incisions as indicated 3 months postoperatively	Lindstrom surgical nomogram for astigmatism[32]	7-8 mm at cornea

Abbreviation: LRI, limbal relaxing incision.

(Reprinted by permission of the publisher from Budak K, Friedman NJ, Koch DD: Limbal relaxing incisions with cataract surgery. *J Cataract Refract Surg* 24:503-508. Copyright 1998 by Elsevier Science Inc.)

in patients with astigmatism greater than 2.0 D. The safety, efficacy, and predictability of limbal relaxing incisions (LRIs) for correcting naturally occurring astigmatism at the time of cataract surgery were prospectively evaluated in 12 eyes of 11 patients.

Methods.—Incisions were made with a guarded diamond knife set at a depth of 600 μm using a modified Gills nomogram to perform LRIs (Table 1). The LRIs were based on preoperative corneal astigmatism as determined by standard keratometry and computerized videokeratography. The goal was a 50% to 75% decrease in astigmatism without overcorrections (Table 4).

Results.—Mean age of 7 female and 4 male patients was 62.8 years. The only patient with a history of ocular disease or surgery had had glaucoma

TABLE 4.—Current Approach to Correcting Astigmatism During Cataract Surgery

Astigmatism (D)	Incisions
<0.5	3.5 mm clear corneal temporal
With the rule	
0.5-1.25	3.5 mm superior limbal or clear corneal temporal plus LRIs
≥1.50	3.5 mm clear corneal temporal plus LRIs (± CRIs after cataract surgery) or 3.5 mm superior limbal plus LRIs or 6.0 mm superior scleral
Against the rule	
0.5-1.25	3.5 mm clear corneal temporal
1.5-1.75	Clear corneal temporal plus LRIs (± CRIs after cataract surgery) or ≥6.0 mm anterior scleral
>2.00	Clear corneal temporal plus LRIs (± CRIs after cataract surgery)

Abbreviations: LRIs, limbal relaxing incisions; *CRIs*, corneal relaxing incisions.

(Reprinted by permission of the publisher from Budak K, Friedman NJ, Koch DD: Limbal relaxing incisions with cataract surgery. *J Cataract Refract Surg* 24:503-508. Copyright 1998 by Elsevier Science Inc.)

surgery with a superior bleb. The mean values for preoperative keratometric cylinder, arithmetic reduction in cylinder at 1 month postoperatively, and vector change in cylinder were 2.46 D, 1.12 D, and 1.47 D, respectively. The with-the-wound (WTW) change was −0.70 D. The target correction, according to the nomogram, was achieved in 3 eyes (25%). The other 9 eyes (75%) remained undercorrected. No eyes were overcorrected. From 1 day to 1 month after surgery, a 0.55 WTW regression was observed without any marked alteration in cylindrical axis. The WTW changes were not associated with age.

Conclusion.—Patients with astigmatism greater than 1.5 to 2.0 D are usually considered candidates for some form of surgical correction. Potential complications of other approaches make LRIs a likely alternative for correcting preoperative astigmatism at the time of cataract surgery. The 6.0 to 8.0 mm incision length allows some flexibility in choosing the proper axis. Patients in this series had a mean decrease in astigmatism of 1.47 D and a mean WTW change of −0.70 D at 1 month postoperatively. Astigmatism may be corrected easily and practically using LRIs. Even though 75% of patients were undercorrected, this is preferable to overcorrection. A larger series of patients needs to be evaluated for a longer period to fully determine the merits of LRIs with cataract surgery.

▶ I have been performing LRIs for the last 3 years. It is a great technique that can treat astigmatism of 2 to 3 D. It is nice in that it does not require any special keratomes or marking devices and can be performed with even a standard metal cataract blade. It should be noted that the results by the authors of this article were obtained using a guarded diamond keratome.

For higher ranges of astigmatism (over 3 D) arcuate incisions are needed. However, these higher degrees of astigmatism are not clinically as common. It is much more typical to encounter a patient who has 2 D or less of astigmatism.

As standard cataract incisions have become smaller and smaller, they tend to exert less of an astigmatic effect. Although surgeons will still typically place 4-mm or smaller incisions on the axis of the steepest astigmatism, they should realize that these incisions are not going to, in any way, lessen the pre-existing astigmatism. In these instances, it is nice to be able to perform LRIs to help deal with any pre-existing astigmatism.

R. Tipperman, M.D.

Liquefied Aftercataract: A Complication of Continuous Curvilinear Capsulorhexis and Intraocular Lens Implantation in the Lens Capsule

Miyake K, Ota I, Miyake S, et al (Miyake Eye Hosp, Nagoya, Japan; Nagoya Univ, Japan)

Am J Ophthalmol 125:429-435, 1998 1–2

Introduction.—Aftercataract may occur after continuous curvilinear capsulorrhexis and posterior chamber intraocular lens implantation. The

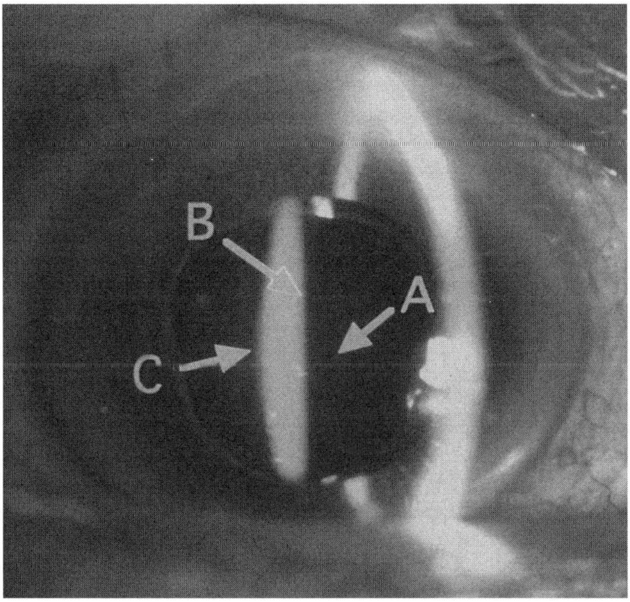

FIGURE 1.—An eye with liquified aftercataract with a large amount of substance. The capsular opening created by continuous curvilinear capsulorrhexis had been occluded by the lens optic, and fibrosis was noted evenly along the entire circumference. **A**, the slit-lamp beam of anterior surface of the intraocular lens optic; **B**, the beam of the posterior surface of the intraocular lens optic; **C**, the beam of the posterior lens capsule. Note that the posterior lens is slightly distorted posteriorly. (Reprinted by permission of the publisher from Miyake K, Ota I, Miyake S, et al: Liquified aftercataract: A complication of continuous curvilinear capsulorhexis and intraocular lens implantation in the lens capsule. *Am J Ophthalmol* 125:429-435. Copyright 1998 by Elsevier Science Inc.)

entire edge of the anterior capsule opening becomes attached to the lens optic in the aftercataract and creates a closed chamber between the lens and the posterior lens capsule in which a liquefied milky white substance accumulates. Reported are the clinical features of 41 eyes with aftercataract.

Methods.—The medical records of 41 patients (41 eyes) with aftercataract were reviewed for data regarding sex, age, preoperative ocular complications, surgical procedure, intraoperative complications, intraocular lens styles and materials, postoperative complications, time of onset of aftercataract and its slit-lamp findings, visual acuity, refractory errors before and after onset of the aftercataract, and management of liquefied aftercataract.

Results.—Ocular diseases before cataract surgery included 14 eyes with diabetic retinopathy; 4 eyes with glaucoma; and 2 eyes with uveitis. Phacoemulsification was done after continuous curvilinear capsulorrhexis while the posterior chamber intraocular lens, composed of polymethylmethacrylate, was securely fixated inside the lens capsule. Fibrosis was observed at 2 months to 6 years after surgery along the entire surface of the intraocular lens optic and the edge of the capsular opening created by continuous curvilinear capsulorrhexis. This caused a closed chamber be-

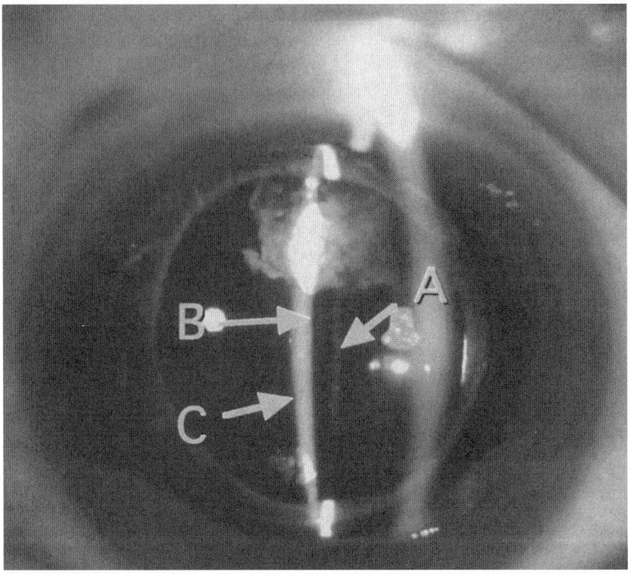

FIGURE 2.—An eye with liquified aftercataract and a small amount of liquified material. **A**, the slit-lamp beam of the anterior surface of the intraocular lens optic; **B**, the beam of the posterior surface of the intraocular lens optic; **C**, the beam of the posterior lens capsule. Note the mass of pearls within the liquified substance at the superior part of the space between the intraocular lens optic and posterior lens capsule. Fibrosis was noted evenly along the entire circumference between the anterior surface of the intraocular lens optic and edge of the capsular opening created by continuous curvilinear capsulorrhexis. (Reprinted by permission of the publisher from Miyake K, Ota I, Miyake S: Liquified aftercataract: A complication of continuous curvilinear capsulorhexis and intraocular lens implantation in the lens capsule. *Am J Ophthalmol* 125:429-435. Copyright 1998 by Elsevier Science Inc.)

tween the intraocular lens and the posterior lens capsule, which accumulated a liquefied, milky white substance (Figs 1 and 2). Liquefied aftercataract was detected along with other types of aftercataract in 23 of 41 eyes: 12 eyes with fibrosis, 11 eyes with Elschnig pearls, and 1 eye with a Soemmering ring. Inflammation was not observed in any eyes. Six eyes had decreased visual acuity caused by the liquefied aftercataract.

Conclusion.—A new type of aftercataract is characterized by a liquefied milky white substance that accumulates between the lens optic and the posterior lens capsule when the anterior capsular opening, originally created by continuous curvilinear capsulorrhexis, is occluded with the lens optic.

▶ This is a really interesting article! It describes a condition that I have seen from time to time and have personally noted as being unusual but have never given as much thought to as these authors have. On several occasions, I have been asked by colleagues to look at a "cloudy" posterior capsule that, in retrospect, was a "liquefied aftercataract" as described by these authors. I have noted it myself in several patients on whom I have performed YAG capsulotomy and, with initial opening of the capsule, have found that the liquefied material flows back into the vitreous. As the authors note, there is never any sign of an inflammatory response, and this condition seems to be unique to patients in whom the anterior capsulorrhexis seals down tightly around the anterior surface of the intraocular lens optic.

I believe that this is a much more common postoperative phenomenon than most surgeons realize. If one examines patients carefully, one can often see a whitish liquefied material in some portion of the capsular bag during the postoperative period. Understanding this phenomenon will allow surgeons to realize that this is a normal postoperative occurrence and not a sign of some unusual inflammatory condition.

R. Tipperman, M.D.

Implantable Contact Lens for Moderate to High Myopia: Phase 1 FDA Clinical Study With 6 Month Follow-up

Sanders DR, Brown DC Martin RG, et al (Ctr for Clinical Research, Chicago; Eye Centers of Florida, Fort Myers; Carolina Eye Associates, Southern Pines, NC; et al)

J Cataract Refract Surg 24:607-611, 1998 1–3

Introduction.—At the end of 1996, there were about 400 cases of implantable contact lens (ICL) implantation worldwide. Reported were outcomes of 10 patients in a United States Food and Drug Administration trial who underwent phase I implantation of ICLs to treat moderate-to-high myopia.

Methods.—Ten patients with myopia of 7.00 to 20.00 D (mean preoperative myopia, 7.75 D) underwent implantation of a single-piece plate-design lens 11.5 to 13.0 mm in length. Horizontal white-to-white measurements were taken. The ICL power was calculated using a formula developed by Staar Surgical that incorporated the patient's refraction, keratometry, measured anterior chamber depth, and corneal thickness. The ICLs were evaluated preoperatively and 1 day, 1 week and 1, 3, and 6 months postoperatively.

Results.—The mean spherical equivalent was −0.025 D at 6 months (a decrease from baseline of 7.725 D). At 6 month follow-up, 5 of 10 eyes had an uncorrected visual acuity (UCVA) of 20/20 or better. All eyes had a UCVA of 20/30 or better and a best spectacle-corrected visual acuity (BSCVA) of 20/20 or better. Six eyes had a BSCVA of 20/15 or better. Six eyes improved by 1 or more lines of BSCVA. All eyes were within ±1.125 D of emmetropia; 8 were within ±0.250 D. There were no intraoperative or postoperative complications or reactions in this series.

Conclusion.—The 6-month outcome of the first 10 patients with ICLs implanted for myopia in the United States was excellent. Future trials will help determine the role of ICL implantation among the various refractive surgery treatment choices.

Staar Collamer Posterior Chamber Phakic Intraocular Lens to Correct Myopia and Hyperopia

Rosen E, Gore C (BMI Alexandra Hosp Cheadle, Manchester, England)
J Cataract Refract Surg 24:596-606, 1998 1–4

Introduction.—The Staar posterior chamber phakic intraocular lens (IOL) was created for the surgical correction of moderate-to-high hyperopia and myopia. Its range of correction ranges from +10.00 to −20.00 D. The IOL is placed in the posterior chamber anterior to the crystalline lens to help retain the accommodation of the crystalline lens. The efficacy, safety, and predictability of implanting a collagen polymer (Staar Collamer) posterior chamber phakic IOL to correct myopia and hyperopia were assessed.

Methods.—Sixteen eyes were myopic and 9 were hyperopic in 14 patients with a mean age of 37.9 years. Patients underwent thorough evaluation that included refractive, general, ocular, social, and personal histories; visual acuity; refraction; tonometry; topography; biometry; biomicroscopy; pupil size in dim illumination; and posterior segment evaluation.

Surgical Technique.—A neodymium:yttrium-aluminum-garnet (Nd:YAG) laser iridotomy was performed before lens implantation in the upper peripheral iris. Two iridotomies were performed 90 degrees apart to avoid pupil block after IOL insertion. The surgical implantation was performed through a clear corneal, sutureless,

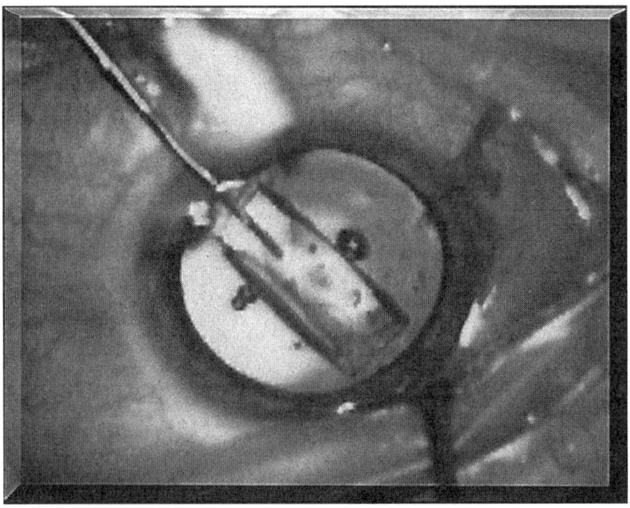

FIGURE 1.—The posterior chamber phakic intraocular lens is delivered from a cartridge nozzle and rolled into a tube in the anterior chamber amid and viscoelastic, which aids the controlled unfolding process. (Reprinted by permission of the publisher from Rosen E, Gore C: Staar collamer posterior chamber phakic intraocular lens to correct myopia and hyperopia. *J Cataract Refract Surg* 24:596-606. Copyright 1998 by Elsevier Science Inc.)

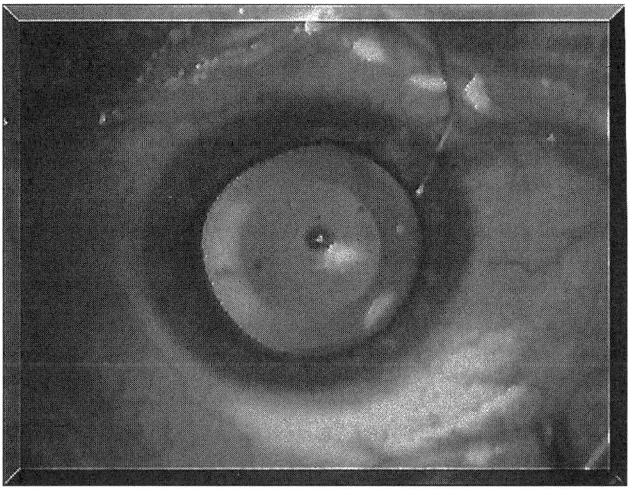

FIGURE 2.—The phakic intraocular lens in situ in the posterior chamber as the Healonid is exchanged for a balanced salt solution. (Reprinted by permission of the publisher from Rosen E, Gore C: Staar collamer posterior chamber phakic intraocular lens to correct myopia and hyperopia. *J Cataract Refract Surg* 24:596-606. Copyright 1998 by Elsevier Science Inc.)

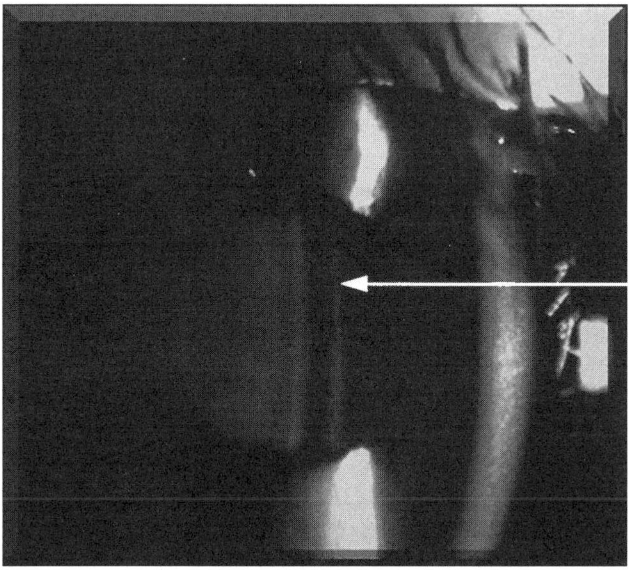

FIGURE 3.—Slit lamp optical section photograph shows the vaulting of the intraocular lens (*arrow*) over the center of the crystalline lens. (Reprinted by permission of the publisher from Rosen E, Gore C: Staar collamer posterior chamber phakic intraocular lens to correct myopia and hyperopia. *J Cataract Refract Surg* 24:596-606. Copyright 1998 by Elsevier Science Inc.)

self-sealing incision 2.6 × 1.5 mm. The 4-foot plates of the IOL lay anterior to the dilated iris diaphragm before being gently levered into position behind the iris through the pupil (Figs 1, 2, and 3).

Results.—All eyes had a significant increase in uncorrected visual acuity at 3-month follow-up. Two patients (3 eyes) were able to perform most activities without glasses. Three weeks after surgery, pupil block glaucoma of the right eye developed in 1 patient. It was caused by functional closure of the laser iridotomies. Emergency surgical iridectomy was performed. Three weeks later, the patient experienced pupil block of the left eye and underwent vitrectomy and lensectomy with removal of the IOL. Six eyes were undercorrected by more than 0.50 D.

Conclusion.—Posterior chamber phakic IOL may be considered safe and efficacious in the correction of myopic and hyperopic refractive errors, with good refractive stability.

▶ Both of these studies (Abstract 1–3 and 1–4) demonstrate excellent early results with an implantable "contact lens." The surgical technique required for the implantation of the lens will be familiar and comfortable to any anterior segment surgeon. This, obviously, represents a tremendous benefit compared with laser-assisted in situ kertatomileusis which definitely has a learning curve for the beginning surgeon. Interestingly, in studies that have compared the results of laser-assisted in situ kertatomileusis with the implantable contact lens, patients who have had both procedures tend to prefer the eye that has an implantable contact lens. Although Food and Drug Administration approval for an implantable contact lens is still at least 3 years away, these articles give reason to believe that this procedure may turn out to be a popular one in the refractive surgeon's armamentarium.

There were no complications in any of the patients reviewed by Sanders et al. In the article by Rosen and Gore, one patient did have significant difficulty with pupillary block and, ultimately, malignant glaucoma developed. It should be noted that this patient had the preoperative peripheral iridotomies performed by a resident physician and it was believed that they were not adequate in size to prevent pupillary block. Although these studies present only a limited clinical follow-up, they do reveal a technology that has tremendous potential for the future.

R. Tipperman, M.D.

Long-term Follow-up of Iatrogenic Phototoxicity

Postel EA, Pulido JS, Byrnes GA, et al (Duke Univ, Durham, NC; Med College of Wisconsin, Milwaukee; Natl Naval Med Ctr, Bethesda, Md; et al)

Arch Ophthalmol 116:753-757, 1998 1–5

Introduction.—Iatrogenic phototoxicity is correlated with duration of surgery. Most earlier trials of iatrogenic phototoxicity have been small, so the prognosis for this condition is not well defined. The long-term outcomes of 24 patients with iatrogenic phototoxicity was reported.

Methods.—Medical records of 24 patients (24 eyes) with iatrogenic phototoxicity from 3 medical centers were analyzed for data regarding visual outcome, type and duration of procedure, and location and size of phototoxic lesions. Fluorescein angiograms and serial photographs were examined.

Results.—The mean patient age was 67 years. Phototoxic injury was observed after anterior segment surgery in 20 eyes and after vitrectomy in the remaining 4 eyes. The mean surgical time was 109 minutes (range, 50-220 minutes). For each type of surgery, the mean surgical time was as follows: 78 minutes for 6 phacoemulsifications, 104 minutes for 13 extracapsular cataract extractions with posterior chamber lens implantation, and 138 minutes for 4 vitrectomies. The difference in duration of surgery for anterior segment procedures and vitrectomies was not significant. The mean final visual acuity for all patients was 20/40 (range 20/15 to counting fingers). The mean final visual acuity for vitrectomized eyes was 20/900. Vision in the immediate postoperative period was positively correlated with final vision. Eight eyes (24%) were symptomatic (decreased vision, metamorphopsia, and soctomata) or had Amsler grid changes observed immediately postoperatively. At final follow-up, 7 of 8 patients continued to be symptomatic or had persistent changes on Amsler grid testing. Two patients had choroidal neovascularization, presumably related to the phototoxic lesions. Phototoxic lesions seem to spare the fovea after anterior segment surgery and involve the foveal center after vitrectomy.

Conclusion.—Most patients with iatrogenic phototoxicity do well. The prognosis is good for persons with extrafoveal lesions. Foveal injury can occur with vitrectomy and is usually associated with worse visual outcome. The development of choroidal neovascularization may have an effect on final visual outcome.

▶ Iatrogenic phototoxicity is a relatively uncommon clinically significant problem after cataract surgery. However It definitely needs to be included in the differential diagnosis of any patient with decreased vision after cataract surgery. For surgeons who participate in resident teaching cases, it is probably much "higher up" on the differential diagnostic list than for surgeons who are performing "speedier" surgery.

This article probably represents one of the largest collated series of patients with phototoxicity with some of the best follow-up data. It shows that, in general, the lesions and vision do tend to improve with time, so patients can be reassured that their symptoms should improve. However, as with many other retinal problems, the ultimate prognosis is definitely linked to the initial level of vision, so patients with poor initial vision tend to have poor outcomes. Because choroidal neovascularization developed in several patients in this series, patients with retinal phototoxicity should be followed closely so that they can be evaluated for this complication.

R. Tipperman, M.D.

The SRKII Formula in the Calculation of Intraocular Lens Power
Nurözler A, Ünlü N, Yalvaç IS, et al (Ankara Hosp, Turkey)
Ophthalmologica 212:153-156, 1998 1–6

Background.—The Sanders-Retzlaff-Kraff (SRK) power formula is now the most widely used formula for implant power calculation. Sanders has modified the formula (the SRKII) to change the A constant depending on axial length. The predictive accuracy of the SRKII formula for eyes of average axial length and long eyes was determined.

Methods and Findings.—The survey included 344 eyes undergoing cataract extraction with implantation of a posterior-chamber intraocular lens. The axial length of the eyes ranged from 22 to 28.9 mm, with a mean of 24.3 mm. Ninety-eight eyes were classified as long and 246 eyes were of average axial length (Fig 1). Ninety-four percent of the average eyes were within 1 of the expected refraction, and 98.8% were within 2 dpt, compared with 58.2% and 84.7%, respectively, in the long-eye group.

Conclusions.—The SRKII formula performs credibly in average-length eyes. In long eyes, the ratio of large refractive deviations was greater than that in the other group.

► Anterior segment surgeons do everything possible to ensure a good result with cataract surgery. When I teach residents, I often stress to them that it does not benefit the surgeon or the patient to do a technically perfect job if the postoperative refraction, based on the implant power calculation, is less than optimal.

Surprisingly, there are still many surgeons who use the SRKII power formula to calculate implant strength. This formula can give relatively good

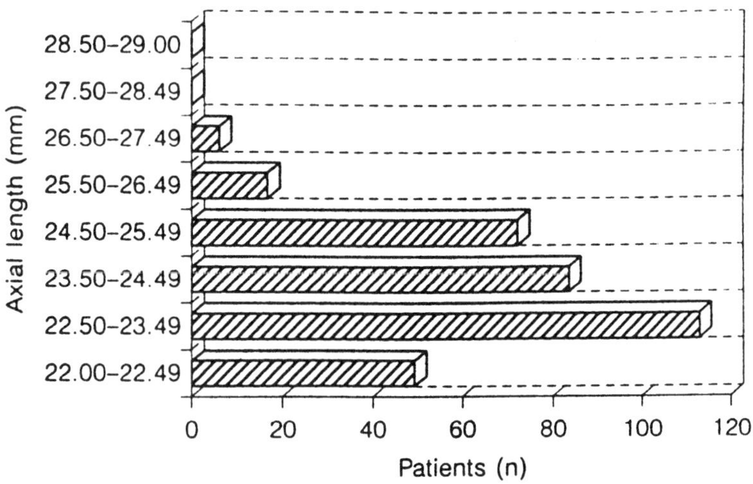

FIGURE 1.—The distribution of eyes according to axial length. (Courtesy of Nurözler A, Ünlü N, Yalvaç IS, et al: The SRKII formula in the calculation of intraocular lens power. *Ophthalmologica* 212:153-156, 1998. Copyright S. Karger AG, Basel.)

results for average-length eyes when an emmetropic postoperative refraction is desired. If, however, a nonemmetropic postoperative refraction is desired, or the surgeon is dealing with a long or short axial length eye, the SRKII formula tends to be inaccurate, compared to modern third generation theoretical formulas.

The importance of this article is its clear demonstration that surgeons who are still using the SRKII formula should update their implant power calculations with one of the newer third generation theoretical formulas, to obtain better overall postoperative results for their patients.

R. Tipperman, M.D.

Relationship Between Intraocular Lens Biomaterials and Posterior Capsule Opacification

Ursell PG, Spalton DJ, Pande MV, et al (St Thomas' Hosp, London; Kings College, London; United Med and Dental Schools, London)

J Cataract Refract Surg 24:352-360, 1998 1–7

Background.—Posterior capsule opacification (PCO) is the most common complication of cataract surgery. A system for objectively measuring the degree of PCO in an individual eye was developed, using high-resolution digital imaging and dedicated image processing software. This system was used to follow the development of PCO in a prospective, randomized, cohort study of patients with a polymethylmethacrylate (PMMA), silicone, or AcrySof intraocular lens (IOL).

Methods.—By random assignment, 99 eyes received a PMMA, silicone, or AcrySof IOL. The lenses had PMMA haptics and 6 mm optics. One surgeon performed a standardized surgical protocol, using an extracapsular method with capsulorrhexis. Patients with surgical complications were excluded from the final analysis. All patients had standardized medication and follow-up. A digital retroillumination camera with a dedicated software program was used to assess posterior capsule opacification. Assessment was based on the analysis of texture in the image, and calculated as the percentage area of opacified capsule.

Findings.—At 2 years, percentage of PCO differed significantly among the 3 lens types. Compared with PMMA and silicone lenses, the AcrySof

TABLE 2.—Percentage of PCO at Each Follow-up

	Percentage of PCO					
	6 Months		1 Year		2 Years	
IOL Type	Median	Range	Median	Range	Median	Range
PMMA	19.90	1.3 to 66.0	26.1	9.5 to 54.1	43.65	3.9 to 67.0
Silicone	20.05	7.7 to 59.4	22.2	5.8 to 61.2	33.50	4.7 to 75.6
AcrySof	8.20	4.1 to 34.7	10.7	1.1 to 34.4	11.75	2.6 to 52.0

lenses were associated with less PCO. No significant differences occurred between PMMA and silicone lenses (Table 2).

Conclusions.—This is the first objective report of decreased PCO associated with an IOL material. There is a significant, beneficial reduction in PCO with AcrySof IOLs, compared with the PMMA and silicone lenses studied.

► A number of factors have been shown to help decrease the incidence of PCO. These include the use of a biconvex lens optic and aggressive polishing of the posterior capsule. This article demonstrates that acrylic material in the Alcon AcrySof lens tends to produce the lowest degree of PCO.

Unfortunately, the authors used an IOLAB LI41U lens as the silicone lens to compare. This lens represents a first generation silicone material, and later generation silicone materials may have a lower incidence of PCO.

If the acrylic lens does produce a lower incidence of PCO than even second generation silicone lenses do, it would represent a significant advantage of acrylic lenses over silicone lenses.

R. Tipperman, M.D.

Staining of the Lens Capsule for Circular Continuous Capsulorrhexis in Eyes With White Cataract

Horiguchi M, Miyake K, Ohta I, et al (Nagoya Univ, Japan; Shozan-Kai Miyake Eye Hosp, Nagoya, Japan)

Arch Ophthalmol 116:535-537, 1998 1–8

Background.—Continuous circular capsulorrhexis (CCC) is often difficult to perform in eyes with a mature cataract and white lens cortex, because anterior lens capsule visibility is poor. To improve visibility of the capsule, a capsular-staining technique was developed using indocyanine green (ICG), which facilitates the CCC.

Methods.—Outcomes of phacoemulsification and intraocular lens implantation in 10 eyes with the capsule stained were compared with the outcomes in 10 eyes treated with standard CCC. None of the patients included had signs of uveitis, glaucoma, or corneal disorders, and none of the cataracts had a liquefied cortex. For the new procedure, 25 mg of ICG was dissolved in 0.5 mL of aqueous solvent mixed in 4.5 mL of irrigating solution, with a concentration of 0.5% and osmolarity of 270 µOsm. After making the sclerocorneal or corneal incision, the surgeon filled the anterior chamber with air and injected a small amount of viscomaterial around the incision to prevent air leakage. One or 2 drops of ICG solution were placed on the anterior capsule. The anterior chamber was then replaced with viscoelastic material. Once the air and redundant ICG were removed, the stained anterior capsule became clearly visible, and the CCC was performed easily.

Findings.—The surgical procedures were completely successful. All patients had excellent visual recovery. None had increased intraocular pressure. On postoperative days 1, 3, and 7, laser flare-cell photometry demonstrated no significant differences between groups. Neither corneal endothelial cell count nor coefficient of variation differed significantly between the 2 groups, before or after surgery.

Conclusions.—This pilot study suggests that ICG in CCC is useful for improving visualization of the anterior capsule in eyes with a mature cataract. Further research is needed to determine the safety of this technique.

► Performing CCC in a patient with a mature white cataract is one of the more difficult surgical problems the anterior segment surgeon can encounter. There are a variety of techniques to help facilitate visualization of the anterior lens capsule. This latest description of using ICG to stain the lens capsule and improve visualization sounds terrific.

Other techniques which I have found to be helpful are using a very high density viscoelastic, which helps tamponade any liquefied cortical material; using indirect illumination from the side with an endo illuminator; and using the irrigation/aspiration instrumentation to remove any liquefied cortex which might enter the anterior chamber once the capsule is punctured.

Although I have not had the opportunity personally to try the technique described in this article, I am planning to use it on my next patient who has a mature lens.

R. Tipperman, M.D.

Outcomes and Ocular Growth Rates After Intraocular Lens Implantation in the First 2 Years of Life

Hutchinson AK, Wilson ME, Saunders RA (Med Univ of South Carolina, Charleston)

J Cataract Refract Surg 24:846-852, 1998 1–9

Introduction.—In recent years, the use of intraocular lenses (IOLs) to correct pediatric aphakia has become increasingly common, and for older children it may represent a standard of care. In children younger than 2 years, however, the use of IOLs remains controversial, because increased tissue reactivity and marked axial length and refractive changes have been cited as contraindications to IOL use in this age group. Few studies have examined this age group. In a group of children younger than 24 months, implantations of IOLs were reviewed.

Methods.—Seventeen patients aged 12 days to 22 months had intraocular lens implantation in 22 eyes. Recordings were taken of change in axial length over time, postoperative complications, the need for additional surgery, predicted versus actual postoperative refraction, and visual outcomes.

TABLE 2.—Actual Versus Target Postoperative Error

Patient	Age at Surgery (Months)	Refractive Error (D): Target Refractive Error	Refractive Error (D): Actual Postop Refractive Error	IOL Calculation Error* (D)
JG	0.4	+15.2	+16.0	0.8
JL	2.4	+10.0	+11.5	1.5
AT	4.2	+8.6	+4.5	−4.1
AT	4.5	+8.0	+4.8	3.2
DD	5.4	+4.0	+8.0	4.0
PO	6.5	+4.8	+4.0	0.8
BT	7.1	+3.9	+4.3	0.4
KP	9.1	+5.4	+5.8	0.4
WL	12.3	+5.0	+3.8	−1.2
JH	14.7	+2.9	+4.5	1.6
ZA	15.5	+3.1	+5.0	1.9
ZA	16.0	+2.9	+4.3	1.4
JS	15.9	+6.2	+6.0	−0.2
TW	17.5	+2.0	+2.9	0.9
TW	18.4	+2.0	+3.3	1.3
CB	18.4	+3.0	+3.0	0
AH	18.4	+3.0	+3.5	0.5
AH	18.8	+3.0	+3.5	0.5
BW	19.9	−0.7	−2.5	−1.8
MH	21.6	+2.4	+3.1	0.7
KB	21.9	+3.0	+5.0	2.0

*Error = predicted postoperative refraction minus actual postoperative refraction.
Abbreviations: D, diopters; *IOL*, intraocular lens.
(Reprinted by permission of the publisher from Hutchinson AK, Wilson ME, Saunders RA: Outcomes and ocular growth rates after intraocular lens implantation in the first 2 years of life: *J Cataract Refract Surg* 24:846-852. Copyright 1998 by Elsevier Science Inc.)

A similar group of age-matched patients who were left aphakic at the time of surgery was used for comparison of complication rates.

Results.—In the majority of operated eyes, visual acuity measurement, which was limited to fixation-preference testing in most patients, revealed amblyopia. No significant difference in growth between the fellow and the operated eyes was found, according to serial axial lengths in 11 patients who had a mean follow-up of 20 months. In all patients, the targeted postoperative refractive error was hyperopic (Table 2). When comparing the pseudophakic patients and the age-matched phakic group, there was no significant difference in complication rates. In 44% of aphakic eyes (14 of 32), it was noted in the chart that the patient had stopped wearing glasses or contact lenses for at least 2 months.

Conclusions.—In children younger than 2 years, IOL implantation appears to be a safe and effective alternative to contact lens or spectacle correction of aphakia. By eliminating periods of uncorrected aphakia, it may aid amblyopia treatment. The complication rate or reoperation rate was not significantly higher in pseudophakic patients than in a similar population having cataract extraction but who were left aphakic at the time of surgery. A downsized 10.0-mm diameter, one-piece all-polymethylmethacrylate, modified C-loop capsular IOL for very young patients is recommended. Downsizing is less necessary with newer IOLs that are more flexible.

▶ The use of IOLs in pediatric patients is becoming increasing commonplace, although it is still not universally accepted. In most case reviews, the patients have been at least 2 years of age. This study represents probably the largest series dealing with IOL implantation in patients younger than 2 years. In addition, this study also evaluated changes in axial length.

In comparing the implanted eye with the fellow eye, there did not seem to be a difference in the growth rate of the eye that received an IOL. The complication rate in this study was acceptable.

Of note was that in patients followed up through the study who were aphakic, 44% of the patients at some point had to stop wearing glasses or contact lenses for at least 2 months' time. Certainly in patients this age, amblyopia is a great concern, and it may turn out that the problems associated with correction of aphakia via a contact lens or spectacles may be greater than the problems associated with IOL implantation.

Although this is still only an early study, it does lend support to the concept that IOL implantation may become a viable approach for children younger than 2 years with cataracts.

R. Tipperman, M.D.

Diagnosis of Infectious Endophthalmitis After Cataract Surgery by Polymerase Chain Reaction

Lohmann CP, Heeb M, Linde H-J, et al (Univ of Regensburg, Germany)
J Cataract Refract Surg 24:821-826, 1998 1–10

Introduction.—After intraocular surgery, the development of infectious endophthalmitis is very rare, with an incidence of less than 1%. Acute endophthalmitis can appear between 2 and 7 days after surgery and is most often caused by *Staphylococcus epidermidis*, *Staphylococcus aureus*, and *Streptococcus* species. Delayed postoperative endophthalmitis occurs 4 weeks to years after intraocular surgery, with a mean onset of 9 months. It is caused by indolent microorganisms such as *Propionibacterium acne*, *Actinomyces israelii*, and *Corynebacterium*. In the case of intraocular infections, traditional identification methods often fail because of the small number of causative infectious pathogens within the eye. The use of polymerase chain reaction (PCR) as evaluated to determine whether identification of the causative agent is improved and whether diagnosis in cases of infectious endophthalmitis is quicker.

Methods.—To detect the infectious agent, microscopy, diagnostic culture, and PCR reaction were used in evaluating the aqueous humor and vitreous of 16 eyes with infectious endophthalmitis (10 acute, 6 delayed).

Results.—In 3 eyes microscopy of the vitreous was positive, and in 7 eyes the culture media results were positive; acute endophthalmitis was present in all of these eyes. In the aqueous humor, significantly fewer positive results were obtained. In the aqueous humor of all 16 eyes and in the vitreous of 14 eyes, an infectious agent was detected using PCR. In 2 eyes with delayed endophthalmitis, the vitreous sample was negative.

Conclusions.—PCR was more successful in detecting the infectious agent than the conventional microbiological tests, especially in the diagnosis of delayed endophthalmitis where, in all eyes, the pathogen was detected in the aqueous humor.

▶ This article demonstrates the ability of PCR to quickly and accurately identify infectious agents in chronic, acute, and late-onset endophthalmitis. I chose this article because the technique of PCR may not be well known to many anterior segment surgeons. Basically, this technique involves a way of identifying DNA sequences specifically for infectious bacteria. It allows for the rapid identification of an infectious agent in several hours. Strikingly, using this technique, the infectious bacteria were able to be identified in all patients from samples of aqueous humor.

Obviously, in treating endophthalmitis, rapid diagnosis and treatment are helpful in trying to obtain the best possible clinical outcome. At present, the technique of PCR may not be available at every institution, but given the extreme effectiveness in its ability to identity infectious agents of all types, it should become a more common clinical test. One potential drawback of the PCR is that it only identifies the infectious agent. It does not give antibiotic sensitivities. This can still only be obtained through culture techniques.

In the last few years, there has been a quiet revolution in the management of endophthalmitis. This has been spurred mostly by the endophthalmitis vitrectomy studies. However, I believe the use of PCR will further improve our ability to manage patients with endophthalmitis.

For instance, one of the more difficult situations is a patient who has postoperative inflammation several weeks after surgery. It can be difficult to discern whether this is just a severe inflammatory response or actually represents an infectious process. If in the long-term the PCR turns out to be as specific as this current article demonstrates, it may be a handy tool in helping to evaluate these patients.

R. Tipperman, M.D.

Phacoemulsification in Eyes With Pseudoexfoliation
Drolsum L, Haaskjold E, Sandvig K (Natl Hosp, Oslo, Norway)
J Cataract Refract Surg 24:787-792, 1998 1–11

Objective.—After undergoing phacoemulsion, patients with pseudoex foliation are at high risk of intraoperative problems such as inflammation. Inflammation, associated with small pupil size, is thought to be caused during manual extraction by the increased trauma resulting from extracting the nucleus through the small pupil. Because endocapsular phacoemulsion stretches the pupil less, it should not lead to inflammation. Intraoperative complications, including inflammation, and postoperative clinical outcomes of phacoemulsion were compared in eyes with and without pseudoexfoliation.

Methods.—Between January, 1994, and June, 1995, extracapsular cataract surgery was performed in 1,197 eyes, 197 (16.5%) of which had pseudoexfoliation. Phacoemulsion was performed in 178 eyes (122 women), average age 80 years, with exfoliation (group 1) and in 974 eyes (605 women), average age 73 years, without exfoliation (group 2). There were 164 group 1 patients and 916 group 2 patients who were followed for 4 months. One-piece poly(methyl methacrylate) intraocular lenses were planted.

Results.—Group 1 patients had a harder lens, smaller pupil, and more phakodonesis than group 2 patients. In group 1, phacoemulsion took longer, and there were more capsular tears and zonular dialysis. Incidence of vitreous loss and frequency of a postoperative inflammatory response were similar between groups. Visual acuity at 4 months was similar to that reported in other studies. Eyes with pseudoexfoliation (86.5%) and eyes without pseudoexfoliation (92.4%) achieved a visual acuity of at least 0.5. Manual extraction in eyes with pseudoexfoliation may result in pigment effusion, sphincter rupture, or a tear in the fragile capsule or zonules.

Conclusion.—Whereas phacoemulsion is safe for most eyes with pseudoexfoliation, intraoperative complication rates were higher than in eyes without pseudoexfoliation. Inflammation accompanying manual extraction was probably the result of trauma caused by manipulation of the nucleus through a small pupil.

▶ This article by Drolsum et al. and one by Scorolli et al.[1] demonstrate a significant increase in complications associated with pseudoexfoliation. In general, patients still have good postoperative results; however, compared to patients who do not have pseudoexfoliation the incidence of capsular or zonular tear and vitreous loss is much greater.

Day in and day out, pseudoexfoliation is the most common problem faced by anterior segment surgeons. When performing cataract surgery on patients with pseudoexfoliation, it is critical to try to obtain the largest pupillary dilation possible to facilitate nucleus removal. With a larger pupil diameter, it is possible to obtain a larger capsulorrhexis. This facilitates nucleus removal and decreases stress on the zonules. Intraoperatively, it is better for the surgeon to go slow and try to avoid any maneuvers that result in significant chamber fluctuations.

As noted in the following review of the capsular tension ring (Abstract 1–12), the use of these devices will, hopefully, simplify the management of patients with pseudoexfoliation and decrease the incidence of complications associated with their surgery.

One would hope that in the future an article will be published showing that when capsular tension rings were used in patients with pseudoexfoliation, the incidence of complications was no greater than for an average patient.

R. Tipperman, M.D.

Reference

1. Scorolli L, Scorolli L, Campos EC, et al: Pseudoexfoliation syndrome: A cohort study on intraoperative complications in cataract surgery. *Ophthalmologica* 212:278-280, 1998.

In Vitro Evaluation of the Efficacy of the Capsular Tension Ring for Managing Zonular Dialysis in Cataract Surgery

Sun R, Gimbel HV (Univ of Calgary, Alta; Loma Linda Univ, Calif; Univ of California, San Francisco)

Ophthalmic Surg Lasers 29:502-505, 1998 1–12

Objective.—Small studies have shown that the capsular tension ring maintains the circular contour of the capsular bag avoiding intraocular lense (IOL) decentration in patients with zonular dialysis. An in vitro model of zonular dialysis was developed to evaluate the function of the tension ring.

Methods.—After capsulorrhexis and lens removal, fresh pig eyes were implanted with posterior capsule (PC) IOLs with and without open polymethylmethacrylate capsular tension rings (Fig 1). Zonules were cut in some eyes to encourage capsular bag decentration. In other eyes, the capsular bag was isolated with forceps.

Results.—Five Morcher (Stuttgart, Germany) and 5 OPHTEC (Groningen, Holland) tension rings were implanted into the capsular bag and 3 Morcher and 3 OPHTEC rings were inserted into isolated capsular bags. The Morcher ring fit well into the bag because it has a smaller opening. Cutting the zonule results in significant IOL decentration. Implantation of the tension ring prevented IOL decentration. Alternatively, implantation of a polymethylmethacrylate capsular tension ring before or during phacoemulsion in 4 patients with extensive traumatic zonular dialysis allowed PC IOL in-the-bag implantation. Four to 10 months after implantation, all IOLs were well centered and patients had excellent vision and no complications. In a clinical study, 14 patients with damaged zonules implanted with capsular tension rings, had no decentration 2 to 11 months after surgery.

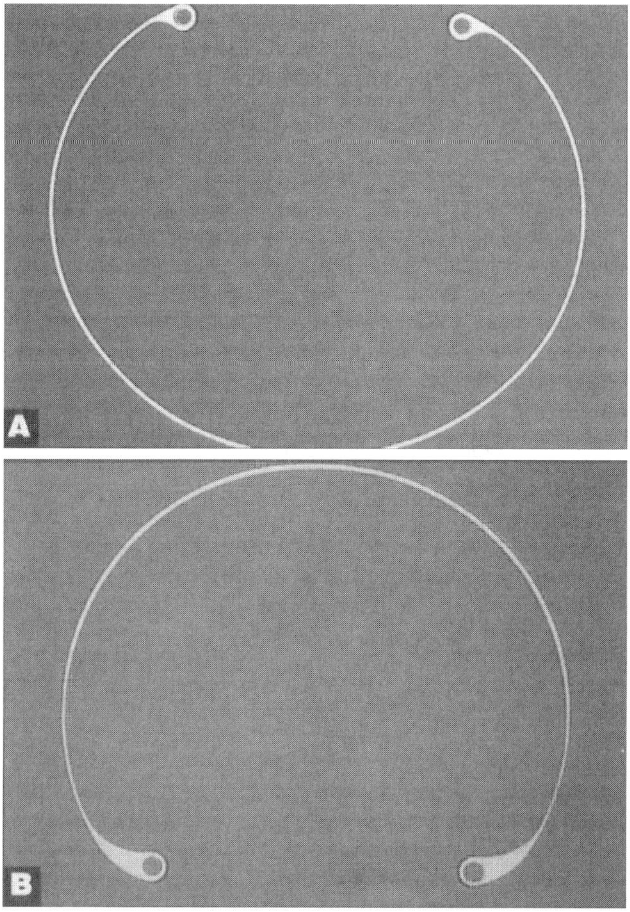

FIGURE 1.—Open polymethylmethacrylate capsular tension rings manufactured by A, Morcher GMBH, Stuttgart, Germany, and by B, OPHTEC, Groningen, Holland. (Courtesy of Sun R, Gimbel AV: In vitro evaluation of the efficacy of the capsular tension ring for managing zonular dialysis in cataract surgery. *Ophthalmic Surg Lasers* 29:502-505, 1998).

Conclusion.—Cutting zonules in 1 quadrant of the meridian resulted in significant decentration of the IOL, whereas implanting a tension ring-in-the-bag resulted in centering of the IOL by maintaining the circular contour of the capsular bag. A capsular tension ring appears to stabilize the capsule and improves the safety and efficacy of phacoemulsion and PC IOL implantation, maintains circular contour, and provides additional support to the bag. This may decrease migration of lens epithelial cells to the posterior capsule, thereby reducing the likelihood of secondary cataract.

▶ This is yet another article demonstrating the ability of the capsular tension ring to help ensure IOL centration in patients with poor zonules. Obviously, another advantage of the capsular tension ring is to allow for removal of the nucleus through phacoemulsification in patients with poor zonular support. (Earlier in this YEAR BOOK [Abstract 1–11] is an article demonstrating the significant increase in complications in patients with pseudoexfoliation owing to a large degree of abnormal zonular integrity.)

Although these capsular tension rings are not currently approved by the Food and Drug Administration in the United States, they are gaining increasing use world wide. It is certainly only a matter of time before this technology becomes widely available. In the long term, they probably will be used in many patients with pseudoexfoliation as well as other forms of zonular instability.

R. Tipperman, M.D.

Intravitreal Gas Injection for Hypotony After Cataract Surgery
Weinberger D, Stiebel H, Lusky M, et al (Tel Aviv Univ, Israel)
J Cataract Refract Surg 24:1490-1492, 1998 1–13

Background.—The safety and efficacy of injecting perfluoropropane gas into the vitreous cavity were evaluated in the treatment of hypotony, after uneventful cataract surgery with posterior chamber intraocular lens (PC IOL) implantation.

Patients and Methods.—Five patients, 4 women and 1 man, aged 61 to 74, who had cataract extraction with PC IOL implantation reported visual acuity of hand motion, pain, discomfort, and redness in the operated eye at 3 to 6 weeks after cataract surgery. In all patients, iridocyclitis with choroidal detachment and serous retinal detachment caused the hypotony. The procedure included a 5.0 mm wide scleral tunnel, nucleus removal with a glide, and in-the-bag PC IOL implantation with a viscoelastic material.

Results.—At 3 to 6 weeks, a deep anterior chamber and the IOL positioned in the bag were seen. There was moderate iridocyclitis with flare and cell in the anterior chamber, but the vitreous was clear. Hypotony was 2 to 4 mm Hg. A wide open angle and deep anterior chamber without cyclodialysis clefts were seen with gonioscopy. Choroidal detachment, choroidal folds, and an exudative peripheral retinal detachment without retinal holes were seen with funduscopy. Examination also showed a swollen optic nerve head with engorged vessels, and with the posterior pole attached. No wound dehiscence or leakage of aqueous in the tunnel was seen. Hypotony, choroidal detachment, and exudative retinal detachment resolved in all patients. Visual acuity also improved. There were no complications. Under peribulbar anesthesia, another procedure was performed. Perfluoropropane gas 0.7 to 1.0 mL was injected through the pars plana into the vitreous cavity. Intraocular pressure and the appearance of the optic nerve were monitored. Patients were then put into a prone position to prevent forward displacement of the gas bubble and pressure on the lens. Patients were positioned face down for the first 2 weeks to prevent the gas bubble from pushing the lens-iris diaphragm forward.

Discussion.—Intravitreal expansive gas injection is easy and relatively safe. The amount of gas required to restore hypotony and the time needed to retain gas in the eye will determine the choice of perfluorocarbons or sulfurohexafluorides. The benefits of this procedure include immediate restoration of intraocular pressure and prevention of complications from chronic hypotony. These benefits outweigh the low risk of complications from intravitreal gas injection.

▶ This article describes 5 patients who had hypotony, caused by inflammation combined with choroidal detachment and serous retinal detachment, who were treated with injection of intravitreal gas. Although this is not a common complication after small incision cataract surgery, I thought this article was worth including because of its novel approach. In the few patients I have seen with hypotony following cataract surgery, the choroidals have usually resolved spontaneously. It is possible that these authors' patients had more significant problems with hypotony, related to having had essentially manual nucleus expression rather than small incision phacoemulsification. The authors, however, report that none of these patients had wound leaks or cyclodialysis clefts.

R. Tipperman, M.D.

Artist's Impression of Endocapsular Phacoemulsification Surgery

Sumich PM, Francis IC, Kappagoda MB, et al (Dalcross Private Hosp, Sydney, Australia; Concord Hosp, Sydney, Australia)

J Cataract Refract Surg 24:1525-1528, 1998 1–14

Background.—It is useful for the ophthalmic surgeon to understand what patients may see during certain surgical procedures when vision is retained. Patients often receive less information about the intraoperative experience than about preoperative or postoperative management, though the procedure itself is the most feared and vivid event for many patients. An artist draws and describes her impressions of endocapsular phacoemulsification and intraocular lens implantation.

Methods.—A 77-year-old woman illustrated and described her visual perceptions of endocapsular phacoemulsification and intraocular lens implantation, in 6 stages arbitrarily chosen by her. Thirty consecutive patients were shown the drawings to determine the drawings' value in helping to inform and prepare patients for surgery.

Results.—The artist's illustrations and descriptions show that she had clear visualization of the surgical instruments, with colorful abstract imagery. The artist's drawings indicate that her surgical experience was generally positive. Among 30 consecutive patients shown the drawings, patients with poorer visual acuity from denser retrobulbar blocks reported seeing fewer colors and felt that the artist's sketches were less useful.

Discussion.—These illustrations and descriptions of endocapsular phacoemulsification surgery may help the surgeon to understand what a patient is likely to see at each stage when vision is retained. With the artist's permission, her illustrations and descriptions are shown to most of these authors' patients to help to prepare them for surgery. Describing the visual experience that patients may have during surgery can help to relieve anxiety in some patients and may provide better informed consent.

▶ I think most anterior segment surgeons will find this article interesting, and it is probably worth reviewing the original article to clearly see the artist's hand-drawn pictures. Many times, patients will ask what surgery will be like or what they will see. This article is nice to have to recommend to our patients, so they can find the experience more pleasant. Interestingly, this patient did have a peribulbar injection, but still saw significant colors and formed images. Obviously, topical anesthesia patients see much more.

I believe there are certain patients who will have much less apprehension regarding their surgery if they are allowed to review the types of pictures generated by the artist in this article.

R. Tipperman, M.D.

Intraoperative Crystallization on the Intraocular Lens Surface

Olson RJ, Caldwell KD, Crandall AS, et al (Univ of Utah, Salt Lake City)

Am J Ophthalmol 126:177-184, 1998 1–15

Background.—Intraoperative crystallization on the surface of intraocular lens (IOL) implants has been reported, but incidence, etiology, and prevention of such crystallization have not been defined. The 4-year results of a physician survey, laboratory studies, and clinical observations of intraoperative crystallization on the surface of the IOL are reported.

Methods.—A survey was sent to all ophthalmologists in 5 western states in the United States. Physicians were asked if they had ever encountered crystallization on the IOL surface in any patient. The physicians were also asked to identify the viscoelastics, IOLs, and other solutions they used. One physician submitted a sample of crystallization on a glass slide, which was analyzed to determine the relative elemental composition. BSS (Alcon Surgical, Fort Worth, Tex) and BSS Plus (Alcon Surgical) were measured and analyzed for precipitation during in vitro studies. Various solutions of Healon GV (Pharmacia/Upjohn, Kalamazoo, Mich) and calcium chloride were also analyzed for precipitation. Silicone IOLs and plate silicone were placed with various BSS and BSS Plus solutions consisting of various viscoelastics and calcium concentrations. Prominent crystallization on an IOL surface was examined, photographed, and studied for a maximum of 3 years in 7 patients.

Results.—The physician response rate was 88%: 206 ophthalmologists returned 181 surveys. These physicians reported more than 29,600 cataract surgeries. Intraoperative crystallization on the IOL surface was reported with IOL implantation in 22 patients and 22 eyes in 1993. A correlation was seen between crystallization and BSS Plus and silicone IOLs. The cation was calcium. Scanning electron microscopy of the specimen showed feathery crystal in a leaf-like pattern. The 7 patients with silicone lenses and crystallization had symptoms of varying degrees. Macular degeneration was seen in 2 patients, but decreased vision (to 20/40) from the deposits was documented in at least 2 patients, in the absence of any other cause of such decreased vision. Most cases cleared spontaneously, but at 3 years some crystallization between the capsule and lens remained.

Discussion.—Crystallization on the IOL surface in cataract surgery occurs rarely; this survey found an incidence of 1 in 1,400 cases. The authors believe the actual incidence may be less than 1 in 10,000 cases, which would explain why so few ophthalmologists encounter the condition. Crystallization may be associated with calcium as the cation, related to an osmotic gradient around the IOL with elevated calcium concentration. If this occurs during surgery, the lens should be immediately exchanged after irrigating the anterior chamber with BSS and filling the capsular bag with a viscoelastic of low molecular weight.

► Prior to reading this article, I believed I had seen, heard, or personally experienced virtually any complication that could occur with cataract surgery. This article, however, demonstrates a new potential problem with cataract surgery and therefore, I felt it was worth including. Although this problem is rare (the authors feel it may occur in only 1 in 10,000 cases), I think it is certainly worth knowing about. Apparently, with certain viscoelastics, and especially with silicone lenses, it is possible for significant crystallization to occur on the optic surface. This would significantly, adversely affect patients' vision.

The authors suggest that in these cases, if crystallization occurs, the lens be removed, the anterior segment and posterior chamber be flushed with BSS, and a different viscoelastic be used when a new lens is placed.

Obviously, if the surgeon is not aware of this potential problem, it will be unclear what was forming on the surface of the lens at the time of surgery. As a result, I feel that although this is a rare complication, it is worth noting.

R. Tipperman, M.D.

Cystoid Macular Edema Associated With Latanoprost in Aphakic and Pseudophakic Eyes

Ayyala RS, Cruz DA, Margo CE, et al (Univ of South Florida, Tampa; Watson Clinic, Lakeland, Fla; Retina-Vitreous Associates of Florida, Tampa; et al)

Am J Ophthalmol 126:602-604, 1998 1–16

Background.—Latanoprost is a phenyl-substituted prostaglandin analogue that lowers intraocular pressure when applied topically to the eye.

This reduction seems to be achieved by increased uveoscleral outflow. Four patients with latanoprost-related cystoid macular edema are described.

Methods.—The medical records of 4 patients (6 eyes) with open-angle glaucoma in whom cystoid macular edema developed were reviewed. Cystoid macular edema developed shortly after treatment with latanoprost was begun. The posterior capsule was absent in patients 1 and 2, had Nd:YAG capsulotomy in patient 3, and was intact in patient 4. The time from start of treatment with latanoprost to diagnosis was 7 to 30 days.

Results.—In 4 patients and 6 eyes (2 aphakic eyes and 4 pseudophakic eyes), topical latanoprost was temporally related to the development of cystoid macular edema. In all patients, the cystoid macular edema resolved after discontinuation of latanoprost. One patient had mild vitritis, but this also resolved after latanoprost was discontinued. Best-corrected visual acuity returned to baseline, in 5 of 6 eyes, by 5 weeks after treatment with latanoprost.

Discussion.—Cystoid macular edema can occur as a complication of treatment with latanoprost. How latanoprost causes cystoid macular edema is unclear. Some evidence indicates that cystoid macular edema can be induced by prostaglandins through the cyclic adenosine monophosphate system. These 4 cases are anecdotal and were not part of a well-controlled epidemiologic study. Further studies are needed to determine how the risk of cystoid macular edema in patients who are pseudophakic or aphakic, and to determine the percentage of cases of cystoid macular edema, related to treatment with latanoprost, that may be irreversible.

▶ Latanoprost has become a widely used glaucoma medication because of its significant safety profile and its ability to lower intraocular pressure. Most anterior segment surgeons are now probably aware of the reported increased incidence of cystoid macular edema occurring with latanoprost, but for those who are not, I felt this article definitely was worth including. I would stress that this association is controversial.

The exact mechanism by which latanoprost induces cystoid macular edema and inflammation is unclear. However, because all cataract patients are at greater risk for developing cystoid macular edema, I believe that, based on these findings, latanoprost is probably not the drug of choice for controlling postoperative pressure spikes.

Perhaps over time, as the mechanism with which latanoprost may induce cystoid macular edema is unraveled, we may be able to develop an effective treatment for cystoid macular edema as well.

R. Tipperman, M.D.

Trabeculectomy Function After Cataract Extraction

Chen PP, Weaver YK, Budenz DL, et al (Univ of Washington, Seattle; Univ of Miami, Fla)

Ophthalmology 105:1928-1935, 1998 1–17

Objective.—Preoperative, intraoperative, and postoperative factors were analyzed retrospectively to identify risk factors related to loss of intraocular pressure control after extracapsular cataract extraction or phacoemulsification with intraocular lens placement. The resolution of post-trabeculectomy hypotony after cataract extraction was also examined.

Methods.—The medical records of 115 consecutive patients (115 eyes) who had extracapsular cataract extraction or phacoemulsification with intraocular lens after trabeculectomy were reviewed in a retrospective, noncomparative case study. The mean age of patients was 68. No patient had bleb revision with cataract extraction. One patient had choroidal effusions drained when extracapsular cataract extraction was performed, and 1 patient had pars plana vitrectomy for retained nuclear fragments on the same day as phacoemulsification. Factors were examined to determine their association with loss of intraocular pressure control needing additional medication, bleb needling, or additional glaucoma surgery. The mean-follow up was 21.1 months. Follow-up after extracapsular cataract extraction was significantly longer than follow-up after phacoemulsification.

Results.—After follow-up, additional medication for glaucoma or needling of the filtering bleb was needed in 35 eyes to maintain control of intraocular pressure. There were significant associations with both intraoperative iris manipulation and early postoperative peak intraocular pressure greater than 25 mm Hg. In all, 11 eyes required additional glaucoma surgery. Factors that were significantly associated with additional glaucoma surgery were a patient age of 50 years or younger, preoperative intraocular pressure greater than 10 mm Hg, and early postoperative peak intraocular pressure greater than 25 mm Hg. The cumulative percentage of patients not needing reoperation for glaucoma was 93% at 1 year and 90% at 2 years. At the last patient visit, mean intraocular pressure had increased to 1.6 mm Hg greater than precataract extraction levels and was similar to levels in the first month after operation. The median time between cataract extraction and additional glaucoma medication or bleb needling was 1.6 months. The median time between nonsurgical intervention and additional glaucoma surgery was 3.6 months. Eleven of 19 eyes with hypotony before cataract extraction still had hypotony after cataract extraction, despite increased intraocular pressure (from a mean of 4.6 to 7.5 mm Hg).

Discussion.—Factors that decrease postoperative intraocular pressure control include cataract extraction performed after trabeculectomy, patients age of 50 or younger, preoperative intraocular pressure greater than 10 mm Hg, intraoperative iris manipulation, and early postoperative intraocular pressure greater than 25 mm Hg. The majority of bleb failures are seen soon after cataract extraction. It is not currently possible to predict resolution of pre-existing hypotony after cataract extraction.

▶ This article reviews risk factors for trabeculectomy failure when cataract surgery is performed in patients who have undergone previous glaucoma filtering surgery. My own perception is that, as glaucoma specialists have become more comfortable with small incision cataract surgery, they have become more aggressive about performing combined cataract and glaucoma filtering surgery. Nonetheless, there are definitely patients who undergo glaucoma surgery alone and then require subsequent cataract surgery. This article shows that patients under 50 years of age who have a preoperative pressure of greater than 10 mm Hg, and who have intraoperative iris manipulation or early postoperative pressure greater than 25 mm Hg are at risk for further trabeculectomy failure. However, the patients in this study had their cataracts removed by large-incision, manual, nuclear expression surgery rather by than small-incision phacoemulsification.

It is likely, however, that the same risk factors which caused bleb failure with large-incision surgery cause greater risk with small-incision surgery as well.

I did find it interesting to note that the authors do not report a complete correlation with resolution of postoperative hypotony from glaucoma filtering surgery following cataract surgery. I have had the personal experience of operating on a moderate number of patients with cataracts and hypotony following glaucoma filtering surgery and have found that, in virtually all cases, the hypotony resolved. I did, however, aggressively discontinue steroids very early in the postoperative period for these patients and tried to induce conjunctival scarring at the time of cataract surgery. This may be the reason why some patients with hypotony have an elevation of their intraocular pressure following cataract surgery.

R. Tipperman, M.D.

Long-term Follow-up of Extracapsular Cataract Extraction and Posterior Chamber Intraocular Lens Implantation in Patients With Uveitis

Krishna R, Meisler DM, Lowder CY, et al (Cleveland Clinic Found, Ohio)
Ophthalmology 105:1765-1769, 1998 1–18

Background.—Cataracts are a complication of uveitis and must often be removed for visual rehabilitation and for evaluation of posterior segment pathology. In the last 20 years, extracapsular cataract extraction with posterior chamber intraocular lens (IOL) implantation has become more common, and ophthalmologists are more often placing IOLs in patients with uveitis. Short-term postoperative results of extracapsular cataract extraction with posterior chamber IOL implantation have been encouraging. Long-term results in patients with uveitis who have had extracapsular cataract extraction and posterior chamber IOL implantation are reported.

Methods.—A series of 28 patients (36 eyes) was reviewed retrospectively. Level of best-corrected Snellen visual acuity, change in visual acuity, length of follow-up, long-term results, and complications were analyzed. The mean follow-up was 81.4 months.

Results.—Preoperatively, the mean best-corrected visual acuity was 20/200. At 81.4 months, visual acuity had improved in 94% of eyes. For all eyes, the average change in visual acuity was an improvement of 6.4 Snellen lines. Postoperatively, the mean best-corrected visual acuity was 20/40, and 75% of eyes were 20/40 or better. There was a 56% prevalence of cystoid macular edema, a 56% prevalence of epiretinal membrane, and a 58% prevalence of posterior capsule opacification.

Discussion.—Macular disorders are the most common postoperative cause of limitations in visual acuity in eyes with uveitis that undergo extracapsular cataract extraction with posterior chamber IOL implantation. An association between epiretinal membranes and ocular inflammation has been reported. Successful long-term visual results can be seen in patients with uveitis who are treated with extracapsular cataract extraction and posterior chamber IOL implantation. Preoperative and postoperative inflammation must be carefully controlled. Between the authors' short-term and long-term studies, Snellen visual acuity decreased by an average of only 1.1 lines, despite increased rates of cystoid macular edema, epiretinal membrane, and posterior capsule opacification.

▶ IOLs have been developed over the past several decades. At first there were many patients in whom their use was felt to be contraindicated. These included pediatric patients and patients with uveitis. Obviously, as experience with implants has grown, surgeons have "pushed the envelope" and have begun using IOLs in both pediatric patients and patients with uveitis.

The value of this study lies in its long-term follow-up of patients with uveitis who have received posterior chamber lens implantation. In general, the patients do extremely well and the lenses do not really seem to play much of a role in altering the course of the patient's uveitis. Obviously, these patients are much better off being left pseudophakic than aphakic. In addition, secondary lens implantation in a patient with uveitis can be quite complicated, because often the patient's posterior capsule will scar to the posterior iris. As a result, I counsel almost all my patients with uveitis that they are probably safer and better off, in the long term, going ahead with posterior chamber lens implantation at the time of cataract removal. I do explain that there is an increased risk, but the potential increase in benefit is enormous.

It is important that the intraocular inflammation be completely controlled prior to cataract surgery. This, at times, requires both topical anti-inflammatories and systemic steroids.

R. Tipperman, M.D.

2 Refractive Surgery

The Year in Refractive Surgery

by Christopher J. Rapuano, M.D.

The biggest developments in the refractive surgery arena as the decade (if not the millennium) draws to a close involve excimer laser surgery. While other lasers and refractive surgery technologies are in development and testing phases, excimer laser photorefractive keratectomy (PRK) and laser in situ keratomileusis (LASIK) dominate the refractive surgery field.

Two new excimer lasers received Food and Drug Administration approval for the treatment of myopia (and one also for astigmatism). Autonomous Technologies Corporation received approval to treat up to −10 D of myopia and up to −4 D of astigmatism (maximum spherical equivalent, −10 D). The Autonomous laser is a scanning slit laser with an integrated eye tracking system. Nidek Co., Ltd. received approval to treat up to −13 D of myopia. The Nidek laser is a flying spot laser.

These two laser systems double the number of FDA-approved excimer lasers in the United States. Not only will they bring added competition (and, hopefully, a decrease in the currently expensive user fees charged by VISX and Summit), but also they should encourage continued innovation by all excimer laser manufacturers.

Summit and VISX are continuing to push forward. In the past year, Summit received FDA approval to treat up to −4 D of astigmatism (maximum spherical equivalent, −6 D). VISX received FDA approval to treat high myopia, up to −12 D at the spectacle plane. VISX also received FDA approval for hyperopic PRK, the first laser approved for the treatment of hyperopia. Even the holmium:YAG laser, which has been in FDA trials treating hyperopia for years, has not yet received FDA approval. The VISX indications are for 1 to 6 D of hyperopia at the spectacle plane in patients 21 years or older. The best results appear to be in presbyopes and pre-presbyopes with under 4 D of hyperopia.

The best "long-term" follow-up study on PRK was published this past year.[1] It included 6-year follow-up data on PRK with the Summit laser using a 4-mm diameter ablation zone. While that size ablation zone is no longer used, the study demonstrated excellent corneal clarity and visual stability over the follow-up period with no intraocular or retinal side effects noted.

PRK is also pushing the envelope. Mild keratoconus may not be the absolute contraindication for PRK it was once thought to be. One small study demonstrated improved uncorrected and best corrected vision after astigmatic PRK in 7 of 8 mild keratoconus patients.[2] Another small study did not detect an increase in corneal haze or scarring in keloid formers after PRK.[3] This finding brings into question the FDA's keloid formation as a relative contraindication to PRK. Although many surgeons considered PRK dead with the advent of LASIK, these new lasers, the new FDA approvals, and the good long-term follow-up data seem to have breathed new life into PRK.

By far the largest increase in refractive surgery interest in the past year has been with LASIK. While several studies comparing PRK and LASIK for low, medium, and high degrees of myopia have demonstrated similar visual results in the two groups after the first few months, the rapid visual recovery, with minimal to no pain, offered by LASIK is what brings patients in.[4]

A large study on one surgeon's first 1,000 LASIK procedures demonstrates excellent visual results with few vision-threatening complications.[5] Additionally, the authors found a definite learning curve to the procedure, with many fewer intraoperative microkeratome-related complications in the last 400 cases than in the first 200 cases.

LASIK is not without complications, however. The first studies on "diffuse lamellar keratitis" or "shifting sands of the Sahara syndrome" were reported.[6] This is an important complication to recognize and treat properly. Delayed treatment can result in thinning (melting) of the stromal bed below the inflammation, with a significant overcorrection. As it can resemble an infection, appropriate diagnosis can avoid unnecessary lifting of the flap and treatment with intensive antibiotics.

With the FDA approval of PRK for the treatment of hyperopia, LASIK for hyperopia was bound to be just around the corner. In fact, given the larger epithelial defect required for hyperopic PRK (8-9 mm) than for myopic PRK (6 mm), there is a potential added benefit to LASIK (with its minimal epithelial defect). Of course, this larger ablation zone requires a larger LASIK flap. Newer microkeratomes can not only achieve larger flaps, but can place the hinge superiorly (for the Chiron Hansatome) or at any position (Moria Carriazo-Barraquer). Additionally, these new microkeratomes are easier to assemble (with less or no chance of allowing the blade to enter the anterior chamber) and use.

Patient selection, always critical before refractive surgery, has also been modified for LASIK. When it was first introduced several years ago, the upper limit of treatment was in the 18 to 25 D range. This high end has steadily declined to around 12 D with the postoperative keratometric reading ideally being no less than 34 to 35 D.

Another aspect of patent selection gaining more attention is pupil size. Surgeons are becoming more and more aware that certain patients with seemingly excellent refractive surgery results who have significant visual complaints (especially at night) have large pupils. While most surgeons measure pupil size in some manner, it has been difficult to reliably measure pupil size in dim illumination. The Colvard pupillometer (I have no financial interest) uses light amplification to accomplish this task in a reproducible fashion.[7] I believe that some method of pupil measurement in dim illumination should be standard before refractive surgery.

As we enter the new millennium, advances in refractive surgery continue at a dizzying pace. Over the next decade, there are sure to be improvements in current techniques and technology, along with new procedures. The intracorneal ring, holmium:YAG, and picosecond and femtosecond lasers are just a few of the technologies we are certain to be learning more about.

References

1. Stephenson CG, Gartry DS, O'Brart DP, et al: Photorefractive keratectomy: A 6-year follow-up study. *Ophthalmology* 105:273-281, 1998.
2. Kremer I, Shochot Y, Kaplan A, et al: Three year results of photoastigmatic refractive keratectomy for mild and atypical keratoconus. *J Cataract Refract Surg* 24:1581-1588, 1998.
3. Tanzer DJ, Isfahani A, Schallhorn SC, et al: Photorefractive keratectomy in African Americans including those with known dermatologic keloid formation. *Am J Ophthalmol* 126:625-629, 1998.
4. Hersh PS, Brint SF, Maloney RK, et al: Photorefractive keratectomy versus laser in situ keratomileusis for moderate to high myopia: A randomized study. *Ophthalmology* 105:1512-1523, 1998.
5. Gimbel HV, Anderson Penno EE, van Westenbrugge JA, et al: Incidence and management of intraoperative and early postoperative complications in 1000 consecutive laser in situ keratomileusis cases. *Ophthalmology* 105:1839-1848, 1998.
6. Smith RJ, Maloney RK: Diffuse lamellar keratitis: A new syndrome in lamellar refractive surgery. *Ophthalmology* 105:1721-1726, 1998.
7. Colvard M: Preoperative measurement of scotopic pupil dilation using an office pupillometer. *J Cataract Refract Surg* 24:1594-1597, 1998.

Photorefractive Keratectomy: A 6-Year Follow-up Study

Stephenson CG, Gartry DS, O'Brart DPS, et al (St Thomas' Hosp, London; Moorfields Eye Hosp, London; Addenbrooke's Hosp, Cambridge, England)

Ophthalmology 105:273-281, 1998 2–1

Background.—The first excimer laser photorefractive keratectomies (PRKs) in the United Kingdom were performed in 1989, using a 4-mm ablation zone. This article describes 6-year follow-up on those patients who participated in that PRK trial.

Study Design.—The study group consisted of 120 patients who had myopic PRK corrections of 2 to 7 D using a 4-mm ablation zone. The surgical technique, the ablation zone size, and the postoperative regimen were the same for all patients. Of the original group, 83 patients were available for 6-year follow-up that included a detailed ophthalmic examination and questionnaire. Induced refractive change, objective corneal

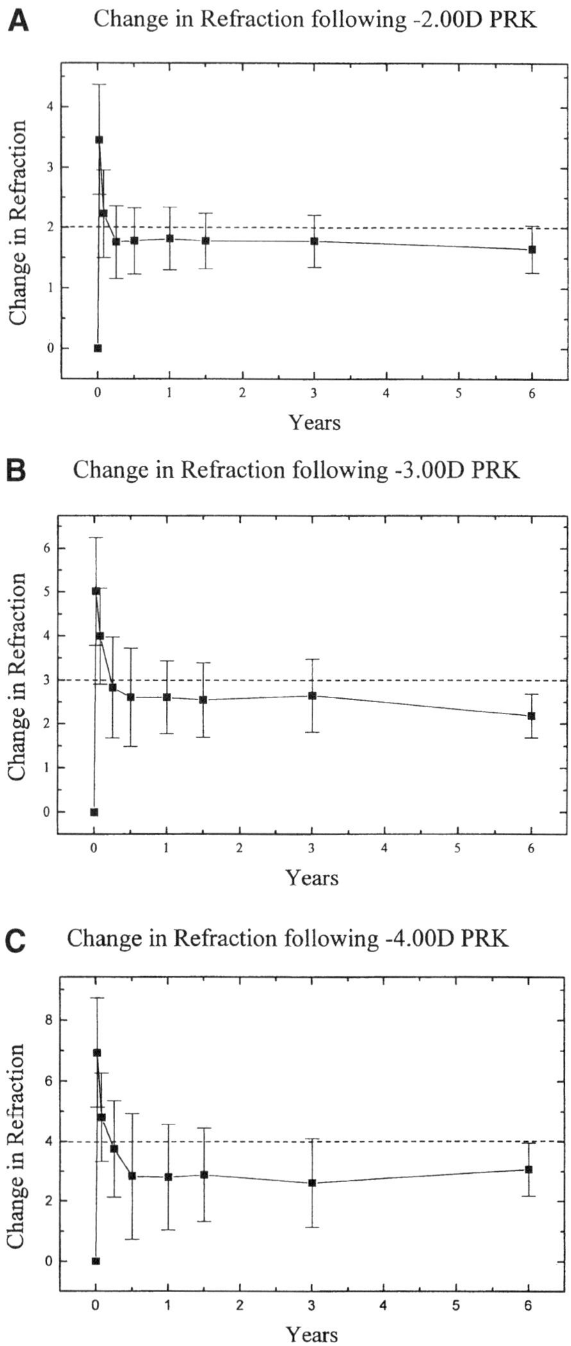
A
Change in Refraction following -2.00D PRK
Change in Refraction
0
1
2
3
4
0
1
2
3
4
5
6
Years
B
Change in Refraction following -3.00D PRK
Change in Refraction
0
1
2
3
4
5
6
0
1
2
3
4
5
6
Years
C
Change in Refraction following -4.00D PRK
Change in Refraction
0
2
4
6
8
0
1
2
3
4
5
6
Years

(Continued)

FIGURE 2 (cont.)

D Change in Refraction following -5.00D PRK

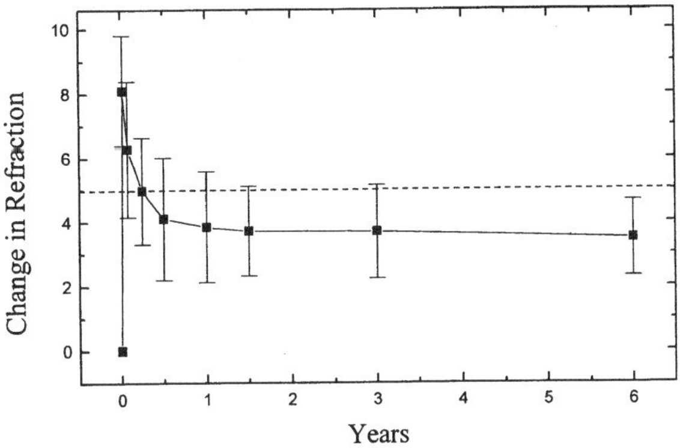

E Change in Refraction following -6.00D PRK

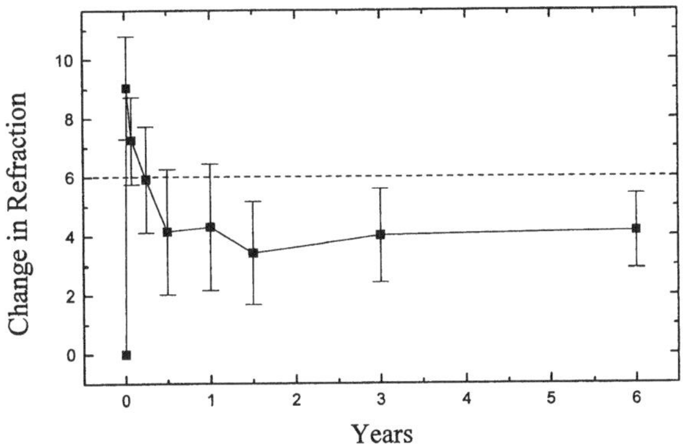

F Change in Refraction following -7.00D PRK

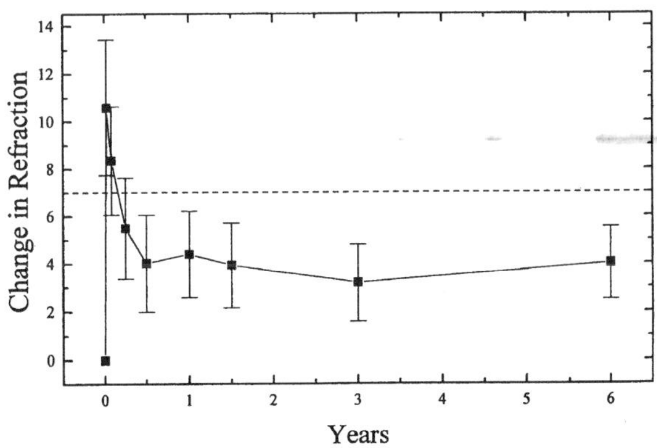

FIGURE 2.—A–F, graphs relating change in refraction to time in the 6 treatment groups. Initial overcorrection in all patients followed by regression to a plateau between 3 and 6 months. The error bars are ± 1 standard deviation. (Published courtesy of *Ophthalmology*, from Stephenson CG, Gartry DS, O'Brart DPS, et al: Photorefractive keratectomy: A 6-year follow-up study. *Ophthalmology* 105:273-281, 1998.)

haze, glare, halo measurements, and long-term complications were assessed.

Findings.—At 6-year follow-up, there were no signs of corneal decompensation, thinning or ectasia of the cornea, epithelial staining or instability, or visually significant cataract, and no significant retinal changes or detachment. None of these patients had elevated intraocular pressure. The average final refraction had remained stable from 1-year to 6-year follow-up (Fig 2). There was no hyperopic shift or diurnal fluctuation of refraction. Haze increased after PRK to a maximum at 3 to 6 months postoperatively and then declined. Nine patients reported a significant halo effect at low light levels.

Conclusions.—The initial group of patients who underwent PRK in the United Kingdom were examined 6 years postoperatively. The average PRK-induced refractive change stabilized after 3 to 6 months and remained stable for the 6-year follow-up visit. There was no long-term refractive hyperopic drift, and haze was minimal. There were no late-phase complications. Night halos remained a problem for a small number of patients from this initial group treated with a 4-mm ablation zone.

► While most of us think that PRK surgery has been around for years and years, and many of us think it may even be past its prime, this 6-year study is the longest, best follow-up study to date. Being a long-term follow-up study, it is plagued by 2 problems. First, it reports on an early technique using a 4-mm diameter ablation zone (6 mm or larger is now standard). Second, the 6-year follow-up was only 68% (good, but not great). Nevertheless, several findings are quite important and should be stressed. No further regression was found after the 6- to 12-month follow-up (the exact time depends on initial manifest refraction). No hyperopic shift was found. No diurnal fluctuation was found. Haze tended to decrease and vision tended to improve over time. No other ocular side effects were noted. These findings bode well for long-term follow-up for newer PRK techniques using larger ablation zones.

C.J. Rapuano, M.D.

Allergic Conjunctivitis as a Risk Factor for Regression and Haze After Photorefractive Keratectomy

Yang H-Y, Fujishima H, Toda I, et al (Tokyo Dental College; Keio Univ, Tokyo; Itoh Hosp, Mobara, Japan)

Am J Ophthalmol 125:54-58, 1998 2–2

Background.—Allergic conjunctivitis may be associated with subepithelial haze in patients who undergo photorefractive keratectomy (PRK). The relationship between allergic conjunctivitis and the results of PRK with a 4.5-mm ablation zone were examined in 57 eyes.

Methods.—The study group consisted of 57 eyes in 57 adult Japanese patients. The eyes were classified as 30 normal, 16 with allergic conjunc-

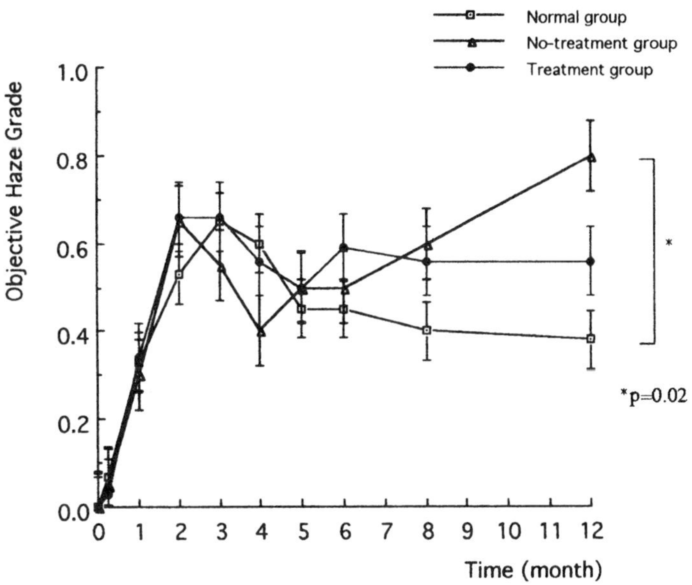

FIGURE 1.—The change in subepithelial haze over time. There was no significant difference in the mean haze score among groups at 3, 6, or 8 months after surgery. At 12 months, the haze score was significantly higher in the no-treatment group than in the treatment and normal groups (unpaired *t* test, $P = 0.02$). There was no significant difference in the haze score between the treatment and normal groups ($P = 0.24$) or the treatment and no-treatment groups ($P = 0.20$). *Symbols: Open square*, normal group; *open triangle*, no-treatment group; *solid circle*, treatment group. (Reprinted by permission of the publisher from Yang H-Y, Fujishima H, Toda I, et al: Allergic conjunctivitis as a risk factor for regression and haze after photorefractive keratectomy. *Am J Ophthalmol* 125:54-58. Copyright 1998 by Elsevier Science Inc.)

tivitis treated with 3 months of fluorometholone and cromolyn sodium 12 weeks after PRK, and 11 with allergic conjunctivitis which were not treated. The patients were followed for 12 to 18 months.

Results.—There was no significant difference in the average haze score among these 3 groups at 3, 6, or 8 month follow-up. At 12 months, the haze score was significantly higher in the no-treatment group (Fig 1). There was no significant change in refraction during the first 3 postoperative months in any of these 3 groups. The no-treatment group had significant regression beginning at 6 postoperative months (Fig 2). Uncorrected visual acuity of 20/40 or better was achieved by all 30 patients in the normal group, 15 of 16 in the treated group, and only 6 of 11 patients in the no-treatment group.

Conclusions.—The results of this study indicate that untreated allergic conjunctivitis is associated with the development of corneal haze and myopic regression after PRK. When allergic conjunctivitis was treated, these adverse effects were significantly decreased. Anti-allergic medication should be considered for PRK patients with allergic conjunctivitis.

▶ This study nicely documents worse outcome after PRK in patients with untreated allergic conjunctivitis. Vision, haze, and refractive regression were worse in the untreated allergic patients than in the normal patients. While

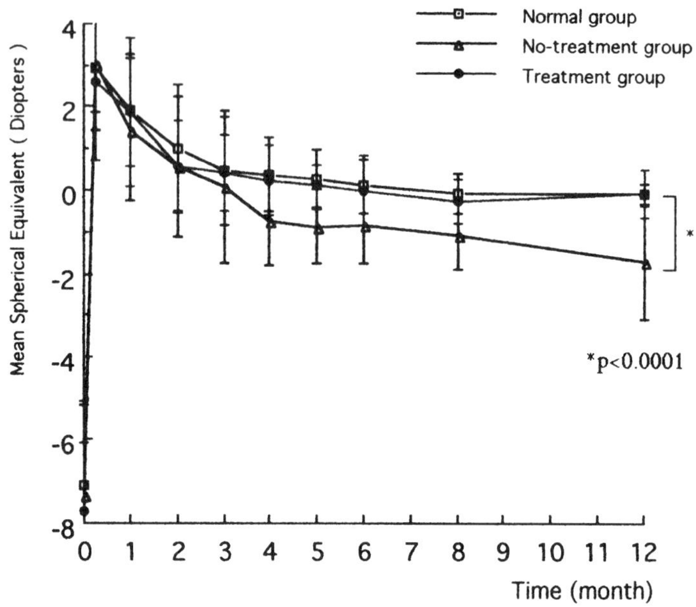

FIGURE 2.—The change in refraction over time. There was no significant change in refraction during the first 3 months in any group, but the no-treatment group showed significant regression at 6 and 12 months after surgery (Scheffe test at 12 months: no-treatment group vs treatment group, $P < 0.0001$, no-treatment group vs normal group, $P < 0.0001$). There was no significant difference between the treatment and normal groups ($P = 0.99$). *Symbols: Open square*, normal group; *open triangle*, no-treatment group; *solid circle*, treatment group. (Reprinted by permission of the publisher from Yang H-Y, Fujishima H, Toda I, et al: Allergic conjunctivitis as a risk factor for regression and haze after photorefractive keratectomy. *Am J Ophthalmol* 125:54-58. Copyright 1998 by Elsevier Science Inc.)

the authors do not give the dates of treatment, it probably occurred 4 to 5 years ago, because a 4.5-mm diameter ablation zone was used. While a 6.0-mm or larger diameter ablation zone is now typical, these findings should not be ignored. I agree with the authors' conclusions that allergic conjunctivitis should be treated aggressively after PRK, but add that the eyes should be free of active allergic inflammation prior to PRK as well.

C.J. Rapuano, M.D.

Contrast Sensitivity and Glare Disability After Radial Keratotomy and Photorefractive Keratectomy

Ghaith AA, Daniel J, Stulting RD, et al (Alexandria Univ, Egypt; Emory Univ, Atlanta, Ga)

Arch Ophthalmol 116:12-18, 1998 2–3

Background.—Most studies examining refractive surgical procedures rely on visual acuity, which is a crude measure of visual performance in everyday life. Contrast sensitivity is the ability to detect luminance differences between adjacent areas. Glare disability is the reduction of visual acuity caused by light elsewhere in the visual field. Both contrast sensitivity and glare disability were assessed in patients who underwent radial keratotomy (RK) and photorefractive keratectomy (PRK).

Methods.—The study group consisted of patients with a total of 30 eyes undergoing RK and 30 eyes undergoing PRK. Preoperatively, a detailed history and complete ophthalmological examination were obtained. Visual acuity was assessed. All patients had ophthalmological examinations at 1, 3, and 6 months postoperatively. Contrast sensitivity and glare disability were evaluated by the CSV 1,000, the Multivision Contrast tester (MCT) 8,000, the Pelli-Robson chart, and the Brightness Acuity Tester (BAT). Patients completed a vision questionnaire.

Results.—Contrast sensitivity decreased after both RK and PRK through the 6 months postoperative follow-up. Glare disability was significantly increased 1 month after PRK, as measured by MCT 8,000 and BAT, and at 3 and 6 months after RK, again by the MCT 8,000. PRK decreased contrast sensitivity significantly more than RK did at 1 month, as assessed by MCT 8,000. There was no significant difference in visual performance between RK and PRK patients up to the sixth postoperative month, as measured by CSV 1,000, Pelli-Robson chart, or BAT. There was no consistent difference when patients were assessed by MCT 8,000. There was no consistent correlation between patient reports on questionnaires and patient scores on these contrast sensitivity or glare disability tests.

Conclusions.—Although both RK and PRK appeared to reduce contrast sensitivity and increase glare disability, according to the 4 assessments used in this study, the relative effect was highly dependent on the timing of assessment and on the instrument. Results of these assessments did not match patient responses to questionnaires. The changes in contrast sensitivity and glare disability detected after RK or PRK do not appear to be clinically significant in the everyday lives of patients undergoing these procedures.

▶ The results of this well-designed study reflect the poor technology available clinically to assess contrast sensitivity and glare disability. Three different instruments were used to test contrast sensitivity, and 2 different instruments were used to test glare. While deficits were found for contrast sensitivity and glare after both RK and PRK, these findings did not correlate well with patients' reported symptoms. It would be interesting to repeat the objective and subjective testing at 1 year or longer after surgery to determine whether these findings persist.

C.J. Rapuano, M.D.

Myopic Picosecond Laser Keratomileusis With the Neodymium–Yttrium Lithium Fluoride Laser in the Cat Cornea

Hanuch OE, Agrawal VB, Bassage S, et al (Univ of Rochester, NY)
Ophthalmology 105:142-149, 1998 2–4

Background.—The advent of laser technology that can selectively remove intrastromal corneal tissue has created new possibilities for modifying the refractive power of the cornea to treat myopia, hyperopia, and astigmatism. The effects of myopic picosecond laser keratomileusis (PLK) were investigated in the cat cornea.

Methods.—Three groups of 4 cats each underwent treatment on 1 eye. The other eye was used for comparison. Group 1 underwent a sham operation; group 2, 100-μm lenticle thickness; and group 3, 150-μm lenticle thickness. The intervention was picosecond laser keratomileusis, a new intrastromal laser method with the neodymium–yttrium lithium fluoride picosecond laser. The procedure was similar to laser keratomileusis in situ, consisting of 2 lamellar ring cuts and 1 vertical ring-shape cut defining a 4-mm-diameter intrastromal lenticle.

Findings.—Group 2 had a mean diopter change of 5.4 at 1 month, which remained stable during 6 months of follow-up. In group 3, the change in diopters was 8.1 at 1 month and 6.8 at 6 months. No significant changes occurred in group 1. Corneal thickness was decreased significantly

A

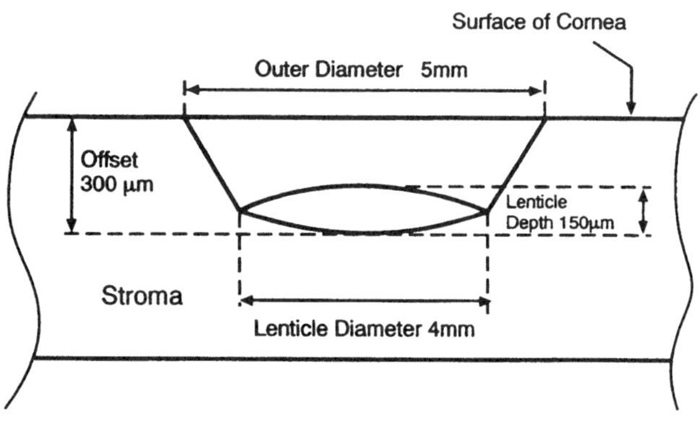

Pattern:	Lens	Lenticule thickness:	100/150μm
Energy:	30μJ	Offset:	300/350μm
Spot Sep:	30μm	Lenticule diameter:	4mm
Rep.Rate:	1000Hz	Outer diameter:	5mm

Total Pattern Time: 150 seconds

FIGURE 1.—A, schematic of picosecond laser keratomileusis intrastromal procedure and laser parameters. (Published courtesy of *Ophthalmology*, from Hanuch OE, Agrawal VB, Bassage S, et al: Myopic picosecond laser keratomileusis with the neodymium–yttrium lithium fluoride laser in the cat cornea. *Ophthalmology* 105:142-149, 1998.)

by 1 month in groups 2 and 3. However, by 3 months it had regressed to near preoperative values. The corneas were clear at 6 months, with no grossly visible scarring. Slit-lamp assessment revealed a faint, thin line of haziness, barely visible in the periphery of the flap. Histologic assessment demonstrated no significant collagen disruption, inflammation, or endothelial irregularities (Fig 1, A).

Conclusions.—Myopic intrastromal PLK has a refractive effect on the cornea. This effect depends on the thickness of the lenticle removed and persists for at least 6 months, with minimal stromal haze and no operative complications. Further research is needed to verify the efficacy of PLK as a valid refractive procedure.

▶ The creation and subsequent healing of the corneal flap in the laser-assisted in situ keratomileusis (LASIK) procedure is not without problems. Intrastromal ablation, where no epithelial break is made at all, has been attempted in the past without great success. The technique reported in this study uses the cutting aspect of the picosecond laser intrastromally to create the anterior and posterior planes of the lenticle to be removed. Then a small incision is made at the edge of the lenticle, and forceps are used to reach in and take the lenticle out.

This study is obviously a small early cat study but demonstrates that the technique is possible. Ideally, it could eliminate many of the potential complications of the current LASIK procedure, but much more research is required.

C.J. Rapuano, M.D.

Laser In Situ Keratomileusis for Moderate and High Myopia and Myopic Astigmatism

Knorz MC, Wiesinger B, Liermann A, et al (Klinikum Mannheim, Germany)
Ophthalmology 105:932-940, 1998 2–5

Background.—Patients with greater than −6 D of myopia undergoing wide-area ablation photorefractive keratectomy are at risk of refractive instability, corneal scarring, night aberration, and loss of visual acuity. There is little information on the use of laser in situ keratomileusis (LASIK) in this situation. The predictability, stability, and safety of a standardized LASIK technique were examined in eyes with myopia and myopic astigmatism.

Methods.—The nonrandomized trial included 93 consecutive eyes of 55 patients: 37 eyes had myopia of −5 to −29 D with corneal astigmatism of less than 1 D (group 1), whereas 56 eyes had myopia of −5 to −25 D with astigmatism of 1 to 4.5 D (group 2). The LASIK procedure was performed using the Automatic Corneal Shaper, with a preset flap thickness of 160 μm, and the Keracor 116 excimer laser. A single-zone and single-pass ablation was used for spherical correction, with pretreatment to prevent central islands. Eye movements were compensated for by use of an active eye-tracking device. Evaluation included refractive predictability and stability, corneal topography, corneal interface scarring and thickness, and patient satisfaction.

Results.—Eyes receiving a lower correction were more likely to be within 0.5 and 1 D; there were significant differences between corrections of −5 to −9.9 D and −15 to −29 D. Group 2 eyes achieved significantly greater stability with corrections for −5 to −9.9 D than with corrections of −15 to −29 D. At most recent evaluation, 4% of eyes had lost 2 lines of corrected visual acuity. These included 1 patient in the spherical group and 1 patient in the toric group undergoing corrections of −10 to −14.9 D, and 1 patient in the spherical group undergoing correction of −15 to −29 D; no patient undergoing correction of −5 to −9.9 D lost 2 or more lines.

The frequency of central islands decreased from 25% at 1 week to 17% at 12 months in group 1, and from 37% to 16% in group 2. Decentrations were found in 6% of group 1 and 4% of group 2 at 1 year. Corneal refraction was highly stable, even in patients with high myopia. Mean endothelial cell counts did not decrease significantly at any attempted correction. For patients with spherical corrections, all were highly satisfied in the −5 to −9.9 D group, as were 90% of those in the −10 to −14.9 D group; of those with corrections of more than −15 D, 22% were unsatisfied or only moderately satisfied. For patients with toric corrections, the percentage of patients who were unsatisfied or only moderately satisfied was 16%, increasing to 50% for corrections of more than −15 D. The intraoperative complication rate was 1%, and the reoperation rate 2%.

Conclusions.—In patients with myopia of up to −10 D, the standardized LASIK procedure used in this study offers stable manifest refraction, adequate uncorrected central visual acuity, and good patient satisfaction. Acceptable results may be achieved in patients with myopia of up to −15 D, though with more visual loss and reduced patient satisfaction. Even with pretreatment, central corneal islands are the most frequent complication. Patient satisfaction is lower with astigmatism correction than with spherical correction.

► The authors present a well-done but small study of 93 eyes, 85 of which were followed up for 1 year. Eyes were divided into myopia with (56 eyes) and without (37 eyes) significant astigmatism and by level of myopia: −5 to −10 D (20 eyes), −10 to −15 D (34 eyes), and −15 to −29 D (39 eyes). Unfortunately, the smallest number of eyes were in the −5- to −10-D group, perhaps the most common level of myopia treated by surgeons performing both photorefractive keratectomy and LASIK. The uncorrected vision, best-corrected vision, refractive stability, and patient satisfaction results were quite good for the 5- to 10-D group, good for the 10- to 15-D group, but relatively poor for the over 15-D group. Patients treated for astigmatism generally did not do as well as those not treated for astigmatism. One intraoperative complication (thin flap) occurred. Two reoperations because of flap complications (one epithelial ingrowth and one dislocated flap) were required. Three other eyes required reoperations for undercorrection and one for a central island.

The peer review data on LASIK is still coming in, but the early results appear to be promising up to 10 to 15 D. However, the authors believe that other options, such as phakic intraocular lens and clear lens extraction should be investigated for myopia greater than 15 D.

C.J. Rapuano, M.D.

Laser Thermal Keratoplasty for the Treatment of Photorefractive Keratectomy Overcorrections: A 1-Year Follow-up

Pop M (Michel Pop Clinics, Montreal and Hull, PQ)

Ophthalmology 105:926-931, 1998 2–6

Introduction.—A common method of correcting myopia is photorefractive keratectomy (PRK). The use of holmium:yttrium-aluminum-garnet (YAG) laser thermal keratoplasty (LTK) when re-treating PRK-overcorrected myopic eyes was evaluated with patients who were overcorrected by at least 1 D.

Methods.—There were 33 patients (36 eyes) who had become hyperopes after myopic PRK treatment; they were given LTK, using a nontouch holmium:YAG laser. Four to 8 spots per ring, up to 3 rings, were applied in concentric circles with a diameter ranging from 6 to 8 mm from the visual axis to correct hyperopia. There was a range of 8 to 24 spots. These patients were compared with a control group with preoperative refraction values not statistically different from the PRK-plus-LTK group.

Results.—The mean refraction was + 1.14 ± 1.09 D at 12 months after the LTK retreatment. From 1 to 12 months, the regression was 0.5 ± 1.1 D. Fifty percent of the eyes were within 1 D of emmetropia at 12 months (Fig 1). Uncorrected visual acuity of 20/40 or better was found in 93% of the eyes. Uncorrected visual acuity of 20/20 or better was found in 24% of the eyes. For 11 eyes (34%) that regained original sphere values or higher, refraction was not stable. The procedure did not increase or decrease haze, nor did it affect best-corrected visual acuity.

Conclusion.—Two thirds of the retreated eyes did not need further retreatment at 12 months after a LTK retreatment after an initial PRK. For PRK overcorrection retreatments, clinical data showed that LTK should be kept for +1 to +2 D of hyperopia.

▶ Dr. Pop, an extremely experienced and innovative PRK surgeon in Canada, reports on noncontact LTK for overcorrection after PRK. He compares the data to LTK for primary hyperopia. Overall, the refractive effects of LTK were somewhat greater after PRK than in primary hyperopia, but the effects were not huge in either group. The good news is that there were very few side effects, including only 1 eye losing 1 line of best spectacle corrected vision at 12 months. Given the unhappiness of many overcorrected PRK patients, LTK is probably worth a try. The author concludes that LTK is best for eyes with less than 2.00 D of overcorrection.

C.J. Rapuano, M.D.

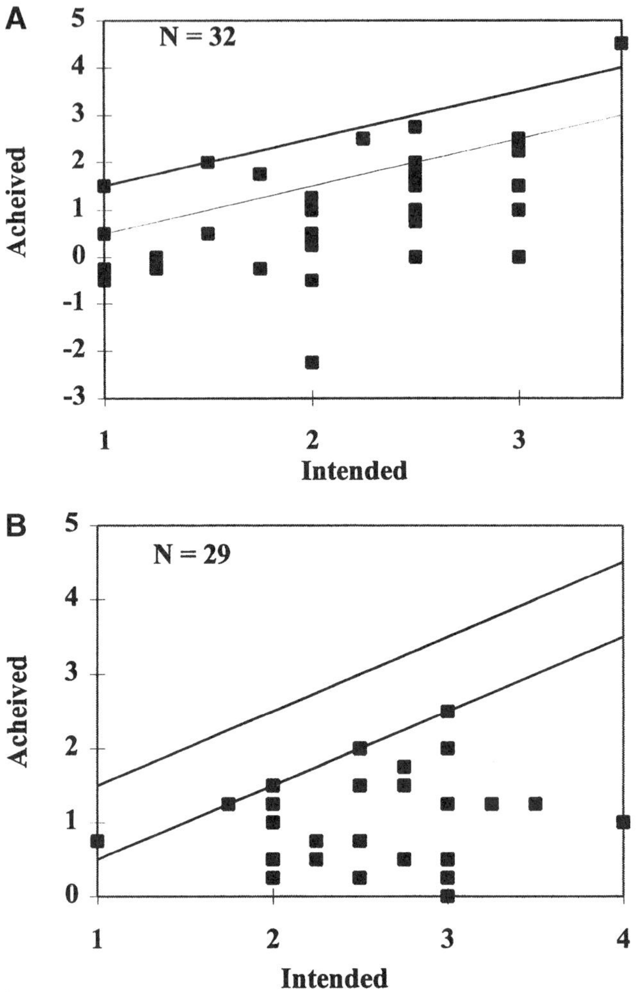

FIGURE 1.—A, scattergram of the sphere values (diopters) before laser thermal keratoplasty retreatment vs. 12 months postoperatively shows achieved vs. intended correction toward emmetropia for the photorefractive keratectomy plus laser thermal keratoplasty group. B, scattergram of the sphere values (diopters) before laser thermal keratoplasty treatment vs. 12 months postoperatively showing achieved vs. intended correction toward emmetropia for the laser thermal keratoplasty group. Straight lines indicate levels within ± 0.5 D of the intended correction. Number of eyes (*n*) is shown. (Published courtesy of *Ophthalmology*, from Pop M: Laser thermal keratoplasty for the treatment of photorefractive keratectomy overcorrections: A 1-year follow-up. *Ophthalmology* 105:926-931, 1998.)

Hyperopic Automated Lamellar Keratoplasty: Complications and Visual Results

Lyle WA, Jin GJC (Eye Inst of Utah, Salt Lake City)

Arch Ophthalmol 116:425-428, 1998 2–7

Introduction.—A new treatment for hyperopia is hyperopic automated lamellar keratoplasty. Fairly good results for eyes with a measurement of under 4.5 D has been found. But there was decreasing accuracy with increasing attempted correction. There has been no peer-reviewed report on the long-term results of hyperopic automated lamellar keratoplasty, even though the procedure has been performed for several years. To examine the long-term safety and efficacy of hyperopic automated lamellar keratoplasty, a prospective study was conducted.

Methods.—Fifty patients (67 eyes) had hyperopic automated lamellar keratoplasty in a 2-year period. There were 25 eyes with primary hyperopia and 42 eyes with consecutive hyperopia after myopic refractive surgery. About 87% (57 eyes) were followed for 6 months and 67% (45 eyes) were followed for at least 1 year, whereas 21 eyes were followed for 2 to 4 years.

Results.—The mean preoperative spherical equivalent was +2.87 ± 1.28 D. At 3 months, the mean postoperative spherical equivalent was −0.03 ± 1.42 D. At 6 months, it was −0.42 ± 2.25 D. At 1 year, it was −0.55 ± 3.00 D, and at 2 years, it was −0.58 ± 1.53 D. At the last follow-up, it was 0.35 ± 1.79 D. Between 3 months and 1 year, the mean myopic shift was 0.50 D. Between 1 and 2 years, the mean myopic shift was 1.00 D. There was meaningful reduction of hyperopia and improvement of visual acuity with hyperopic automated lamellar keratoplasty, particularly for patients with primary hyperopia. With this procedure, however, long-term refractive instability is a serious problem. Iatrogenic keratoconus occurred in 11 of 42 eyes (26%) in which hyperopic automated lamellar keratoplasty was performed.

Conclusion.—The use of hyperopic automated lamellar keratoplasty should be discouraged because of its long-term instability and high incidence of iatrogenic keratoconus after the procedure. This is especially true for consecutive hyperopia after radial keratotomy.

► The authors performed hyperopic automated lamellar keratoplasty on 67 eyes. This is a procedure in which a deep lamellar incision (300-425 microns, 50%-72% corneal depth) is made with a microkeratome across most of the cornea, leaving the nasalmost aspect uncut, creating a hinge. Twenty-five eyes underwent correction for primary hyperopia, 41 procedures followed overcorrected radial keratotomy, and 1 followed overcorrected myopic automated lamellar keratoplasty. For primary hyperopia, 84% of eyes achieved 20/40 or better uncorrected visual acuity and only 1 eye lost 2 lines of best spectacle-corrected vision. For overcorrected radial keratotomy, iatrogenic keratoconus developed in 41 eyes, with decreased vision, progressive myopic shift, and inferior steepening requiring penetrating keratoplasty.

Interestingly, there were no significant differences in the corneal thickness or depth of incision in the eyes in which keratoconus developed, compared with the eyes in which it did not. Of course, those eyes may develop iatrogenic keratoconus in the future. Hyperopic automated lamellar keratoplasty is not a good procedure for overcorrected radial keratotomy.

On a separate note, in multiple places in the paper, the authors discuss results at different time periods but then end with results "at last follow-up" as if the last follow-up occurred after the 2-year mark. However, follow-up ranged from 3 to 49 months, so "at last follow-up" is relatively meaningless.

C.J. Rapuano, M.D.

A Prospective Randomized Trial of Topical Soluble 0.1% Indomethacin Versus 0.1% Diclofenac Versus Placebo for the Control of Pain Following Excimer Laser Photorefractive Keratectomy

Assouline M, Renard G, Arne JL, et al (Univ of Paris VI; CHU Purpan, Toulouse, France)

Ophthalmic Surg Lasers 29:365-374, 1998 2–8

Introduction.—For the correction of low-to-moderate myopia, photorefractive keratectomy (PRK) has become widely accepted, and refractive results have been comparable to or better than those observed after radial keratotomy. Most patients, however, complain of intense ocular pain after PRK, and occasionally they complain of headache, tearing, photophobia, or foreign body sensation. After the procedure, the pain usually begins within 30 to 60 minutes. Within 4 to 6 hours, it becomes severe and decreases gradually after the first postoperative day. As soon as the corneal re-epithelialization is complete, the pain resolves. The efficacy and safety of 2 nonsteroidal anti-inflammatory drugs, 0.1% indomethacin solution and 0.1% diclofenac solution, were compared with a placebo in reducing pain for patients who had PRK.

Methods.—There were 120 patients who were randomly assigned to receive either 0.1% indomethacin solution, 0.1% diclofenac solution or placebo. Pain, subjective symptoms, and epithelial wound healing after the procedure were measured for 2 days.

Results.—On the day of surgery, 0.1% indomethacin solution significantly reduced pain compared with the placebo, whereas 0.1% diclofenac did not reach a significant level of efficacy. In the placebo group, analgesic intake by the oral route was significantly greater on the day of surgery. In the group treated with 0.1% indomethacin, severe photophobia was significantly less frequent. In the patients treated with 0.1% diclofenac, corneal wound healing was significantly delayed when compared with the other groups.

Conclusion.—The pain induced by excimer laser photoablation can be controlled by topical 0.1% indomethacin solution without any detrimental effect to corneal epithelial wound healing. A significant delay in the re-epithelialization process was seen with topical diclofenac. The differences observed in pain reduction on the operative day, although statistically significant, are small.

▶ This well-designed and well–carried out study demonstrates a small advantage of indomethacin over diclofenac in pain reduction during the first 24 hours after PRK. Additionally, the authors found less delay in re-epithelialization with indomethacin than with diclofenac. Still, all eyes were re-epithelialized by postoperative day 3. I believe the bottom line is that every little bit helps. If indomethacin is a little bit better for pain control and re-epithelialization, it may supplant the much more commonly used diclofenac after surface PRK.

C.J. Rapuano, M.D.

Photorefractive Keratectomy Versus Laser In Situ Keratomileusis for Moderate to High Myopia: A Randomized Prospective Study

Hersh PS, Brint SF, Maloney RK, et al (UMDNJ-New Jersey Med School, Newark; Eye Surgery Ctr of Louisiana, New Orleans; Univ of California Los Angeles Laser Refractive Ctr; et al)

Ophthalmology 105:1512-1523, 1998 2–9

Objective.—Results of a randomized, multicenter, clinical study of photorefractive keratectomy (PRK) versus laser in situ keratomileusis using the Summit Apex excimer laser (LASIK) in 220 myopic eyes of 220 patients with moderate-to-high myopia were reported.

Methods.—Patients with myopia (−6.0 to −15.0 D), aged 21 to 64 years, were randomly assigned to the PRK (n = 105; 47% women) or to the LASIK procedure (n = 115; 58% women) using a Summit laser and the Automatic Corneal Shaper microkeratome. Patients were evaluated before surgery and at 1, 3, and 7 days and at 1, 3, and 6 months after surgery. The diameter of the treatment zone for all patients was 6.0 mm.

Results.—Whereas uncorrected visual acuity at early time points was better with the LASIK procedure than with PRK, at 1 month and later the difference had disappeared (Fig 2; Table 1). The mean predictability for uncorrected vision for the PRK group was −0.77 D, and for the LASIK procedure it was −1.43 D. The loss of visual acuity with glasses of 2 Snellen lines at 6 months was similar for both groups. The odds ratio of 3.98 suggests that there is less likelihood of loss of visual acuity with glasses after the LASIK procedure than after PRK. Three LASIK patients had flap-related complications which were corrected without adverse outcomes.

Conclusion.—Whereas early results indicated superiority of the LASIK procedure over PRK, by 6 months the difference had disappeared, al-

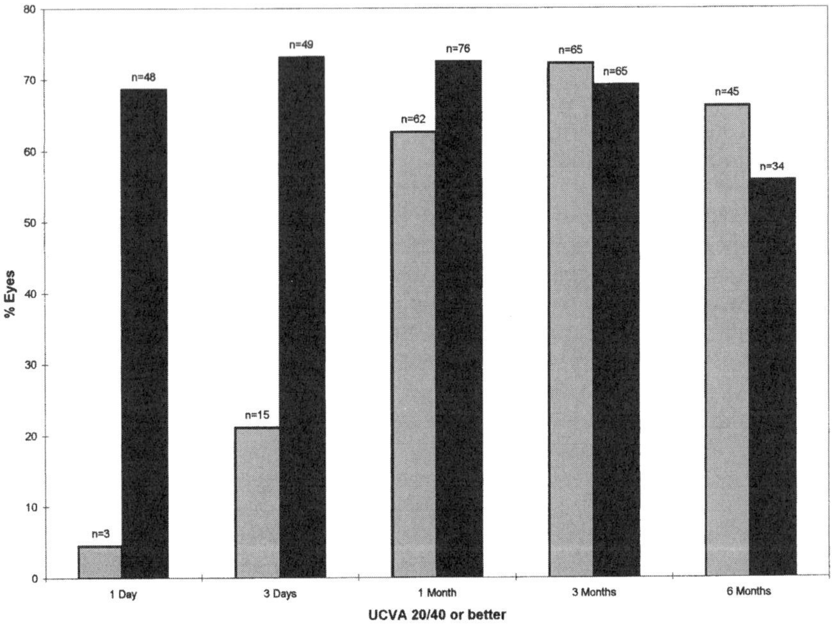

FIGURE 2.—Percentage of patients with uncorrected visual acuity of 20/40 or better after PRK and laser in situ keratomileusis (LASIK) at different timepoints. *Gray columns* indicate PRK; black columns indicate LASIK. *Abbreviation: UCVA*, uncorrected visual acuity. (Published courtesy of *Ophthalmology*, from Hersh PS, Brint SF, Maloney RK, et al: Photorefractive keratectomy versus laser in situ keratomileusis for moderate to high myopia. *Ophthalmology* 105:1512-1523, 1998.)

though there was a trend toward better uncorrected visual acuity with PRK at 6 months. Flap complications occurred in the LASIK group only. Whether differences in visual acuity between the 2 procedures occur beyond 6 months remains to be seen.

▶ This study is the first randomized, prospective comparison of PRK and LASIK. The authors randomized 120 eyes of 120 patients with −6 to −15 D of myopia to receive PRK or LASIK. Although many investigators believe that LASIK is a better procedure than PRK for all levels of myopia, most believe it is a better procedure for the higher myopes, that is, over −6 D. In fact, the authors demonstrated that from 1 month to 6 months postoperatively there were no significant differences in the uncorrected or best corrected visual acuity results between the PRK and LASIK groups. As expected, the visual results were far better for LASIK than for PRK during postoperative days 1 to 3.

Although the study was well-designed and well carried out, it is important to note that there was only a 65% follow-up for PRK and a 53% follow-up for LASIK at 6 months. The results also revealed 2 unexpected findings: (1) there was a trend toward better 20/40 uncorrected vision with PRK than with LASIK and (2) there was a trend toward less loss of best corrected vision with LASIK. It should always be kept in mind that all these results are for 1

TABLE 1.—Uncorrected Visual Acuity After Photorefractive Keratectomy and Laser-Assisted In Situ Keratomileusis

UCVA	1 Day		3 Days		1 Mo		3 Mos		6 Mos	
	PRK (n = 67)	LASIK (n = 70)	PRK (n = 71)	LASIK (n = 67)	PRK (n = 99)	LASIK (n = 105)	PRK (n = 90)	LASIK (n = 94)	PRK (n = 68)	LASIK (n = 61)
≥20/20	0 (0.0)	7 (10.0)	0 (0.0)	9 (13.4)	9 (9.1)	19 (18.1)	14 (15.6)	20 (21.3)	13 (19.1)	16 (26.2)
20/25 to 20/40	3 (4.50)	41 (58.5)	15 (21.1)	40 (59.7)	53 (53.5)	57 (54.3)	51 (56.7)	45 (47.9)	32 (47.1)	18 (29.5)
20/50 to 20/80	8 (11.9)	20 (28.6)	30 (42.3)	13 (19.4)	36 (36.4)	18 (17.1)	19 (21.1)	22 (23.4)	14 (20.6)	15 (24.6)
20/100 to 20/200	30 (44.8)	2 (2.9)	23 (32.4)	5 (7.5)	1 (1.0)	11 (10.5)	6 (6.7)	7 (7.4)	9 (30.2)	12 (19.7)
≤20/200	26 (38.8)	0 (0.0)	3 (4.2)	0 (0.0)	0 (0.0)	0 (0.0)	0 (0.0)	0 (0.0)	0 (0.0)	0 (0.0)

Note: Figures are number of eyes with percentages in parentheses.

Abbreviations: UCVA, uncorrected visual acuity; *PRK,* photorefractive keratectomy; *LASIC,* laser-assisted in situ keratomileusis.

(Published courtesy of *Ophthalmology* from Hersh PS, Brint SF, Maloney RK, et al: Photorefractive keratectomy versus laser in situ keratomileusis for moderate to high myopia. *Ophthalmology* 105:1512-1523, 1998.)

specific excimer laser, 1 nomogram and 1 type of microkeratome. Given the suboptimal follow-up and the 2 seemingly contradictory findings, more work needs to be done to determine which of these procedures is best for our patients.

Numerous questions remain. Does the clear advantage of faster visual recovery outweigh the potential flap complications? Does better long-term follow-up reveal similar results? Do different lasers, nomograms and microkeratomes affect these results? Additional investigations are required to answer these important questions.

C.J. Rapuano, M.D.

Diffuse Lamellar Keratitis: A New Syndrome in Lamellar Refractive Surgery

Smith RJ, Maloney RK (Jules Stein Eye Inst, Los Angeles; Univ of California, Los Angeles)

Ophthalmology 105:1721-1726, 1998 2–10

Objective.—After lamellar refractive surgery, infectious keratitis can occur. This infection can be confused with the self-limiting syndrome, diffuse lamellar keratitis. Factors distinguishing the 2 were discussed retrospectively, and 13 cases were presented.

Methods.—Infiltrates developed in 13 eyes in 12 patients after lamellar surgery using a microkeratome (Automatic Corneal Shaper; Chiron Vision, Irvine, Calif) to create the flap. A photorefractive ablation of 6.0 mm was performed in the stromal bed using an excimer Summit Apex laser (Summit Technology, Waltham, Mass). The flap was repositioned and allowed to settle in place for 5 minutes.

> *Case Report.*—Man, 42, with a preoperative refraction of −8.00 + 0.25 × 100° and a postsurgical correction of 20/20 after laser in situ keratomileusis, was comfortable, with a clear cornea and no epithelial defect on the first postoperative day. At 4 days, he reported soreness. Fine granular opacities were scattered throughout the flap interface, with infiltrates confined to the interface. The condition resolved within 2 days.

Results.—Diffuse lamellar infiltrates after lamellar procedures appear 2 to 6 days after surgery, causing pain or photophobia. The infiltrate is confined to the interface but is scattered and diffuse with multiple faint foci. The infiltrates may be more concentrated around surgical debris, but there is little or no anterior chamber reaction, no overlying epithelial defect, and no involvement of the conjunctiva. The cause is unknown. No bacteria, fungi, or mycobacteria have been found. In this series of patients, the condition resolved within 2 weeks.

Conclusion.—Noninfectious diffuse lamellar keratitis, a syndrome of unknown origin appears after lamellar refractive surgery. The condition begins 2 to 6 days after surgery with pain or photophobia and resolves within 2 weeks.

▶ Although this condition has been discussed anecdotally in refractive surgery circles, the authors present the first series regarding "diffuse lamellar keratitis." It is also called "sands of the Sahara syndrome." It is extremely important to recognize this condition to treat it appropriately. Severe cases of diffuse lamellar keratitis have led to stromal loss and mild scarring, with secondary flattening and overcorrection. It is not infectious and the flap should not be lifted, the interface should not be cultured and intensive antibiotics should not be started. The condition appears to be inflammatory and the treatment of choice is an increase in topical steroids and close follow up.

C.J. Rapuano, M.D.

Laser Vision Correction for Low Hyperopia: An 18-Month Assessment of Safety and Efficacy

Jackson WB, Casson E, Hodge WG, et al (Univ of Ottawa, Ont; Ottawa Gen Hosp, Ont)

Ophthalmology 105:1727-1738, 1998 2–11

Objective.—The safety and efficacy of hyperopic photorefractive keratectomy (PRK) using the refined, larger zone ablation architecture and the VISX STAR Excimer Laser System and the influence of other factors on clinical outcome—including epithelial removal technique and certain postoperative patient management parameters—were evaluated in a prospective, nonrandomized, open-label clinical trial.

Methods.—Thirty-eight patients, with an average age of 51.49 years, with hyperopia of +1.0 to +4.0 D with +1.00 D cylinder or less underwent PRK with the VISX 193-nm, broad-beam STAR Excimer Laser System. The system was fitted with the hyperopic module operating at 6 Hz with an optical zone set to 5 mm, with the ablation gradually tapering peripherally to 9.0 mm and centrally toward a 0.9-mm–diameter central

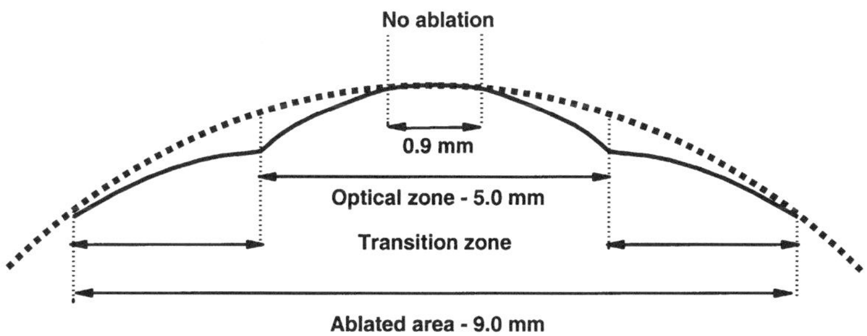

FIGURE 1.—Hyperopic ablation profile of the VISX STAR Laser. (Published courtesy of *Ophthalmology*, from Jackson WB, Casson E, Hodge WG, et al: Laser vision correction for low hyperopia: An 18-month assessment of safety and efficacy. *Ophthalmology* 105:1727-1738, 1998.)

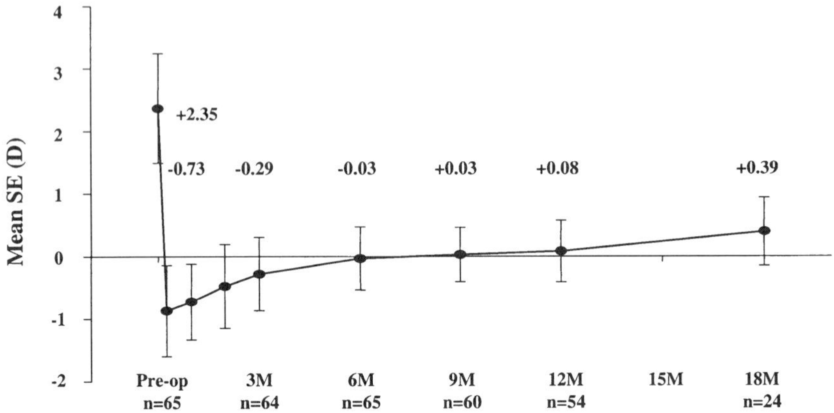

FIGURE 3.—Mean manifest spherical equivalent (diopters) over time. (Published courtesy of *Ophthalmology*, from Jackson WB, Casson E, Hodge WG, et al: Laser vision correction for low hyperopia: An 18-month assessment of safety and efficacy. *Ophthalmology* 105:1727-1738, 1998.)

zone that remained unablated (Fig 1). The deepest ablation, 8 µm/D of correction, was performed at the 5-mm–diameter zone. The first 11 patients had the epithelium removed by means of a Paton spatula, and the remaining patients had epithelium removed by a 7-mm Merocel sponge and an Amoils epithelial scrubber. Patients were followed for at least 6 months.

Results.—The average cycloplegic refraction was +2.47 D. Epithelial healing occurred in 4 days in 50 eyes and in 6 days in 5 eyes. The longest healing period was 9 days. The average spherical equivalent at 1 month was −0.73 D (Fig 3). At 1 and 3 months, there was a trace haze in 48% and 37% of eyes, respectively. In 1 patient, a grade 1.0 haze developed at 12 months in the left eye and at 18 months in the right eye. Compared with eyes with hyperopia exceeding +3 D, eyes with a preoperative hyperopia of +3 D or less were more likely to be within ±0.5 D of the intended spherical equivalent at 6 months and within ±1.0 D at 18 months.

At 1 year 80% of eyes were within ±0.5 D of the desired spherical equivalent. Only 1 eye was not within ±1.0 D at 1 year. At 1 week, near uncorrected visual acuity was better than distance uncorrected visual acuity because of overcorrection. The eyes regressed in the first 6 months, remained stable to 12 months, and regressed further by 18 months by +0.31 D for a small number of patients. Although at 1 month 17 of 65 eyes had lost 2 lines or more because of epithelial irregularities, best spectacle-corrected visual acuity improved gradually until at 6 months, only 1 eye had lost more than 1 line. Eyes that had the epithelium removed using the brush technique had a better outcome than eyes that had the epithelium removed using the Paton spatula.

Conclusion.—Hyperopic PRK is safe and effective, although recovery of best spectacle-corrected visual acuity an uncorrected visual acuity is slower than with the myopic procedure, and some regression of spherical equivalent appeared at between 12 and 18 months.

► This article was published a few months before VISX Inc. received Food and Drug Administration approval to treat hyperopia with PRK. This study, although on the small side with only 65 eyes of 38 patients, had excellent follow-up of 100% at 6 months and over 80% at 1 year. There was moderate overcorrection at 1 month, with regression at from 6 to 12 months. With more limited follow-up, there appeared to be additional regression at from 12 to 18 months. Compared with PRK for myopia, there is a larger epithelial defect with a slightly longer time to re-epithelialization but, surprisingly, less pain. There was also a slower recovery of uncorrected and best-corrected vision compared with myopic PRK.

Overall, the patients were very pleased both in the early postoperative period (with good reading vision) and the later postoperative period (with good distance vision). The authors found that the refractive results were significantly better for hyperopia treatments under +3.00 D than for between +3.00 and +4.00 D. I find it very interesting that the Food and Drug Administration approved the VISX laser for hyperopic correction up to +6.00 D given the more limited data over +3.00 to +4.00 D.

C.J. Rapuano, M.D.

Laser In Situ Keratomileusis for Hyperopia

Argento CJ, Cosentino MJ (Instituto de la Visión, Buenos Aires, Argentina; Univ of Buenos Aires, Argentina)

J Cataract Refract Surg 24:1050-1058, 1998 2–12

Objective.—The stability, predictability, and safety of laser in situ keratomileusis (LASIK) for mild and moderate hyperopia were assessed.

Methods.—LASIK was performed by 1 surgeon using the Chiron Technolas Keracor 116/117 excimer laser on 679 eyes in 321 patients (38.8% men). Based on preoperative spherical equivalent, patients were divided into 3 groups: group A, 2.00 D or less (n = 203); group B, 2.00 to 3.00 D (n = 225); and group C, more than 3.00 D (n = 251). The optical zone ranged from 4.2 to 5.5 mm with a total ablation diameter of 8.1 to 9.5 mm (Fig 1). The diameters of keratectomies, performed with Chiron microkeratomes, were approximately 8.5 mm.

Results.—At 6 months, uncorrected visual acuity was 20/40 or greater in 94.1% of group A, 100% of group B, and 87.8% of group C; it was 20/20 to 20/25 in 70.3%, 75.0%, and 45.3%, respectively. The inflammatory infiltrate at the interface seen in 3.1% of eyes disappeared within 4 weeks. Folds, generally the result of poor handling, occurred in 6.8% of eyes and decentration of the treatment in 3.5%. Both complications generally led to loss of lines. Stability was observed 3 to 6 months after surgery.

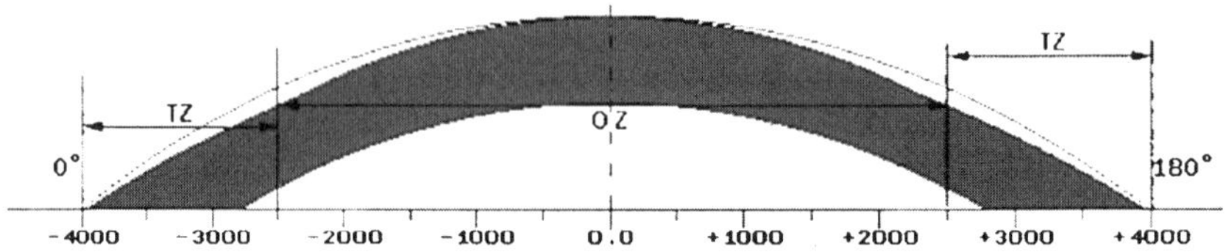


```
Last name......................:
Eye............................: R
Sph Refraction (dptr)..........: 2.0
Cyl Refraction (dptr)..........: 2.0      Axis cyl.............: 90°
Zone diameter..................: 5.0 mm
Zone (Cyl) diameter............: 5.0 mm
Ablation.......................: 4.0 µm
Pulses.........................: 1992
```

FIGURE 1.—PlanoScan ablation parameters along the flat (180 degree) meridian for the treatment of +2.00 +2.00 × 90. The diameter of the optical zone (*OZ*) is 5.0 mm, and the transition zone (*TZ*) extends to 8.1 mm. (Reprinted by permission of the publisher from Argento CJ, Cosentino MJ: Laser in situ keratomileusis for hyperopia. *J Cataract Refract Surg* 24:1050-1058. Copyright 1998 by Elsevier Science Inc.)

Conclusion.—LASIK is safe, effective, and predictable for correcting mild-to-moderate hyperopia.

► Photorefractive keratectomy was approved by the Food and Drug Administration for myopia several years before LASIK became widely used. Consequently, most refractive surgeons started with PRK for myopia, and many have converted to LASIK. However, as Food and Drug Administration approval of excimer laser PRK for hyperopia has just recently occurred, many surgeons are not interested in hyperopic PRK but rather are interested in hyperopic LASIK. The authors demonstrate very good refractive results for eyes with less than +3.00 D of hyperopia and fair results for hyperopia greater than +3.00 D. They found stability between 3 and 6 months postoperatively with good follow-up to 6 months.

However, with only 38% follow-up at 1 year, long-term stability has been established. Additionally, the authors found 2.9% free caps, and 3.1% of eyes had diffuse lamellar keratitis. In 6.8% of eyes, folds developed in the flap, and 3.5% of eyes had significant decentration, both conditions generally causing decreased best-corrected visual acuity.

In contrast to the situation with myopic LASIK, a larger flap needs to be created to encompass the larger ablation. The larger flap may be associated with the relatively high incidence of flap-related complications. A randomized study comparing hyperopic PRK and LASIK would be very useful.

C.J. Rapuano, M.D.

Incidence and Management of Intraoperative and Early Postoperative Complications in 1000 Consecutive Laser In Situ Keratomileusis Cases

Gimbel HV, Penno EEA, van Westenbrugge JA, et al (Gimbel Eye Centre, Calgary, Alta)

Ophthalmology 105:1839-1848, 1998 2–13

Background.—Laser in situ keratomileusis (LASIK) surgery gains high marks from surgeons and patients alike for the correction of myopia, hyperopia, and astigmatism. These authors reported the experience of 1 surgeon in performing 1,000 of these procedures and provide recommendations for preventing and managing complications.

Methods.—Retrospective review of charts from April 1995 to February 1997 identified the first 1,000 cases of myopic LASIK surgery performed by 1 surgeon. The 523 patients had a mean age of 33 years, and their preoperative spherical equivalent ranged from −1.00 D to −23.00 D. The surgeon used an NIDEK Excimer Laser and (in all but 1 case) a Chiron microkeratome to incise the cornea to a depth of 160 μm. After surgery, enhancements, if needed, were performed as early as 1 week (average, 5 months) after surgery. The results given below were noted at 1 month or more after the last enhancement.

Findings.—After surgery, the mean spherical equivalent was −9.56 D (range, −1.00 to −23.00 D). Lateral canthotomy procedures were required for 87 eyes. There were 32 intraoperative complications, (3.2%), 19 related to the microkeratome and 13 related to the surgery (Table 3). All but one of the 19 microkeratome-related complications occurred on a steeper-than-average cornea. LASIK preceded as scheduled in 19 of the cases with complications. In the 13 cases in which LASIK was discontinued, 9 (69.2%) of the patients successfully underwent the procedure at a later date. Flaps had to be repositioned in 18 eyes 24 hours or less after surgery because the flaps shifted or microwrinkles or edge folds developed. The incidence of intraoperative microkeratome complications decreased substantially as the surgeon gained experience (Fig 1); for the first 200 eyes the complication rate was 4.5%, whereas for the last 200 eyes, it was 0.5%.

TABLE 3.—Microkeratome Complications and Surgical Events

Microkeratome Complications (n = 19)	Surgical Events (n =13)
Incomplete pass 12	Insufficient suction 5
Thin flap 3	Bleeding pannus 3
Button hole 3	Epithelial bullae 2
Free cap 1	Flap dislodged 2
	Flap shrinkage 1

(Published courtesy of *Ophthalmology*, from Gimbel HV, Penno EEA, van Westenbrugge JA, et al: Incidence and management of intraoperative and early postoperative complications in 1000 consecutive laser in situ keratomileusis cases. *Ophthalmology* 105:1839-1848, 1998.)

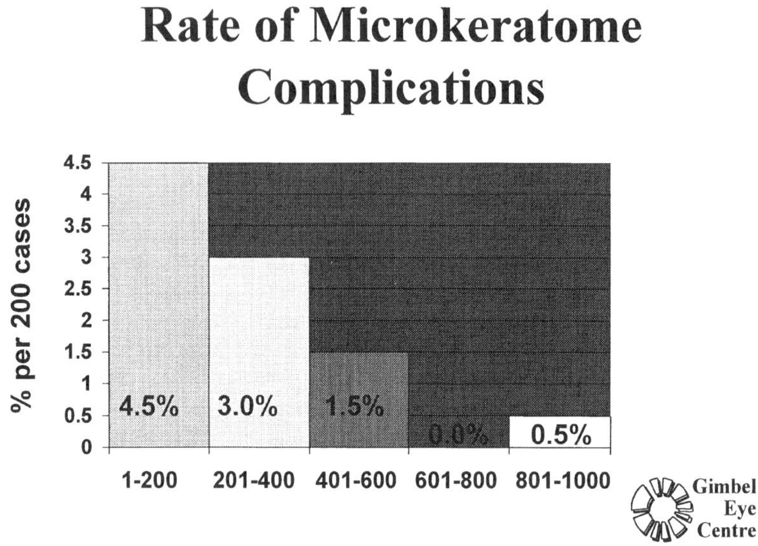

FIGURE 1.—The quarterly rate of intraoperative microkeratome complications declined over the first 1000 myopic laser in situ keratomileusis cases. (Published courtesy of *Ophthalmology*, from Gimbel HV, Penno EEA, van Westenbrugge JA, et al: Incidence and management of intraoperative and early postoperative complications in 1000 consecutive laser in situ keratomileusis cases. *Ophthalmology* 105:1839-1848, 1998.)

Of the 950 eyes with uncomplicated LASIK surgery, 290 (30.5%) needed to be retreated (Table 7), mainly for undercorrection (79.3%) or overcorrection (9.7%). Best-corrected visual acuity 6 months after LASIK remained the same or improved slightly (1 line) in 26 (81.3%) of the 32 eyes that experienced microkeratome or surgical complications, although

TABLE 7.—Retreatment Rates for 1000 Cases of Myopic Laser In Situ Keratomileusis

Group	n	No. of Eyes Needing Re-treatment	%	Mean Time to Re-treatment (Mos)
Uncomplicated LASIK	950	290	30.5	5.1
Microkeratome complications	19	2	10.5	7.5
Intraoperative events	13	3	23.0	8.0
Perioperative flap repositionings	18	6	33.3	3.7

Note: In the group with other intraoperative events recorded, 3 of 13 (23%) had re-treatments with a mean time to re-treatment of 8 months; 2 of these were for undercorrection and 1 was for overcorrection; 6 of 18 cases (33.3%) that required postoperative flap repositioning underwent re-treatment with a mean time of 3.6 months; re-treatment was done for 1 case each of astigmatism, irregular astigmatism, interface debrise, halos, undercorrection, and overcorrection. (Published courtesy of *Ophthalmology*, from Gimbel HV, Penno EEA, van Westenbrugge JA, et al: Incidence and management of intraoperative and early postoperative complications in 1000 consecutive laser in situ keratomileusis cases. *Ophthalmology* 105:1839-1848, 1998.)

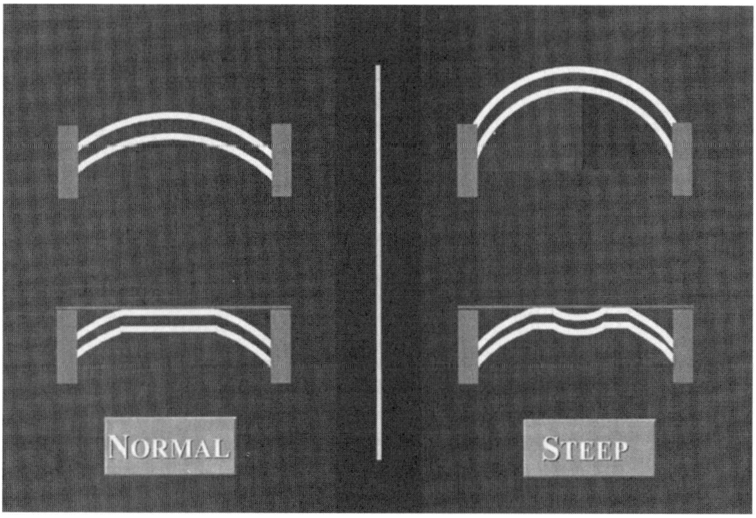

FIGURE 4.—A schematic showing applanation of normal and steep cornea by microkeratome. The steep cornea buckles under the microkeratome foot plate. (Published courtesy of *Ophthalmology*, from Gimbel HV, Penno EEA, van Westenbrugge JA, et al: Incidence and management of intraoperative and early postoperative complications in 1000 consecutive laser in situ keratomileusis cases. *Ophthalmology* 105:1839-1848, 1998.)

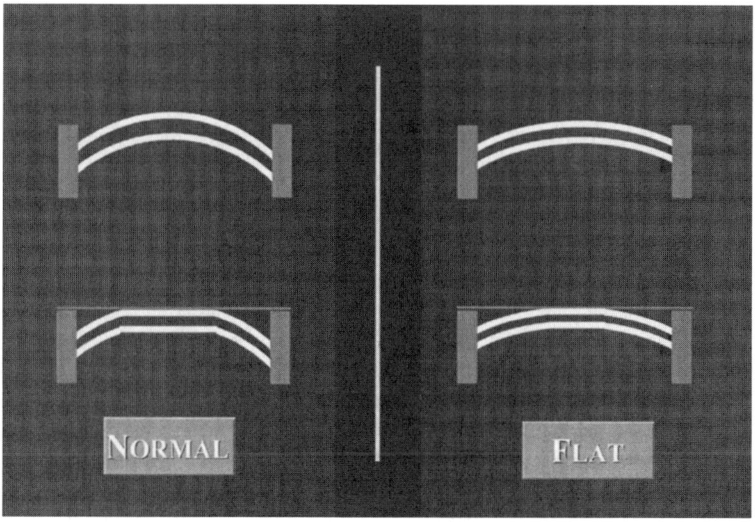

FIGURE 5.—A schematic showing applanation of normal and flat corneas by microkeratome. The flat cornea produces a free cap in with a small diameter. (Published courtesy of *Ophthalmology*, from Gimbel HV, Penno EEA, van Westenbrugge JA, et al: Incidence and management of intraoperative and early postoperative complications in 1000 consecutive laser in situ keratomileusis cases. *Ophthalmology* 105:1839-1848, 1998.)

6 eyes (18.7%) lost 1 line. Of the uncomplicated cases, 16 (1.77%) lost 2 lines or more.

Conclusion.—The safety of LASIK is excellent, but complications can occur. Yet even if complications do occur intraoperatively, with proper management LASIK can be successfully performed at a later date. Steeper-than-average corneas were associated with microkeratome-related complications; thin flaps (average, 45.7 D) and buttonholes (average, 46.7 D) had the steepest corneas, and there was 1 free cap with a very flat cornea (average, 40.9 D). The authors hypothesize that these complications occur because the keratome foot plate compresses excess tissue beyond applanation, causing buckling (Figs 4 and 5).

▶ The authors present an excellent study on the first 1000 LASIK procedures by 1 surgeon. He used a Chiron microkeratome and NIDEK laser. Overall, the authors report a low complication rate and excellent visual results. Important conclusions are that with proper management, even intraoperative microkeratome-related complications can result eventually in an excellent visual outcome. Additionally, the authors document a significant decrease in intraoperative microkeratome complications over the first 1000 cases, with a complication rate of 4.5% in the first 200 cases which decreases to 0.5% in the last 200 cases.

The Discussion section includes a "must read" portion on avoiding complications for all LASIK surgeons. The authors found that the majority of complications were caused by 1 or more of the following: (1) failure to achieve adequate exposure, (2) failure to achieve adequate suction, (3) loose epithelium, (4) wrinkles or debris under the flap, (5) flap shrinkage, and (6) dislodged flap. They also discuss their theory on free caps and flap buttonholes. They discuss each of these complications in detail, with tips on avoiding them.

They stress a few points. Small palpebral fissures and deep orbits predispose to difficulty in obtaining adequate suction. Flat corneas are at greater risk for free caps. Steep corneas are at greater risk for buttonholes. I, personally, have found that anterior basement membrane dystrophy increases the risk of problems from loose epithelium. It is important to note that many of these issues can be identified preoperatively, allowing the surgeon to take precautions to avoid surgical complications.

C.J. Rapuano, M.D.

Transepithelial Photorefractive Keratectomy for Treatment of Thin Flaps or Caps After Complicated Laser In Situ Keratomileusis

Kapadia MS, Wilson SE (Cleveland Clinic Found, Ohio)

Am J Ophthalmol 126:827-829, 1998 2–14

Background.—Laser in situ keratomileusis (LASIK) can be complicated by an irregular flap or cap of corneal tissue resulting from microkeratome malfunction or surgeon error. In 2 patients with irregular LASIK caps or flaps, transepithelial photorefractive keratectomy (PRK) was used to ablate the flap from the central cornea and restore central corneal clarity and more normal visual function.

Case Reports. Woman, 27, sought treatment for a thin superficial cap associated with a central corneal scar 3 months after LASIK. A thin cap in the central cornea was found in association with superficial scarring overlying the entrance pupil where the microkeratome blade exited the cornea. A transepithelial PRK was performed and repeated, with complete phototherapeutic keratectomy ablation of the epithelium done under dim illumination until the ablated zone was completely black, indicating that all epithelium was removed. Two months after this second procedure the central cornea was clear and the previous cap was not visible.

Man, 47, underwent LASIK in the left eye. After the microkeratome was passed, a thin, donut-shaped flap resulted from blade exit and re-entry in the central cornea overlying the pupil. The flap was repositioned without applying the excimer laser. Ten days after this procedure, the flap was in position, but epithelium was discovered in the superficial stroma where the microkeratome had exited the cornea, overlying the pupil. Transepithelial PRK was performed and all epithelium was removed. Four months later, the central 6 mm of cornea overlying the pupil was clear. A portion of the original flap was in the periphery.

Conclusions.—Transepithelial PRK appears to be effective in the treatment of central corneal thin cap or flap abnormalities associated with LASIK. This technique is especially effective in eyes with associated central corneal scarring or with epithelial ingrowth that causes doubling or ghosting of the image or loss of best-corrected visual acuity.

▶ The authors present 2 cases of 1 of the most feared complications of LASIK, the buttonhole flap. This untoward event can result from inadequate suction and/or a steep cornea. Should this complication occur, it is best to replace the flap without excimer laser treatment. Most surgeons recommend allowing the flap to heal for several months and then proceeding with repeat LASIK and cutting a new, deeper flap. However, some patients develop a superficial corneal scar in the central area of the buttonhole, which can adversely affect vision. Repeat LASIK will not remove this scar.

The authors treated 2 such patients with transepithelial PRK with very good results. The fear has been that PRK after a buttonhole LASIK flap will result in excess scarring. While these 2 patients were followed for only 2 and 4 months, the corneas were clear at last follow-up, with no residual scar from the LASIK complication. Although longer follow-up is needed on more patients, transepithelial PRK may be a viable option for this problem.

C.J. Rapuano, M.D.

Photorefractive Keratectomy in African Americans Including Those With Known Dermatologic Keloid Formation

Tanzer DJ, Isfahani A, Schallhorn SC, et al (Univ of Southern California, Los Angeles; Naval Med Ctr, San Diego, Calif)

Am J Ophthalmol 126:625-629, 1998 2–15

Background.—Because of the perceived risk of a visually significant corneal scar, known dermatologic keloid formation is generally considered a contraindication to photorefractive keratectomy (PRK). The incidence and severity of corneal scarring after PRK in African American patients were evaluated, and whether a history of keloid formation correlated with poor surgical outcomes was determined.

Methods and Findings.—Twelve African American patients with 19 affected eyes were included in the study. Three patients with 6 affected eyes had a history of keloid formation. Preoperatively, the mean manifest spherical equivalent was −4.9 D. Three excimer lasers were used: the Summit Omnimed (Summit Technology, Inc, Waltham, Mass) and the VISX Twenty/Twenty "B" and "C" lasers (VISX, Inc, Santa Clara, Calif). Postoperatively, all eyes had an uncorrected visual acuity of 20/40 or better. Seventy-four percent of the eyes had an uncorrected visual acuity of 20/20 or better. Eight of 19 eyes studied for a mean 13.8 months had trace to 1+ corneal haze at the last examination. Only 1 eye from 1 patient known to form keloids showed corneal haze 18 months after surgery.

Conclusions.—Darkly pigmented persons may have excellent visual outcomes after PRK. Postoperatively, all eyes obtained an uncorrected visual acuity of 20/40 or better, and three fourths of the eyes had an uncorrected visual acuity of 20/20 or better. PRK can be successful in patients with a history of keloid formation.

► This study is interesting but small, including only 19 eyes of African American patients. Only 6 of these eyes were in known keloid formers. All eyes did very well after PRK, with no eye demonstrating excessive scarring. The most fascinating part of this article for me was learning that the Food and Drug Administration based its recommendations that keloid formation be a relative contraindication to PRK on 2 patients in the Summit study who had excessive scarring but were *not* keloid formers and on 2 known keloid formers who had perfectly clear corneas after PRK. Although it does not appear that keloid formation is a contraindication to PRK, the small size of the study should be kept in mind.

C.J. Rapuano, M.D.

Three Year Results of Photoastigmatic Refractive Keratectomy for Mild and Atypical Keratoconus

Kremer I, Shochot Y, Kaplan A, et al (Ein Tal Eye Ctr, Tel Aviv, Israel)
J Cataract Refract Surg 24:1581-1588, 1998 2–16

Background.—The increasing use of computerized videokeratoscopy had shown that keratoconus is more common than previously believed. As many as 8% of patients with myopia who are seeking refractive surgery reportedly have features that may indicate keratoconus on topographic analysis. Because of the potential for progression of this ectatic disease in eyes with mild or subclinical keratoconus, ophthalmologists have become uncertain about the outcome of photorefractive keratectomy (PRK) on keratoconus. Long-term outcomes of PRK on eyes with a mild keratoconus were reported.

Methods.—Six patients with 8 eyes with stable compound myopic astigmatism and topographic features of keratoconus underwent VISX (Santa Clara, Calif) Twenty-Twenty excimer laser treatment. The width of the laser beam slit ranged from 4.8 to 5 mm, according to the degree of cylinder. No significant thinning, ectasia, or scarring was seen on preoperative slitlamp examination. Astigmatisms ranged from −2.00 to − 7.50 D. The patients were studied from 36 to 48 months.

Findings.—In 7 eyes, uncorrected visual acuity ranged from 6/30 to finger counting before PRK and from 6/9− to 6/15 after PRK. Patients could perform most of their daily activities without wearing spectacles. The final uncorrected visual acuity was 6/15(−) and 6/15, respectively, in 2 eyes. Uncorrected visual acuity was unimproved and keratoconus progressed in 1 eye.

Conclusions.—In this series, photoastigmatic keratectomy was somewhat effective in eyes with mild, stable keratoconus. However, the progesssion of corneal thinning and ectatic disease may affect long-term outcomes. Further research is needed.

▶ Keratoconus has almost universally been considered an absolute contraindication to PRK. (Rarely, a superficial corneal nodule is amenable to phototherapeutic keratectomy [PTK].) The authors present their results of PRK for "mild and atypical keratoconus." It appears that what they mean by this inclusion criterion is corneal topographic evidence of inferior steepening. Slitlamp examination revealed no Fleischer rings, only 1 with Vogt's striae, and 4 with inferior steepening. Three eyes had completely normal slitlamp examinations. It is debatable whether some of these eyes should be considered to have keratoconus.

Seven of the 8 eyes did quite well after PRK, with very good uncorrected and best corrected vision. The eighth eye, the only one with Vogt's striae, did not gain improved vision and in fact had progression of keratoconus in the follow-up.

The length of follow-up (36 months) is excellent, but keratoconus can be a slowly progressive condition. While I agree that so far the 7 eyes with mild keratoconus (at most) are doing well at 3 years, I have serious concerns regarding using excimer laser PRK to further thin corneas in which the underlying pathology is related to corneal thinning.

C.J. Rapuano, M.D.

Preoperative Measurement of Scotopic Pupil Dilation Using an Office Pupillometer

Colvard M (Ctr for Ophthalmic Surgery, Encino, Calif)

J Cataract Refract Surg 24:1594-1597, 1998 2–17

Background.—Patients with pupils that dilate widely at low illumination levels may not be satisfied with the quality of their vision after keratorefractive surgery. The preoperative measurement of scotopic pupil dilation, using an office pupillometer, was reported.

Methods.—One hundred patients, aged a mean of 28 years, underwent pupil measurement at 15 and 3 lumens. A Rosenbaum pocket-card gauge, a millimeter ruler, and the pupillometer were used for measurement at about 15 lumens. Three technicians chose this illumination level as the lowest at which the pupil of a brown eye could be determined using the Rosenbaum card. The light-amplification pupillometer was then used to measure pupil size at about 3 lumens, an illumination level comparable to that of right-driving conditions.

Findings.—Mean pupil diameter was 5.1 mm at 15 lumens. The measurements obtained with the 3 instruments at this level of illumination did not differ. Pupil diameters at 3 lumens could not be confidently measured using the Rosenbaum card or millimeter ruler. Pupil size ranged from 3 to 9 mm, with a mean of 6.2 mm, as determined by the pupillometer. The mean difference between pupil diameters at 3 and 15 lumens was 1.1 mm, with a range of 0 to 3 mm.

Conclusions.—Pupil dilation at 3 lumens is difficult to predict reliably by measuring pupil size at 15 lumens. The light-amplification pupillometer can be used to determine pupil size at an illumination level comparable to that of night-driving conditions. This device may help surgeons to identify candidates for refractive surgery who are more likely to be unsatisfied with their postoperative vision.

► First, I have no financial interest in this instrument. However, I am absolutely convinced that pupil size affects patient satisfaction after refractive surgery. In general, the larger the pupil, the more visual aberrations patients note. For a given pupil size, the greater the degree of myopia treated, the more visual distortions (due to a smaller effective optical zone) there are. I believe that standardized pupil measurements in dim illumination can alert surgeons (and patients) to which patients have abnormally large pupils and are at higher risk of optical aberrations. Pupil measurements (using 1 of many methods) should be a standard part of the preoperative refractive surgery evaluation.

C.J. Rapuano, M.D.

3 Glaucoma

Introduction

by George L. Spaeth, M.D.

In the field of glaucoma, this past year was characterized, by a lot of hoopla and some substance. Most of the hoopla was in the area where there was little substance. Some of the contributions of real substance went remarkably unnoticed.

Hoopla

Leading the hoopla camp is the whole area of neuroprotection. From all the excitement generated, one would think that the idea was new and proven. Bernard Becker was investigating the possible neuroprotective benefit of Dilantin about a quarter of a century ago.[1] Largely ignored, also, is the almost complete lack of clinical success regarding neuroprotective agents in any field. Spinal cord damage can be lessened by use of corticosteroids, but it is unlikely that the mechanism is truly "neuroprotective." There are a few suggestions of benefits in some other areas—but nothing to write home about yet.

One of the problems in the field of glaucoma is the extremely slow evolution of the common forms of glaucoma and the lack of good animal models. The only experimental models for glaucoma at the moment relate to relatively acutely elevated intraocular pressure. Although the elevation of intraocular pressure certainly is a pathogenetic factor in the development of some types of glaucoma, and although it is important to understand much more about what controls intraocular pressure, nevertheless, one of the most important questions that needs to be answered has to do with why some nerves are *sensitive* and other nerves are *resistant* to the damaging effects of intraocular pressure. If the siren song of "neuroprotection" leads us away from spending time trying to figure out why it is that certain people's nerves are sensitive or resistant to intraocular pressure, patients will have been ill-served. It seems that some of the good work that was being done regarding the pathogenesis of optic nerve damage in glaucoma has been put on hold, and that is a pity.

Another strong contender for hoopla in this past year is the entry of image analyzers into the commercial market. One instrument, for example, the GDx, which individually measures the thickness of the retinal nerve fiber layer is being promoted by its manufacturer as a tool to use in screening for glaucoma. None of the instruments presently available is sufficiently specific to be used in a meaningful way for glaucoma screening of normal populations. For example, consider the usefulness of an instrument that is 99% specific when screening for a disease that affects 1% of the people screened. In such a situation a positive test from the screener would be right only 50% of the time. That is, 50% of the time somebody who was told that he or she had glaucoma would not have glaucoma. Yet ophthalmologists are being advised to use image analyzers to rule in, or rule out, a diagnosis of glaucoma where the ophthalmologists are unsure and where the specificity of the instrument is about 80% or so. This is not just hoopla; it is dangerous and expensive hoopla.

Similarly inflated claims are attributed to new surgical procedures that may, in fact, have some promise, but are as of yet still unproven. A paraphrase of a classic quote comes to mind: "The time to try a procedure is before it is shown not to be effective." Innovation is critically important to the well-being of patients and to the medical profession. Research is a vital part of providing better care. But research also carries with it a responsibility to make sure that patients are protected and that the results of the research can be interpreted in a way which is meaningful. It is possible that viscocanulostomy, "the wick procedure," and pneumatic trabeculectomy may be beneficial procedures. But it is not fair to patients, or to physicians, to hold these procedures out as if they were proven to be the treatments of choice, when it has not been determined that they work at all.

The final entry on the balance side of hoopla relates to most of the comments about how glaucoma affects the "quality of life." We are told that patients are being given "validated" surveys about visual function. The results of these surveys are used to obtain "validated" outcome measures about the course of glaucoma and how medications or surgery affect glaucoma. But none of these surveys has been *validated* in any true sense of the word. For something to be valid means that it corresponds with reality. What those using the word *valid* mean, however, is that the surveys are reproducible. All clinicians know that there is a poor correlation between people's perception of their function and their actual function. Some patients with far-advanced glaucomatous damage which has resulted in vision limited to the ability to see a hand moving in both eyes are vibrant individuals who live busy lives and are, in one sense of the word, "functioning" beautifully. Other individuals with glaucoma who are bothered by the stinging of the eye drops that they use but have no damage, spend their time turning themselves into victims and literally become incapacitated. The first group of patients would do well on quality of life–visual function surveys, whereas the second would do poorly; in fact, however, the visual function of the first group is far *worse* than that of the second. To be valid a survey must show that the findings are in line with what is actually the case. And as far as visual function goes, no survey can do this, because to date there is virtually no information whatsoever about how glaucoma affects actual visual function. Questionnaires cannot obtain that information. For an understanding of how glaucoma affects visual function, investigations must be done into actual visual function. We desperately need such studies.

Substance

On the substance side, a variety of departments have continued to add information about the genetic nature of glaucoma. This is tremendously exciting stuff! Clinicians may wonder at another paper describing LOD scores (the mathematical method of estimating how genes are linked to each other); the truth, however, is that these studies will eventually have an enormous impact on how glaucoma is diagnosed and treated.

One way in which the diagnosis and management of glaucoma will be affected by new genetic discoveries is by changing the classification of glaucoma. For example, we continue to use the label "primary open-angle glaucoma," as if it means something specific, whereas the diagnostic phrase encompasses people with normal or low intraocular pressure whose optic nerves are so sensitive to the damaging effects of pressure that nothing can be done to prevent them from deteriorating. It is conceivable, to cite another example, that one type of what we now call "pigmentary glaucoma" will affect a person who has the gene that affects the pigment epithelial layer of the iris and the retina, whereas another person with "pigmentary glaucoma" has that same gene, but in addition a gene that predisposes to myopia; yet another person will have both those two genes, and yet another that affects the functioning of the trabecular meshwork, predisposing to elevated intraocular pressure. The first of these individuals would be predisposed to developing the signs of pigment dispersion and retinal detachment, and probably would not develop "glaucoma." The second would be more likely to develop optic nerve damage, and the third would be more likely to develop a progressive glaucomatous optic neuropathy. Good clinicians make this type of distinction today, but having a better idea about the fundamental genetic structure of an individual will help separate that person from all the others who look somewhat similar, but are really quite different.

An additional benefit to be garnered from the harvest bin of genetic studies will be a vastly improved understanding of how the environment affects glaucoma (as well as other conditions). Most of us still have an infantile understanding of how genes work. We think, for example, that if one has the gene for the pigment dispersion syndrome that one will show the signs of the pigment dispersion syndrome. But it is far more complex than that. The expression of a gene is affected by the presence or absence of other genes, as well as by environmental conditions. For example, it may well be that the gene for the pigment dispersion syndrome will not express itself unless another gene is activated; activation of that other gene may require something highly specific, such as the presence of glucose. Thus, two people, both of whom have the same gene for the pigment dispersion syndrome, may look very different and act very differently depending upon whether they are brought up with a diet primarily of milk, fruit, and other foods with little glucose, or whether they are fed foods full of cane sugar. Knowing a person's genotype will *not* fully explain the person's phenotype! But knowing a person's genotype (i.e., the person's nature) will provide critically useful information to permit an understanding of how the environment (i.e., nurture) molds that nature into the actual manifestation of the creature.

Also on the substance side of the balance are the studies that have been looking at retinal ganglion cells, counting them, and relating them to other characteristics, such as nerve fiber layer thickness. How welcome it is to see such articles, in contrast to yet another uncontrolled "study" lauding the benefits of some new and unproven surgical procedure.

Not Quite Substance, But Moving Toward It

One of the most important questions about glaucoma that needs to be answered is: "Why do some people with glaucoma lose visual function?" It is disturbing that there have been, quite literally, only a handful of investigators who have looked at this issue seriously. Among those was the seminal paper of Grant and Burke in 1982 entitled "Why do some people go blind from glaucoma?"[2] More recently, studies from the Mayo Clinic and the Wilmer Eye Institute have been addressing the same issue. There are serious flaws in the designs of the studies from both institutions, but the investigators are well aware of those flaws and have done the best they can with the data available to them. What is needed, of course, is a prospective study, and while it would not give us the information we need for 15 or perhaps 30 years, there is no more important question that needs answering. Unfortunately, few investigators are willing to invest the time and effort to develop a study that will provide information so far in the future, and few funding agencies are willing to expend the resources necessary to support such a project. This reluctance, both from the point of view of the investigators and the funding agencies, is short-sighted and unfortunate. Perhaps the American Glaucoma Society, under the direction of the new chair of the research director, Robert Weinreb, can start developing such long-term studies.

References

1. Becker B, Stamper RL, Asseff C, Podos SM: Effect of diphenylhydantoin on glaucomatous field loss: A preliminary report. *Trans Am Acad Ophthalmol Otolaryngol* 76:412-422, 1972.
2. Grant WM, Burke JF Jr: Why do some people go blind from glaucoma? *Ophthalmology* 89:991-998, 1982.

Glaucoma's Impact on Quality of Life and Its Relation to Clinical Indicators: A Pilot Study

Sherwood MB, Garcia-Siekavizza A, Meltzer MI, et al (Univ of Florida, Gainesville; Natl Ctr for Infectious Diseases, Atlanta, Ga)

Ophthalmology 105:561-566, 1998 3–1

Background.—To date, no one has documented the subjective aspects of visual function and quality of life of patients with glaucoma. In addition, no correlation has been established between quality-of-life measures and clinical indicators. These issues were investigated in the current study.

Methods.—Fifty-six patients with glaucoma and 54 control subjects participated in a sex- , race- , and age-stratified, cross-sectional study. Participants completed the Medical Outcomes Study short form (MOS-20) and the Activities of Daily Vision Scale (ADVS). Data were also obtained on glaucoma and the adverse effects of treatment.

Findings.—Compared with the control group, the glaucoma patients scored significantly lower on all MOS-20 categories except pain. Differences were noted in physical (−20%), role (−43%), mental health (−10%), general health (−22%), and social (−9%) measures. Differences also occurred between white and nonwhite patients on MOS physical, role, social, pain, and health subscales and on ADVS near vision. In the patient group, current medication and previous surgery were associated with the ADVS subscales night vision, near vision, and glare. Visual acuity and fields correlated with MOS physical, role, and health subscales and all ADVS subscales. A multiple regression model that included visual acuity and fields, urban residence, and female sex explained 61% of the variability in ADVS overall score.

Conclusions.—Quality of life differed significantly between patients with glaucoma and control subjects. In the patient group, activities of daily vision were correlated with increased field loss, reduced visual acuity, and treatment complexity.

▶ One of the positive outcomes of the "managed care revolution" has been a redefinition of the purpose of care. Although this redefinition has been more negative than positive because the emphasis has shifted toward cost rather than quality, the changes have forced physicians to reevaluate what they are trying to accomplish with their patients, and what they should be trying to accomplish with their patients. For example, physicians typically think in biologic terms, such as weight, or, with respect to glaucoma, the intraocular pressure, the nature of the visual field, and so forth. However, patients are more likely to think in terms of whatever makes them feel good. That is, unless "miseducated" by the physicians, patients do not really care about the level of their intraocular pressure. Rather, patients care only about whether they can see well enough and feel well enough to do whatever they would like to do and must do. Recognizing this, physicians have developed an intense interest in what is frequently referred to as "quality-of-life."

To assess quality of life in a relatively scientific manner, it is necessary to develop methods of obtaining information. And almost all of these have been in the form of questionnaires. Sherwood and his colleagues have used quality-of-life questionnaires to evaluate the effect of glaucoma on the patient's quality of life. Approximately 10 years ago, I performed a pilot study using a questionnaire that we had developed on the Glaucoma Service of the Wills Eye Hospital. What became apparent was that (1) questionnaires that would provide truly meaningful information were difficult to construct and to administer; (2) the variability of patient response was enormous, partially related at least to variable interpretation of words used on the questionnaire; and (3) some commonalities of response could be found. For example, some individuals stated that learning that they had glaucoma resulted in an immediate deterioration in their quality of life, whereas others believed that it resulted in an improvement. People in the former group no doubt were dismayed to learn they had a condition that was generally considered to be a serious ailment, whereas those in the latter group presumably were glad they could put a specific label on their symptoms, believing that the label would then permit them to address the issue appropriately, with consequent long-term benefit.

Sherwood and colleagues in a much better done study using 2 different survey instruments found a deterioration in the quality of life of glaucoma patients. They also found a correlation between various aspects of the patients' glaucomas and the patients' assessment of their own visual function. This would seem, intuitively, to make sense; that is, the more serious the glaucoma, the worse would be the visual field, the more complex would be the medication schedule, and the more likely would be the patient to have difficulties managing his or her own life. However, it is not yet clear whether the questionnaires used to assess quality of life at the present time are any better than the intuitive hunch just mentioned. Humans have a remarkable difference in their ability to cope. Some can handle adversity well and seem to grow in the face of difficulty. Others cope less well, and small changes in their visual capacity can result in dramatic changes in their sense of well-being. Some patients with bilateral hand movements vision lead rich and productive lives, whereas others who have suffered a decrease in visual acuity from 20/20 to 20/30 without any other apparent problem become incapacitated for life.

Health and quality of life are, obviously, subjective perceptions. Health is the sense of feeling whole. Quality-of-life assessment methods can, in fact, provide an impression of how a person feels about his or her own health. At present there are no methods of objectively assessing visual function; that is, how well does a person use a train schedule, how easy is it for a person to find the food on his or her plate, how skillfully can a person match his or her clothes in a way that would present the appearance he or she wants, how able is a person to perform repetitive work in an assembly line, and so forth.

It is still not clear in this reader's mind whether the sophisticated methods used to assess quality of life are any better than a sensitive person asking the patient "How are you?" The questionnaires provide harder, more quantifiable information. However, whether that information is a valid assessment of "how the patient is doing" is another matter.

G.L. Spaeth, M.D.

Patient Noncompliance in the Managed Care Setting: The Case of Medical Therapy for Glaucoma

Gurwitz JH, Yeomans SM, Glynn RJ, et al (Meyers Primary Care Inst, Worcester, Mass; Univ of Mass, Worcester; Harvard Med School, Boston)

Med Care 36:357-369, 1998 3–2

Background.—Although the potentially adverse consequences of patient noncompliance with treatment have long been recognized, accurately identifying which patients are most likely to be noncompliant is still a challenge. Demographic and clinical characteristics associated with noncompliance in patients beginning medical treatment for glaucoma in a managed care setting were studied retrospectively.

Methods and Findings.—Of 616 eligible patients, 152 (24.7%) met the criteria for noncompliance. During the 12-month study, the mean number of days without treatment was 103.9, compared with 6.8 for those categorized as compliant. The variable most strongly associated with noncompliance was fewer visits to an ophthalmologist. Intraocular pressure was comparable in noncompliant and compliant patients.

Conclusions.—Noncompliance with prescribed medical therapy for glaucoma was common in this series. Identifying who is most likely to be noncompliant using demographic and clinical data remains difficult.

▶ The most important single factor influencing the likelihood that a patient with glaucoma will become blind is the biological nature of the disease affecting the particular individual. The second most important factor influencing the course of glaucoma is the patient's ability to care for himself or herself. The patient must be evaluated periodically by a knowledgeable ophthalmologist and must develop a lifestyle compatible with controlling the damage that glaucoma could cause. For example, medicinal therapy is obviously of no help unless the medicines are used.

Two words usually describe a patient who does not use medications as ordered: delinquent or noncompliant. These are unfortunate words. "Delinquent" is clearly inappropriate, because it carries a sense of criminality. "Noncompliant" is also a poor term, because it describes a relationship between the patient and the physician who is totally in charge, and makes all decisions for the patient. In the "compliant-noncompliant" model, the physician orders the patient to do something. If the patient does not follow the physician's orders, the patient is labeled "noncompliant."

However, a patient may have excellent reasons for choosing not to follow a physician's recommendations, including cost, convenience, side effects, poor understanding, or lack of trust. However labeled and whatever the causes the fact is a substantial portion of patients do not use their medications as suggested by their physician. The likely consequence is a substantial number of patients with glaucoma become worse who would not have if they used their medications appropriately. Identification of those who choose not to use their medications as ordered is difficult. The authors suggest a novel way of determining whether patients are filling the prescriptions for their medications. Clearly those patients who do not fill their prescriptions cannot be using their medications appropriately. If such patients could be identified, the physician could then discuss with the patient why the patient chose not to use his or her medications. Such a discussion should lead to a better understanding of the issue, both from the patient's and the physicians point of view, with better care provided. The method, however, does raise some confidentiality concerns. Does the pharmacist or the insurance company or, for that matter, the physician really have any right to know whether or not a patient is using medications? If the insurance company knew and the patient became worse, could the insurance company refuse coverage, anticipating that the patient was responsible for the worsening of the condition? Patients may elect to obtain their medications from sources other than those known to the insurance company. Patients may purchase their medications but fail to use them.

"Compliance" will continue to be a problem when patients do not believe it is in their best interest to use their medications, or more generally, to follow their physician's recommendations. It remains important to identify possible ways to reduce this problem, and the authors' suggestion is certainly worthy of consideration.

G.L. Spaeth, M.D.

Central Corneal Thickness and Intraocular Pressure in a Mongolian Population

Foster PJ, Baasanhu J, Alsbirk PH, et al (Inst of Ophthalmology, London; Med Univ, Ulaanbaatar, Mongolia; Hillerød Hosp, Denmark)

Ophthalmology 105:969-973, 1998 3–3

Background.—Estimates of intraocular pressure (IOP) by applanation tonometry assume that the force with which the cornea resists flattening is equal to the capillary attraction of the tonometer's tear film, and, thus, these opposite forces cancel each other out. Some researchers have begun to doubt these assumptions, however, as differences in central corneal thickness (CCT) have been shown to affect tonometric estimates of IOP. These authors examined the correlation between IOP measurements and CCT in a Mongolian population.

Methods.—The subjects were 1,244 residents of Hövsgöl Province, Northern Mongolia from 10 to 87 years of age. All subjects were examined by an optical pachymeter to measure CCT. Readings were performed only once for each eye and were made by the "touch method," i.e., the reading was taken when the posterior surface of the corneal epithelium in the upper image just touched the anterior epithelial surface of the lower image. All subjects 40 years of age and older were examined by a Goldman-type applanation tonometer to measure IOP. Three IOP readings were made in each eye, and the median of these readings was reported.

Findings.—CCT measurements differed significantly between the right and left eyes in both men (493 ± 32 and 512 ± 32 μm, respectively) and women (496 ± 31 and 515 ± 31 μm, respectively). However, CCTs in men and women did not differ significantly. A significant age-related decrease in CCT was found for both men (4.8 μm/decade for right eyes, 4.9 μm/decade for left eyes) and women (6.2 μm/decade for right eyes, 5.2 μm/decade for left eyes). In contrast, mean IOPs did not differ significantly between the right and left eyes in either men (12.8 ± 3.4 and 12.6 ±3.4 mm Hg, respectively) or women (12.4 ± 3.1 and 12.6 ± 2.7 mm Hg, respectively), nor did IOP decrease significantly with age. Linear regression analysis showed a highly significant positive correlation between CCT and IOP: for subjects 40 to 80 years of age, each increase in CCT of 10 μm was associated with an increase in IOP of 0.18 mm Hg in right eyes and 0.24 mm Hg in left eyes. In other words, IOPs would be increased by 1 mm Hg by only a 55 μm increase in CCT in the right eye, and by only a 42 μm increase in CCT in the left eye.

Conclusion.—These data suggest that variations in CCT account for changes in IOP estimates of 2.3 mm Hg (from right eye data) to 3.1 mm Hg (from left eye data). When the additional effect of age on CCT is considered, even more variation in IOP (up to 3.6 mm Hg) can be accounted for by CCT. Thus, when IOP is being assessed as a risk factor for glaucoma in east Asians, CCT should also be measured and taken into consideration in the interpretation of elevated IOPs.

▶ This article is interesting for a variety of reasons. In the first place, it reminds us of the real differences that exist between different ethnic groups. It has become unfashionable or "politically incorrect" to suggest that biological differences can exist in groups on the basis of ethnic diversity. There is a reason for this; specifically, differences between individuals usually exceed the similarities, even within similar populations. Labels are often applied in a way that suggests they are universally applicable, as a result of which individuals are incorrectly considered and, when those individuals are patients, are incorrectly diagnosed and treated.

Having said that, however, it is important to remember that there are, in fact, biological differences which, while not characteristic of everybody within the group, do provide helpful guidelines for thinking. Young, male, Caucasian myopes are far more likely to have pigmentary glaucoma than acute primary angle–closure glaucoma, which would not be the case for elderly, Jewish, far-sighted females! There simply is not time enough to run through the possibilities presented in every diagnostic situation, and it is essential to home in on the most likely probability, while at the same time remembering that that probability is only that, a probability, and not a certainty. The old saw says it so well, "When you hear hoof beats in Wyoming, don't think of zebras."

The second point worth considering is almost exactly the opposite of the point just made; specifically, although it is prudent to assume that people in whom IOP is found to be elevated do in fact have elevated IOP, it is by no means a certainty that they do. Science deals with measurements, and accuracy of measurement is critical to good science. But all measurements are, to some extent, indirect, based on suppositions that may or may not be valid. Something as apparently simple and direct as measurement of length has considerable possibility for error. For example, the measurement of corneal diameter requires accurate calibration and use of a calipers. With regard to measurement of IOP, the problem is compounded, because pressure is not directly measured but rather estimated by measuring the ease with which the shape of the globe is changed.

One of the major problems in this regard relates to language. We would be less likely to make errors such as the one described in this paper were we to characterize what we do, when we determine how hard we must press against the globe in order to flatten it or indent it a certain amount, in terms of what is actually being done, rather than the assumed outcome. That is, what we are really measuring is corneal compliance, which is related to, but not the same thing as, the pressure within the globe. Were we to do this, our patients would likely benefit, because we would be less likely to think that we really know the pressure within the globe when we push on it with an instrument, and we would probably be more careful in interpreting the meaning of the measurement.

In the broader context, the problem of substituting a method of estimating value for the actual value should make us think of the problem of substituting the means used to achieve an end in place of the actual end. Specifically, we physicians frequently substitute the means of achieving health for the actual goal of health. We become obsessed with lowering IOP and forget that the only purpose for lowering IOP is to enhance or improve the patient's health.

Foster and colleagues' study is a lovely one, which provides important specific information. It also serves as a model for promoting broader understanding.

G.L. Spaeth, M.D.

The Accuracy of Finger Tension for Estimating Intraocular Pressure After Penetrating Keratoplasty

Rubinfeld RS, Cohen EJ, Laibson PR, et al (Wills Eye Hosp, Philadelphia)
Ophthalmic Surg Lasers 29:213-215, 1998 3–4

Background.—When used immediately after a penetrating keratoplasty, Goldmann tonometry is not an accurate estimator of intraocular pressure (IOP). Thus some corneal surgeons use a finger tension technique for estimating IOP in such patients. The accuracy of this technique was determined.

Methods.—Three experienced corneal surgeons performed finger tension estimates on 68 patients the first and second day after penetrating keratoplasty. MacKay-Marg (MM) tonometry readings were also obtained for comparison.

Findings.—The mean pooled finger tension measure was 22.6 mm Hg, compared with 17.6 mm Hg for the MM reading. For the most accurate surgeon, the mean finger tension exceeded the MM reading by 3.9 mm Hg. Lid edema and globe tenderness significantly reduced the finger tension accuracy of all examiners. The finger tension underestimated the MM reading by more than 10 mm Hg in only 1 patient (2%).

Conclusions.—For some patients and surgeons, the finger tension method for estimating IOP after corneal transplantation can be useful. Its utility relies on proper technique and the absence of substantial lid edema and patient discomfort.

► Measuring IOP with a tonometer is a standard part of ophthalmologists' evaluation of patients. About 150 years ago, Bowman introduced the idea of trying to quantify IOP by determining the firmness of the globe with tactile tensions. Development of instrumentation followed from many areas and in many different forms: Maklatov in Russia, Weber in Germany, Schiotz in Scandinavia, Goldmann in Switzerland, MacKay, Marg, and Langham in the United States. Campbell and others have done good work in validating the accuracy of some of these methods. Why would one publish, now, a report about what is probably the most primitive and approximate method of measuring IOP, specifically, finger tension? Why would I choose to discuss this article at this point?

The points that need to be made include the following: (1) no present technique is totally valid; (2) no present method is totally objective and free from the effect of the person using the technique; (3) we tend, erroneously, to attribute validity to techniques in direct relationship to the mechanical complexity of the methods, and (4) expense is a factor that always must be considered.

Some years ago I performed a study in which I compared the reproducibility of various methods of measuring IOP and compared the measurements with each other. We studied finger tension, Goldmann applanation tension, and Shiotz indentation IOPs. Participants were an elderly, experienced member of the attending staff at the Wills Eye Hospital, a Fellow who had taken his training in India, me, and one of the Residents. The correlation between applanation IOP and finger tension was remarkably high for the Indian Fellow and the senior ophthalmologist, fair for me, and nonexistent for the Resident. The correlation between finger tension and applanation tonometry was actually higher than the correlation between Schiotz and applanation tonometry for the Indian Fellow. The conclusion was clear, namely, that the accuracy of "finger tension" depended upon who was performing the test.

Tonometers are typically calibrated by comparing the instrument's measurement with the measurement as determined manometrically in an enucleated eye. It would be surprising if this mimicked exactly the measurement in a living eye. Several authors have compared tonometric readings with manometric determinations in living patients, usually at the time of surgery. Results showed marked variability, with some systematic error. IOP measured as 15 mm Hg with a tonometer could actually be considerably higher or lower than the tonometric determination. A tonometer reading of 15 mm Hg could be found in patients with intraocular pressures of 10 or 20 mm Hg. Tonometers are used in an even less controlled setting, specifically, the outpatient clinic, where the variability is surely greater. The matter of validity, then, that is, the actual agreement between the IOP as determined by the tonometer and the real IOP within the eye is important; it cannot be assumed that the validity of tonometric measurements is great. This is especially true for instruments such as the Tonopen or the Goldmann tonometer, in which a specific figure is read off the screen or off the dial. But we should remember that the cornea may be thicker or thinner than the eye against which the tonometer was calibrated, and therefore the IOP is spuriously higher or lower. The epithelium of the cornea may be edematous or thin, and therefore the IOP may be higher or lower. Or the anterior chamber may be so shallow that the cornea is pressed against the intraocular lens by the tonometer, giving a reading that is much higher than is actually the case.

Laibson's article is an important one that we should read and heed. We all should practice taking "finger tensions" frequently so that when pressure must be estimated and an instrument is likely to be inaccurate, we have some way of knowing what the IOP actually is.

G.L. Spaeth, M.D.

Relationship of Optic Disc Topography to Optic Nerve Fiber Number in Glaucoma

Yücel YH, Gupta N, Kalichman MW, et al (Univ of California, San Diego; Univ of Toronto; Allergan Inc, Irvine, Calif)

Arch Ophthalmol 116:493-497, 1998 3–5

Background.—The association between optic-disc topography and optic-nerve fiber loss in glaucomatous eyes has not been determined. Understanding this relationship is important to the use of topographic parameters to diagnose and monitor glaucoma. Measures of optic-disc topography were compared with the number of surviving optic-nerve fibers in glaucoma.

Methods.—Ten monkeys with laser-induced glaucoma in the right eye were studied. A confocal scanning laser ophthalmoscope was used to measure optic-disc topography in vivo. Histomorphometry was done on optic-nerve cross-sections, using bright-field microscopy with camera lucida. Nerve-fiber number was estimated for each sector and compared with each of 13 global optic-disc topographic parameters.

Findings.—Neuroretinal measures in the glaucomatous eyes showed that optic-nerve fiber number was significantly associated with rim area, retinal-nerve fiber layer (RNFL) cross-sectional area, rim volume, and RNFL thickness. Nerve-fiber count differences between control and glaucomatous optic nerves were most strongly related to mean height contour differences, followed by RNFL cross-sectional area, RNFL thickness, rim volume, and differences in rim area. Nerve-fiber number in glaucomatous eyes was significantly associated with cup volume below reference, cup area, mean cup depth, the ratio of cup area to disc area, and cup shape. Differences in nerve-fiber number between control and glaucomatous optic nerves were most strongly associated with differences in cup shape, followed by mean cup depth, cup volume below reference, ratio of cup area to disc area, cup area, and difference in cup volume below surface. Optic-nerve fiber number was not associated with optic-disc area in glaucomatous eyes.

Conclusions.—In this model of glaucoma, most optic-disc topography measures were significantly associated with optic-nerve fiber number. These data support the use of confocal scanning laser ophthalmoscopy to assess optic-nerve damage in glaucoma.

▶ This is an important study. It does not answer the question of whether topographic changes in the optic disc or the loss of neurons and glia comes first. It was not designed to answer that question. However, this study does establish a clear relationship between morphologic changes in the optic disc and the number of neurons passing from the retina through the optic nerve. The model allowed the optic nerve to be subjected to elevated intraocular pressure for over a year. This is a "pure" model, which undoubtedly is not fully representative of all patients with all types of glaucoma. The glaucoma damage in these cases was caused by the elevated intraocular pressure affecting nerves that were presumably normal before the laser treatment that caused the monkey eyes to develop an intraocular pressure elevation. In some human beings, factors other than elevated intraocular pressure almost certainly play a role. The authors have demonstrated, however, that a variety of morphologic changes correlate well with the loss of neurons.

I found it especially interesting that the authors included, among the parameters of morphology studied, the characteristic of the Heidelberg Retinal Tomograph called "cup shape." This is one of the hardest characteristics to quantify, because it involves patterns rather than simply a measurement (such as millimeters, millimeters squared, or millimeters cubed) which would apply to the thickness of the nerve-fiber layer, the rim area, or the cup volume, respectively. These latter measurements are relatively easy to quantify, though not so easy to validate. It is relatively easy to make a measurement, but it is not always clear whether the measurement represents exactly what is being measured. More importantly, the measurement may not be clinically important, because the "reference plane" may have been placed at a level that could not provide the type of information needed to allow the clinician to make the judgment about whether the nerve is damaged, and if so, how extensively.

To determine the shape of the cup is a new capability of image analysis. It represents a major step forward in programming, although it is still a relatively primitive analysis. Perhaps the most important conclusion of this lovely article is the extremely high correlation between the shape of the cup and the decrease in optic-nerve fibers. There is a vast amount of work about image analysis machines still to do, but this article proves that it is worth doing. Clinicians should be able in the future to do with these machines what we can now do with an ophthalmoscope but cannot do with an image-analysis device. Specifically, it may be possible to determine whether an optic disc is glaucomatous, not on the basis of the size of the optic disc or the thickness of the nerve-fiber layer, but rather on the basis of the disc's pattern of appearance. That would be a great step, because it might enable clinicians to make a diagnosis on the basis of a single evaluation, without a second determination demonstrating change.

G.L. Spaeth, M.D.

Retinal Nerve Fibre Layer Polarimetry: Histological and Clinical Comparison

Morgan JE, Waldock A, Jeffery G, et al (Univ Hosp of Wales, Cardiff; Bristol Eye Hosp, England; Inst of Ophthalmology, London; et al)
Br J Ophthalmol 82:684-690, 1998 3–6

Background.—Clinical examination of the retinal nerve fiber layer is useful in diagnosing glaucoma but remains an essentially subjective method. Using the Mark II Nerve Fiber Analyzer, histologic thickness of the retinal nerve fiber layer was compared with retardation measures obtained in vivo.

Methods.—Both eyes of a healthy primate were studied by scanning laser polarimetry. Retinal nerve fiber layer thickness was determined with the best polarimetry image. A nerve fiber layer thickness map was then scaled and aligned to a retardation map.

Findings.—At 216 locations, retinal nerve fiber layer thickness measures were aligned satisfactorily with corresponding retardation values. The overall correlation coefficient for thickness and retardation was 0.70. The best correlation was observed inferior to the optic disc. Correlations seen superiorly and temporally were less positive but still highly significant. The poorest correlation occurred at the nasal aspect of the disc.

Conclusions.—Retinal nerve fiber layer thickness in the primate eye is positively correlated with retardation measures obtained with the nerve-fiber analyzer. However, the correlation coefficient varied around the optic disc, indicating that further assessment of the device is needed before routine clinical use.

► In this study the histologic thickness of the retinal nerve fiber layer in a monkey was compared with the thickness of that same layer as estimated by the Mark II Nerve Fiber Layer Analyzer (Laser Diagnostic Technologies, San Diego, Calif). This is an important validation experiment. The authors are to be congratulated for not using a monkey for this study only, and for using, instead, an animal believed unsuitable for long-term preservation.

The authors found a correlation between the thickness of the retinal nerve fiber layer as determined histologically and the thickness as determined with the polarimetric device, the "nerve fiber layer analyzer." However, in Figure 5 in the original article the comparison of the 2 measurements shows that there is a great deal of variability. Although it is possible to draw a statistically significant line that relates the 2 variables, the spread is marked. The range of thickness also varied, from 6.7 to 26 nm. Other authors have shown that the pattern of thickness varies from patient to patient, both in amplitude and in shape. The authors properly caution against the use of this device in a clinical setting until there has been further evaluation.

G.L. Spaeth, M.D.

Factors Affecting Image Acquisition During Scanning Laser Polarimetry

Hoh ST, Greenfield DS, Liebmann JM, et al (The New York Eye and Ear Infirmary; New York Med College, Valhalla; Singapore Eye Research Inst; et al)

Ophthalmic Surg Lasers 29:545-551, 1998 3–7

Background.—Scanning laser polarimetry (SLP), a noninvasive technique, enables quantitative measurement of peripapillary retinal-nerve fiber layer (RNFL) thickness, using the birefringent properties of retinal ganglion cell axons. The artifacts that may be observed during RNFL measurement with SLP were described.

Methods.—Four hundred twenty-six patients who had received various ocular diagnoses underwent RNFL measurement with SLP between June 1996 and April 1997. Two examiners performed the scanning.

Findings.—Acquiring images was difficult in eyes with corneal grafts or edema, keratic precipitates, anterior uveitis, posterior subcapsular cataract, vitreous opacity, peripapillary atrophy, posterior staphyloma, and high axial myopia. In such cases, clinical correlation with visual-field tests and optic-nerve examination was poor, image reproducibility was poor, and images were unreadable.

Conclusions.—Anterior and posterior segment abnormalities, especially those localized to the cornea and lens, may cause spurious RNFL measurements. Clinicians should carefully consider such abnormalities.

► SLP has been suggested as a way of accurately determining the thickness of the nerve-fiber layer of the retina. The technique offers the opportunity to measure directly the effects of glaucoma damage. Recently it has been reported (see Abstract 3–5) that there is a correlation between the appearance of the optic nerve and nerve-fiber layer, as determined by Heidelberg Retinal Tomography and the number of neurons present. Others have also demonstrated a histological correlation between thickness of the nerve-fiber layer and retinal ganglion cells. Thus, it should be possible to get an idea of glaucoma damage by estimating nerve-fiber layer thickness. However, as this article points out, and as we need to be reminded, there are differences between reproducibility and validity. It may be possible to acquire images in a relatively reproducible way, but those images may not be representing what we think they are representing. In selected individuals, image-analysis devices may provide sufficiently valid measurements for clinically useful information to be garnered. However, this has not yet been demonstrated convincingly. What is apparent is that there are still many hazards to using image-analysis techniques.

G.L. Spaeth, M.D.

Pressure-dependent Neuroretinal Rim Loss in Normal-Pressure Glaucoma

Jonas JB, Gründler AE, Gonzales-Cortés J (Friedrich-Alexander-Univ Erlangen-Nürnberg, Germany)

Am J Ophthalmol 125:137-144, 1998 3–8

Background.—The criteria for glaucoma have in the past, included increased intraocular pressure (IOP). However, patients can have glaucomatous optic nerve damage in association with normal IOP. The current study studied whether the level of IOP in patients with normal-pressure glaucoma is correlated with the degree of glaucomatous optic nerve damage.

Methods and Findings.—Color stereo optic disk photographs of 98 eyes with the focal type of normal-pressure glaucoma, 17 eyes with the highly myopic type of normal-pressure glaucoma, and 36 eyes with age-related atrophic primary open-angle glaucoma were obtained. Morphometric measures of these photographs in all 3 groups showed that the neuroretinal rim area significantly decreased as maximal IOP increased.

Conclusions.—Among patients with different types of open-angle glaucoma with normal IOP, eyes with relatively high IOP have more marked optic nerve damage than those with relatively low IOP. These findings suggest that an IOP in the low-normal range may be less likely to be associated with glaucoma damage than an IOP in the upper-normal range.

► Jonas and colleagues have compiled convincing information that progressive glaucoma damage in patients who have glaucoma in association with "normal" IOP is in fact related to the pressure itself. If this is the case, then, lowering pressure an appropriate amount should eliminate or slow the rate of deterioration in patients who have glaucoma and who also have normal IOPs. However, glaucoma is a mixed bag of conditions, and that heterogeneity applies to patients with "normal pressure glaucoma," as well as patients with glaucoma in association with higher IOP. The heterogeneity of pathogenesis may be even greater in glaucoma patients with lower IOPs. When IOP is elevated, there is a fairly clear-cut model applied to understanding the damage caused by the elevated pressure: specifically, the pressure pushes on the lamina cribrosa, the lamina cribrosa bows posteriorly, the nerves are kinked, and there is an interference with axoplasmic transport, leading to neuronal cell death. If the pressure is markedly elevated, above the level of systolic artery pressure, then the mechanism is acute ischemic optic neuropathy. In individuals with IOPs in the normal range there may well be a variety of different mechanisms, including neurotoxicity, ischemia, support of the lamina, vasospasm, and so forth. Heterogeneity is important to recall, because, if a population of patients with "normal-pressure glaucoma" are studied, it is virtually certain that whatever characteristic is being evaluated will apply to some of the patients but not to all of them. Jonas and colleagues have divided normal-pressure glaucoma into several different entities and have found that there is a pressure-dependent loss of the neuroretinal rim in those types of glaucoma studied. This would suggest that lowering the IOP in these particular patients would result in slowing down the rate of damage caused by glaucoma. This article provides convincing theoretical support, justifying the practice of trying to lower IOP in patients who have progressive glaucoma, even when their pressure is normal at the beginning.

This leads to a concern I have about this article, and indeed to all those in which "normal" is used to describe an IOP that causes damage but which is in the average range. Originally, "normal" meant "average," but with the development of statistical techniques, "normal" has come to mean "healthy." If glaucoma is at least partially related to IOP, then the pressure associated with further deterioration is too high for that particular person. Thus, a person who has an IOP of 15 mm Hg, which is average, and who is getting worse with an IOP of 15 mm Hg, has an IOP which in fact may be average, but is certainly not normal. Were it normal, the person would not be having progressive glaucoma damage. "Normal" has become such a confusing term that it is best to use it with great care, and only when it means "average and healthy." In that way, the term would not be misleading. My advice, then, would be to eliminate the use of "normal" completely in describing the relationship between IOP and a particular patient, unless one was absolutely sure that the pressure played no role whatsoever in the person's glaucoma.

Another point in this regard has to do with the use of the term "pressure" instead of "tension." Tonometers measure the "tenseness" of the globe, though that is not the characteristic that really concerns the ophthalmologist. The ophthalmologist wants to know the pressure inside the eye. The advantage of using "tension" is that it indicates that the measurement is not really a direct indication of pressure, and therefore may be inaccurate. The advantage of using "pressure" is that the term represents more accurately what the ophthalmologist really wants to know and what one thinks one is measuring when using a tonometer. Though the terminology is cumbersome, probably the best phrase to use is "glaucoma in association with average intraocular pressure."

G.L. Spaeth, M.D.

Pseudoexfoliation Syndrome for the Comprehensive Ophthalmologist: Intraocular and Systemic Manifestations

Naumann GOH, Schlötzer-Schrehardt U, Küchle M (Univ of Erlangen-Nürnberg, Germany)

Ophthalmology 105:951-968, 1998 3–9

Introduction.—Pseudoexfoliation syndrome is not only an ocular disease but also a generalized disorder involving abnormal production and/or turnover of extracellular matrix material. All tissues of the anterior segment in the eye and extraocular tissues are involved in this disorder. The findings on the anterior lens capsule are used to base clinical classification of the various stages. This syndrome should be suspected when one sees the existence of circular or segmental posterior synechiae without any other obvious cause. The intraocular and extraocular manifestations, as well as the resulting clinical complications of this common but poorly understood disorder, were reviewed.

Methods.—Biomicroscopy, biocytology, and laser-tyndallometry are used for clinical diagnosis. Light and electronic microscopy, immunohistochemical and molecular biological approaches are used as the laboratory research methods.

Observations.—The focus of clinical-histopathologic correlations are on the involvement of the zonular apparatus (zonulopathy) (Fig 7), the lens (pseudoexfoliation-phacopathy), iris (iridopathy), ciliary body (cyclopathy), cornea (corneal endotheliopathy), and trabecular meshwork (trabeculopathy). Complications that are reviewed include phacodonesis, lens dislocation, and increased incidence of vitreous loss in extracapsular cataract surgery caused by alterations of the zonular apparatus and its insertion into the ciliary body and lens; open-angle glaucoma as well as angle-closure glaucoma resulting from pupillary and ciliary block; early diffuse corneal endothelial decompensation explained by a damaged and numerically reduced endothelium; and blood-aqueous barrier breakdown (pseudouveitis), anterior chamber hypoxia, iris stroma hemorrhage, pigment epithelial melanin dispersion, poor or asymmetric pupillary dilatation, and formation of posterior synechiae resulting from involvement of all cell populations of the iris (Table 6).

Conclusions.—Pseudoexfoliation is of relevance to comprehensive ophthalmologists, including specialists in glaucoma, cataract, cornea, neuro-ophthalmology, and retina, in view of the multitude of clinical complications. It is advisable to pay special attention to the risks associated with pseudoexfoliation before, during, and after surgery.

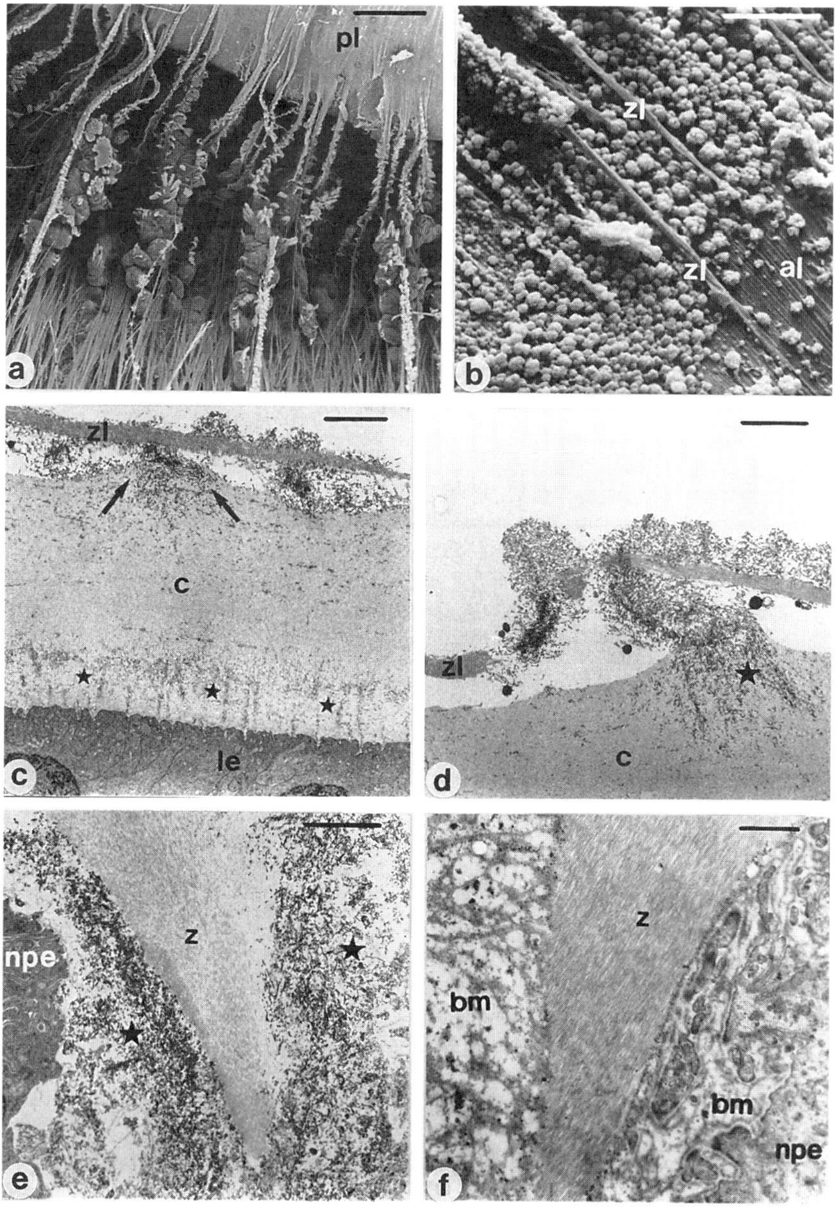

FIGURE 7.—Pseudoexfoliation (PEX)-zonulopathy. **A**, scanning electron micrograph showing accumulation of PEX material on ciliary processes and zonular fibers in the region of the pars plicata (*pl* = posterior lens equator; *bar* = 300 µm). **B**, scanning electron micrograph showing loosened zonular lamella (*zl*) on the anterior lens capsule (*al*) by accumulation of nodular PEX aggregates (*bar* = 100 µm). C, transmission electron micrograph showing separation of the zonular lamella (*zl*) from the capsular (*c*) surface by PEX material (*asterisk*) produced by the lens epithelium (*le*) and erupting through the capsular surface (*arrows; bar* = 5 µm). **D**, rupture of zonular lamella (*zl*) at sites of PEX material (*asterisk*) infiltration (bar = 5 µm). **E**, loosened zonular (*z*) insertion into the disrupted basement membrane of the nonpigmented ciliary epithelium (*npe*) due to accumulating PEX masses (*asterisk*) (*bar* = 5 µm). **F**, regular insertion of a zonular bundle (*z*) into the basement membrane (*bm*) of the nonpigmented ciliary epithelium (*npe*) of a control specimen (*bar* = 1 µm). (Published courtesy of *Ophthalmology*, from Naumann GOH, Schlötzer-Schrehardt U, Küchle M: Pseudoexfoliation syndrome for the comprehensive ophthalmologist: Intraocular and systemic manifestations. *Ophthalmology* 105:951-968, 1998.)

TABLE 6.—Intraocular Complications of Pseudoexfoliation (*PEX*) Syndrome

	Clinical Complications	Causal Mechanisms
Glaucomas and ocular hypertension	Chronic open-angle	Exo- and endotrabecular PEX material, increased aqueous proteins, melanin dispersion (corneal endothelial proliferation)
	Angle-closure	Pupillary block, ciliary block
	Acute pressure rises	"Melanin shower" in mydriasis, pupillary/ciliary block
Lens complications	Phakodonesis, (sub)luxation	Zonular instability
	Extracapsular cataract surgery	Zonular dialysis, vitreous loss ↑, iridopathy, synechiae, secondary cataract ↑, late decentration of posterior chamber lens
	Nuclear cataract	
Iridopathy	Pseudouveitis	Blood-aqueous barrier defect
	Posterior synechiae	
	Poor mydriasis, asymmetric pupillary action	Iris rigidity, stromal atrophy
	Melanin dispersion	Pigment epithelial atrophy
	Capillary hemorrhage	Vasculopathy
	Anterior chamber hypoxia	Reduced capillary flow
Keratopathy	Early endothelial decompensation	Reduced cell count, local PEX production
	Corneal endothelial proliferation	? Anterior chamber hypoxia
Retina	Central retinal vein occlusion	
	Retinal detachment	Vitreous loss, YAG-iridotomy

(Published courtesy of *Ophthalmology*, from Naumann GOH, Schlötzer-Schrehardt U, Küchle M: Pseudoexfoliation syndrome for the comprehensive ophthalmologist: Intraocular and systemic manifestations. *Ophthalmology* 105:951-968, 1998.)

► The authors of this comprehensive, informative, and beautifully illustrated review of the pseudoexfoliation syndrome have made many of the important new observations about the syndrome that are described herein. The association between pseudoexfoliation and glaucoma is well known. In the era of extracapsular cataract surgery, ophthalmologists must be equally aware of the pseudoexfoliation syndrome's effect on the zonule and its contribution to instability and lens dislocation.

In recent years it has become apparent that the pseudoexfoliation syndrome actually is a systemic disorder of elastic tissue. Whether the pseudoexfoliation syndrome has nonocular complications warrants further study. Initial data from Germany suggest that there may be an association between pseudoexfoliation and aortic aneurysms.

R.C. Eagle, Jr., M.D.

► This article on the exfoliation syndrome is a superb review, containing new material as well. My preference is to call the entity "exfoliation syndrome" rather than "pseudo-exfoliation syndrome" because there is nothing "pseudo" about the exfoliation that occurs. The pathology is surely not related merely to exfoliation, as is pointed out by the authors, but an important part of the condition is the sloughing of pigmented and nonpigmented debris into the anterior chamber. I feel especially passionate about this condition, and I am thankful to the authors for preparing a superb article and the editors for publishing it, because despite the continuing contributions of individuals such as Barbara Streeten and Robert Ritch, the condition is egregiously underdiagnosed. Additionally, the most important help in diagnosing the exfoliation syndrome, gonioscopy, is not even considered by the American Academy of Ophthalmology to be a part of a comprehensive ocular examination. The importance of both the exfoliation syndrome and gonioscopy are vastly underestimated.

Here is a brief quiz:

1. What is usually the first sign indicating the presence of the exfoliation syndrome?
2. Is the anterior chamber angle narrow in the exfoliation syndrome?
3. What are the characteristic differences between a routine "narrow anterior chamber angle" (such as that seen in a hyperopic patient with relative pupillary block) and the narrow anterior chamber angle that occurs in patients with the exfoliation syndrome?
4. Is the course of glaucoma in a patient with glaucoma caused by the exfoliation syndrome similar or different to that in a patient with "primary open-angle glaucoma" (idiopathic open-angle glaucoma)?

The answers:

1. The first visible sign in the patient with the exfoliation syndrome is usually a black deposit of pigment within and on the surface of the posterior trabecular meshwork inferiorly. Unlike pigmentary glaucoma, the pigmentation

in the exfoliation syndrome is much more prominent inferiorly than superiorly. It is not unusual for a patient to have 3 or more pigmentations of the posterior trabecular meshwork at the 6 o'clock position and 1 or more pigmentations of the posterior trabecular meshwork at the 12 o'clock position. In contrast, patients with the pigment dispersion syndrome have pigment that is equally dense superiorly and inferiorly. The pigmentary changes precede the visible changes on the lens surface. A Sampaolesi line is highly characteristic, and when present, virtually diagnostic. The Sampaolesi line consists of a deposit of black pigment anterior to Schwalbe's line, limited to the inferior portion of the angle, and present in a scalloped pattern. However, the pigmentary changes in the angle recess and in the area of the trabecular meshwork frequently precede the Sampaolesi line.

2. The anterior chamber angle definitely tends to be narrow in patients with the exfoliation syndrome.
3. In patients with a narrow angle associated with a small anterior segment and relative pupillary block the angle is invariably narrower superiorly than inferiorly. In patients with a narrow angle associated with the exfoliation syndrome, the angle is narrower inferiorly than superiorly. The exact cause for the narrow angle in the exfoliation syndrome is probably an increase in the axial depth of the lens, which would be expected to produce symmetrical narrowing in all quadrants. The cause for the selective narrowing inferiorly is not known but may be a reflection of the characteristic weakness of the zonules in patients with the exfoliation syndrome and the tendency of the lens to move inferiorly in the upright position because of gravity.
4. The course of glaucoma in a patient with the exfoliation syndrome is typically very different from that of a patient who has ordinary "primary open-angle glaucoma." The glaucoma in the patient with the exfoliation syndrome appears to be either of almost no concern or of great concern. Many patients with the exfoliation syndrome never develop elevated intraocular pressures. Most of these people never need any treatment to lower their intraocular pressure because they characteristically do not develop glaucoma damage. The development of optic nerve damage in the absence of elevated intraocular pressure appears to be rare in patients with the exfoliation syndrome and much more common in patients with ordinary primary open-angle glaucoma. However, in some patients with the exfoliation syndrome the intraocular pressure does become elevated. In some of these, the elevation is mild and can often be controlled with an argon laser trabeculoplasty. But in others intraocular pressure becomes highly unstable, with marked spikes to pressures in the 30s or even 40s. This last group of patients, with unstable and elevated intraocular pressures, is the group in whom intraocular pressure damage can occur with disturbing rapidity. In some of these patients it seems as if the optic disc just melts away. This group of patients needs to be monitored with extreme care to prevent the rapid development of far-advanced glaucoma damage. In summary, then, regarding the course of glaucoma in patients with the exfoliation syndrome, the patients by and large do "better" or "worse" than patients with standard primary open-angle

glaucoma; the former group tends to be overtreated and the latter group undertreated.

Surely every surgeon who performs a cataract extraction is aware of the hazards associated with the exfoliation syndrome. It is prudent, then, to make sure that the diagnosis is not missed. This article points out some of the many clues that should alert the surgeon before surgery.

G.L. Spaeth, M.D.

Axon Deviation in the Human Lamina Cribrosa

Morgan JE, Jeffery G, Foss AJE (Univ Hosp of Wales, Cardiff; Univ College London; Univ Hosp, Nottingham, England)

Br J Ophthalmol 82:680-683, 1998 3–10

Background.—Detailed information about the axon paths through the lamina cribrosa is essential to an understanding of the mechanisms underlying axon compression. The course of individual retinal ganglion cell axons through the human lamina cribrosa was investigated.

Methods.—Two normal human eyes removed during treatment for extraocular disease were examined. Retinal ganglion cell axons were labeled with the retrograde tracer horseradish peroxidase applied directly to the optic nerve.

Findings.—Most axons took a direct course through the lamina cribrosa. However, 8% to 12% deviated to pass between the cribrosal plates in both central and peripheral parts of the optic disc.

Conclusions.—These data provide new support for the belief that mechanical axonal compression is a factor in diseases such as glaucoma. The cause of axon misdirection is still not clear. Further research on axon trajectory in the lamina cribrosa, and its relation to susceptibility of the optic nerve to become damaged, is indicated.

► This is an important article for several reasons. It highlights the serious lack of information presently available about pathological changes in the optic nerve in patients with glaucoma. This lack of information is the result of difficulty in obtaining glaucomatous eyes for examination. The Glaucoma Research Foundation continues to emphasize the goal of assisting physicians in obtaining glaucomatous eyes. Globes from patients with glaucoma in different stages of the disease, and with different types of glaucoma, are needed. It is a mistake to be reluctant to discuss this matter with patients who are seriously ill. We may believe that a patient who is facing death may not want to be reminded of that reality, and our concern is probably justified. However, most patients also like to believe that there has been some purpose to their having lived. For some individuals, being able to contribute their eyes for corneal transplantation is helpful and reassuring. Most patients with glaucoma are aware that there is still a huge amount to learn about the condition. It is likely that a thoughtful, nonthreatening discussion with selected patients would allow them to think more positively about their coming death. Globes can also be obtained from patients in whom the eyes will be removed as part of a surgical procedure. Indeed, in the study described in this article, the 2 eyes that serve as the basis of the evaluation were removed at the time of surgery for an orbital tumor. However, it is rare that such surgical procedures are performed on patients with glaucoma.

Because of the rapidity with which postmortem changes occur, plans to harvest the globe and proceed with a method of fixation must be made before the patient's death. Thus, it is likely that only patients dying in a hospital are suitable candidates. The method of fixation depends upon the goals of the study.

What Morgan et al. demonstrate in the present investigation may be very important to understanding the pathogenesis of optic nerve damage in patients with glaucoma. It is not known whether these 2 patients were typical of other patients. It is reasonable to assume that considerable variability exists. Is sensitivity of the optic nerve to change in intraocular pressure related to variability in optic nerve structure? It has already been suggested that in glaucoma the optic nerve may show preferential damage in the inferotemporal area because the laminar pores in that area are larger. This article should stimulate other studies that will lead to a better understanding of why there is such marked individual difference in sensitivity of optic nerves to intraocular pressure.

G.L. Spaeth, M.D.

Echographic Measurements of the Retrobulbar Optic Nerve in Normal and Glaucomatous Eyes

Beatty S, Good PA, McLaughlin J, et al (Birmingham and Midland Eye Centre, Birmingham, England)
Br J Ophthalmol 82:43-47, 1998 3–11

Background.—The diagnostic potential of orbital optic nerve measures in glaucoma has been hindered by the poor resolving power of B-scan US in the retrobulbar region. These authors used a new-generation B scanner to measure orbital optic nerve dimension in eyes with glaucoma and ocular hypertension.

Methods.—Forty-nine patients with glaucoma and 90 control participants were studied. Five repeated echographic measures of the maximal interpial diameter and cross-sectional area of the orbital optic nerve were obtained in 1 eye of each participant on 2 occasions.

Findings.—The mean optic-nerve diameter in the control group was 2.86 mm. This value was independent of height, axial length, spherical equivalent, sex, and race; however, it was inversely associated with age. The reproducibility of optic-nerve diameter measures was 0.149 mm in the control group. The test-retest variability of the interpial diameter was −0.02 mm. The average interpial diameter of the optic nerve was significantly shorter in eyes with glaucoma than in healthy eyes. In addition, glaucomatous optic nerves had a significantly smaller cross-sectional area.

Conclusions.—Echocardiographic measures of the orbital optic nerve are very reproducible. Eyes with glaucoma have reduced optic-nerve interpial diameters and cross-sectional areas, indicating nerve-fiber loss. This method may be helpful in distinguishing normal from glaucomatous eyes when optic-disc morphometry is inconclusive or impossible because of opaque media.

► These authors provide yet another way of distinguishing between glaucomatous and nonglaucomatous eyes. The question is whether this method will be of any use. For example, one can distinguish between population of glaucomatous and nonglaucomatous eyes using tonography, cup disc ratio, and a variety of other findings. The problem, however, is such large variability that the findings, taken by themselves, are usually of little help.

The authors show that the diameter of the retrobulbar optic nerve decreases with increasing age, and is shorter in eyes with glaucoma than in eyes with ocular hypertension or eyes believed to be normal. The ease of measuring the optic-nerve thickness with US recommends the technique for further study. Even now, it may be clinically useful to obtain an estimate of the optic-nerve thickness when evaluating a patient in whom ophthalmoscopic evaluation of the optic nerve is impossible because of opacities in the media.

G.L. Spaeth, M.D.

Flow Velocity of Central Retinal Artery and Retrobulbar Vessels During Cardiovascular Operations

Orihashi K, Matsuura Y, Sueda T, et al (Hiroshima Univ, Japan)

J Thorac Cardiovasc Surg 114:1081-1087, 1997 3–12

Background.—Blood flow and blood pressure must be monitored during cardiovascular surgery to avoid inadequate cerebral perfusion. Transcranial Doppler ultrasound does not provide a consistently good signal, particularly during cardiopulmonary bypass. The current study assessed the blood flow through the central retinal artery, which has been shown to reflect an obstruction of the carotid artery.

Methods.—A 5- or 7.5-MHz conventional echocardiographic probe was used in 28 consecutive patients to determine the relationship between the maximal velocity at the central retinal artery and systolic blood pressure. Assessment of the blood flow of the central retinal artery and retrobulbar vessels was performed during selective or retrograde cerebral perfusion of intra-aortic balloon pumping.

Findings.—Blood flow was visualized clearly in each patient, but it disappeared after dropping below a certain pressure. Systolic blood pressure was correlated with maximal velocity. The mean blood pressure-axis intercept, or *critical closing pressure*, was 35.8 mm Hg. This pressure varied among individuals and between bilateral eyes. After cardiopulmonary bypass, the pulsatility index increased. The blood flow during anastomosis of the ipsilateral artery confirmed the patency of the circle of Willis. Blood flow was seen at the retrobulbar vessels during retrograde cerebral perfusion. Balloon inflation augmented the central retinal artery flow during intra-aortic balloon pumping.

Conclusions.—Orbital vessel monitoring helps to establish the critical closing pressure of the central retinal artery and confirms circle of Willis patency. During cardiovascular operations, the eye can serve as "an acoustic window" to intracranial blood flow.

► The authors describe a method of monitoring blood flow to the retina and suggest that the technique may provide a sensitive measure for assessing adequacy of blood flow to the brain, particularly during cardiovascular surgery. The article has relevance for ophthalmologists. For many years there have been suggestions that insufficiency of blood flow plays a role in glaucoma. The evidence has been both anecdotal and experimental. It can be demonstrated that in many patients with glaucoma, blood flow to the optic nerve and retina is insufficient. However, there have been few clear-cut studies that showed that insufficiency of blood flow preceded damage to the optic nerve and retina. Unfortunately for those interested in establishing the proper role of blood flow in the pathogenesis of glaucomatous damage, the present study will not provide an answer. What it does do, however, is prove that lowering systemic blood pressure can cause acute insufficiency of ocular blood flow. This in itself is an important step ahead, in that it is a confirmation of previous work, the relevance of which has been doubted by some. Many of us who specialize in the practice of glaucoma have cases in which the occurrence of a hypotensive or ischemic episode appears to have been unquestionably associated with a sudden progression of glaucoma damage, such as the patient with moderately advanced glaucoma damage who developed rapid worsening of cupping and field loss unilaterally when the carotid artery was clipped for treatment of an internal intracranial aneurysm. These cases gain added weight in light of the authors' demonstration of insufficiency in response to the hypotension that can occur in association with surgery.

G.L. Spaeth, M.D.

Reversal of Endothelin-1–induced Ocular Hemodynamic Effects by Low-dose Nifedipine in Humans

Strenn K, Matulla B, Wolzt M, et al (Univ of Vienna)

Clin Pharmacol Ther 63:54-63, 1998 3–13

Background.—Evidence suggests that calcium channel blockers may be beneficial in patients with normal-tension glaucoma and vasospastic reactions. Thus, calcium channel blockers may increase ocular blood flow and have a functional antagonism with endothelin-1 (ET-1) in the ocular vasculature.

Methods.—Twelve healthy patients participated in a randomized, double-blind, 3-way crossover study comparing placebo, 2 ng/kg/min ET-1, and 4 ng/kg/min ET-1 and in a randomized, double-blind study comparing placebo and 5 mg nifedipine. Ocular hemodynamics were assessed by laser interferometric measurement of fundus pulsation amplitude (FPA) in the optic disc and by 2-dimensional scanning laser Doppler flowmetry in the optic disc.

Findings.—Endothelin-1 resulted in a dose-dependent decline in FPA and flow. A dose of 4 ng/kg/min caused a reduction of −18% on FPA and −17% in "flow." Nifedipine completely reversed this effect. However, after placebo infusion, nifedipine did not influence ocular hemodynamics.

Conclusions.—Although nifedipine does not increase optic nerve head blood flow during baseline conditions, it reverses ET-1–induced constriction in ocular vasculature at doses that do not affect systemic hemodynamics. This suggests an association between the therapeutic effect of calcium channel blockers and the endothelin system in patients with normal-tension glaucoma. The current findings also provide a rationale for studying low-dose nifedipine as a supplementary medication in patients with glaucoma.

► Strenn and coworkers have performed a lovely study investigating the control of blood flow in humans. To use human subjects in a clinical experiment is difficult. However, human characteristics are not the same as those of other animals, and insights gained from human experimentation can be especially valuable.

This study was carefully performed and showed quite conclusively that the group of normal males studied have a particular type of vessel contraction blocked by a specific pharmacological agent, nifedipine. They also found that nifedipine did not affect ocular hemodynamics. The authors conclude, "The present study provides a strong rationale for a study of low-dose nifedipine as a supplementary medication in glaucoma patients." Although the report is a significant contribution, it is a long way from an isolated pharmacologic study in normal patients to "treatment of glaucoma." Several issues need to be considered that would place this paper in proper perspective.

First, the authors do not demonstrate that nifedipine has no effect on ocular blood flow. They simply did not find any change in blood flow using the methods in the study. Failure to observe an effect does not mean that an effect has not occurred. The authors' method of studying "blood flow" uses the Doppler principle and employs laser as the instrument. The laser is focused on a blood vessel, and an estimate of flow in the vessel is determined, based on the Doppler effect. The instrument does not really measure flow, but rather velocity. The fundamental assumption is that the caliber of the vessel tested does not change. Furthermore, the test is not instantaneous, and during the period that the beam is testing the velocity within the specific vessel, the eye position cannot change significantly. The test is quite reproducible, although reproducibility and validity are not the same thing. One concern relates to the suggestion that nifedipine should be studied as a possible treatment in patients with glaucoma. The authors are to be congratulated in that they very specifically say "study" rather than treat. What do they mean by "glaucoma"? Glaucoma is as diverse as cancer. For example, it would seem virtually certain that nifedipine would have no use in the treatment of glaucoma in which the intraocular pressure ranges 50 or 60 mm Hg, and the damage occurs to the neurons secondary to a compression type of injury, either directly to the neuron or mediated through compression of the blood vessels. For this study to be undertaken, the patients included must have a type of glaucoma in which there is a reasonable chance that abnormality of the regulation of blood flow plays a pathogenetic role.

G.L. Spaeth, M.D.

Complications of Baerveldt Glaucoma Drainage Implants

Nguyen QH, Budenz DL, Parrish RK II (Univ of Miami, Fla)
Arch Ophthalmol 116:571-575, 1998 3–14

Background.—The reported outcomes of the Baerveldt implant, an aqueous humor drainage device used in the surgical management of complicated glaucoma, have been encouraging. However, the incidence of complications associated with this implant is unclear. The incidence of complications and factors associated with complications after Baerveldt glaucoma drainage implantation were investigated.

Methods and Findings.—One hundred three patients undergoing implantation of a Baerveldt glaucoma drainage device in a total of 107 eyes were reviewed. Suprachoroidal hemorrhage occurred in 4% of eyes 3 to 33 days after implantation. Two percent of the eyes had choroidal effusions requiring surgical drainage. Nineteen percent of the eyes had low choroidal effusions needing close observation. Tube blockage occurred in 5% of the eyes, aqueous misdirection in 4%, corneal decompensation in 2%, endophthalmitis in 1%, tube migration in 1%, corneal ulcer in 1%, hyphema in 1%, and implant migration in 1%. Risk factors for suprachoidal hemorrhage were older age, postoperative choroidal effusions, low intraocular pressure immediately after the tube opened, hypertension, and atherosclerosis.

Conclusions.—The incidence of serious postoperative complications associated with Baerveldt implantations in the current series was lower than that reported previously. Risk factors for such complications were similar to those associated with trabeculectomy.

▶ Guarded-filtration procedures (previously called trabeculectomies) remain the second most commonly performed surgical procedure to control intraocular pressure in patients with glaucoma, and argon laser trabeculoplasty remains the first. Because guarded-filtration procedures have resulted in intraocular pressures which were sometimes believed to be higher than ideal, and because the procedures tended to fail in patients with certain types of glaucoma (such as pseudophakic inflammatory glaucoma), many surgeons have tried to modify the procedures or to develop new ones that would work better. Antimetabolites such as a 5-fluorouracil and mitomycin C resulted in a higher success rate in patients with risk factors for failure, and in lower intraocular pressures in patients without risk factors. Ophthalmologists were quick to recognize those advantages, and many ophthalmologists started using antimetabolites quite routinely. Not surprisingly, there was a significant problem; the type of bleb developed with an antimetabolite is similar to that developed with a full-thickness procedure, and there had been many years' experience with the complications associated with full-thickness procedures. Indeed, it was because of these complications associated with full thickness filtering procedures that trabeculectomy was greeted with such overwhelming enthusiasm. But the romance of guarded-filtration procedures performed in association with antimetabolites has, fortunately, worn off. Surgeons are again seeking other ways to lower intraocular pressure, ways that may be associated with fewer complications. Perhaps there will be other antimetabolites that work better. Perhaps modifications of the present antimetabolites will become more satisfactory. Or perhaps a totally new procedure will be developed. But clearly the situation at present is not ideal. Shunting fluid from the anterior chamber to the outside of the globe is a relatively old idea, but only recently have methods been developed that worked in a sufficiently high percentage of cases to be acceptable to surgeons or patients. One of the third-generation types of these procedures used an implant developed by Baerveldt.

This article is a retrospective review of complications that occurred in approximately 100 patients who had a Baerveldt implant placed. The authors compare the complications of such surgery with the complications reported in other studies of tube-shunt procedures and guarded-filtration procedures. However, populations in these studies, varied, as is well known by the authors. Such a difference makes meaningful comparison difficult. Nevertheless, the rate and type of complications associated with placement of a Baerveldt implant are not out of line with the results from similar studies. It is likely that the patients selected for surgery with a Baerveldt implant were more "difficult" than the patients selected to have a standard guarded-filtration procedure. Thus, one would have expected a higher complication rate in the Baerveldt group. That such was not seen is reassuring. However, the authors do not report the long-term results of Baerveldt implant surgery. It is my impression that a patient having a satisfactory postoperative intraocular pressure after a guarded-filtration procedure performed without an antimetabolite is likely to have continuing control of intraocular pressure. This impression is not supported by all long-term studies. However, those studies which did not support it included patients with less-than-ideal results and patients with surgery in association with antimetabolites. Because tube-shunt implants have not been performed extensively in patients who would be expected to have a favorable outcome, it is not possible to determine whether such long-term satisfactory results would be associated with glaucoma surgery using drainage implants. It is almost time to perform a randomized, prospective study comparing primary guarded-filtration procedure with primary tube-shunt procedure.

Development of such a study will not be easy. There is much disagreement about how best to perform a guarded-filtration procedure and also much disagreement about the ideal tube-shunt procedure. If 1 type of procedure works better than the other, is that merely an indication that researchers chose the wrong way to do 1 of the procedures and a better way to do the other procedure? Are there substantive differences among the various glaucoma drainage implants?

Many questions remain unanswered, but this article suggests that the Baerveldt glaucoma drainage implant represents a satisfactory alternative for lowering intraocular pressure surgically in selected patients with glaucoma.

G.L. Spaeth, M.D.

Management of Large, Leaking, and Inadvertent Filtering Blebs With the Neodymium:YAG Laser

Geyer O (Tel Aviv Univ, Israel)
Ophthalmology 105:983-987, 1998 3–15

Introduction.—The widespread use of antimetabolites for treating glaucoma is accompanied by complications, the most frequent and alarming being the formation of large, irritating blebs. Reported is the prospective use of a neodymium:yttrium-aluminum-garnet (Nd:YAG) laser in the treatment of 14 patients with leaking and overfiltering irritating blebs and blebs in surgical wounds after cataract surgery.

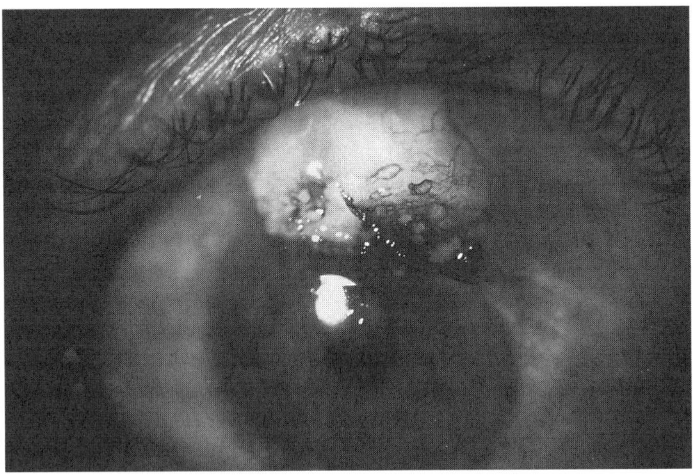

FIGURE 1.—Filtering bleb immediately after Nd:YAG laser treatment. The treated area is "painted" with methylene blue. Note the conjunctival laser. (Published courtesy of *Ophthalmology*, from Geyer O: Management of large, leaking, and inadvertent filtering blebs with the neodymium:YAG laser. *Ophthalmology* 105:983-987, 1998.)

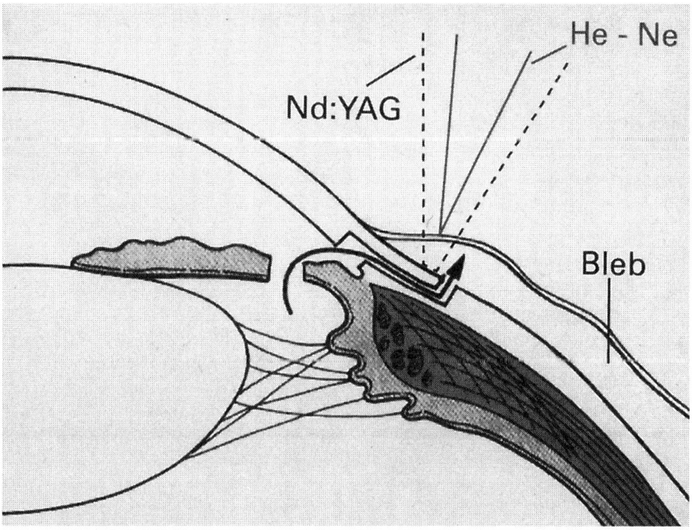

FIGURE 2.—Neodymium:YAG laser treatment of filtering blebs. The aiming beam is focused on the conjunctiva and the laser beam is offset 0.9 to 1.5 mm, 4 to 5 on the Lasag, according to the height of the bleb, to selectively treat the internal surface of the bleb. (Published courtesy of *Ophthalmology*, from Geyer O: Management of large, leaking, and inadvertent filtering blebs with the neodymium:YAG laser. *Ophthalmology* 105:983-987, 1998.)

Methods.—Patients were grouped according to the nature of their bleb problem: group 1, 5 patients with leaking blebs; group 2, 5 patients with large, irritating blebs; and group 3, 4 patients with inadvertent filtering blebs in the surgical wound after cataract surgery. Filtering blebs were treated with the thermal mode of the Lasag Microupter II Nd: YAG laser. The treatment area of the bleb was "painted" with methylene blue and exposed to the Nd:YAG laser using an energy level of 2.5 to 3.75 J in a grid pattern. Flattening, whitening, and wrinkling of the treatment area was achieved using 70-μm–diameter laser burns, with a pulse duration of 20 msec (Fig 1). To selectively treat the internal surface of the bleb, the aiming beam was focused on the conjunctiva with the laser beam offset according to the height of the bleb (offset of 0.9-1.5 mm, 4-5 on the Lasag) (Fig 2). Patients were followed for symptomatology, intraocular pressure (IOP), and complications.

Results.—Patients in all 3 groups had significant increases in IOP that appeared to decrease over time, with the major decrease occurring within the first month after laser treatment. Satisfactory IOP control was sustained in almost all patients (13 of 14) who received either 1 or no antiglaucoma medication.

All eyes had severe conjunctival injection 1 day after laser treatment. At 1 week, the conjunctival injection persisted and the bleb was smaller and was pigmented in the area of treatment (Fig 3). At 1 month after treatment, the bleb was smaller and pigmentation persisted (Fig 4). At follow-up, leaks healed for group 1 patients, symptoms disappeared for group 2

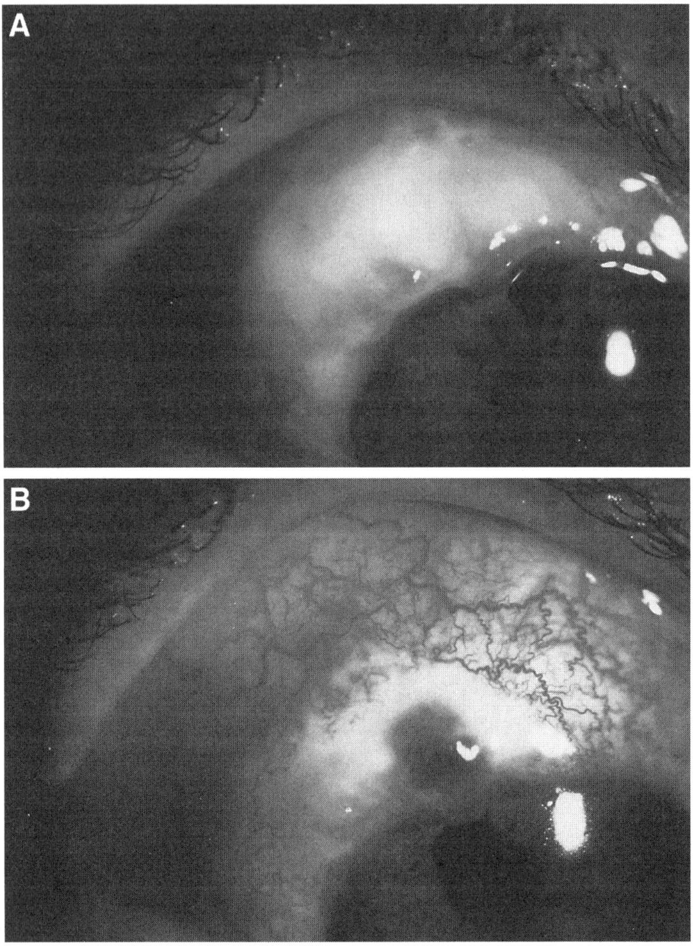

FIGURE 3.—Case 10. A 46-year-old man with pigmentary glaucoma. **A**, a large and irritating bleb developed 1½ years after trabeculectomy with mitomycin C. **B**, 1 week after the laser treatment, the conjunctiva showed marked injection, and the bleb was low with evidence of pigmentation along the treatment site. Note the retraction of the iris toward the bleb. The patient was asymptomatic during a follow-up of 6 months. (Published courtesy of *Ophthalmology*, from Geyer O: Management of large, leaking, and inadvertent filtering blebs with the neodymium:YAG laser. *Ophthalmology* 105:983-987, 1998.)

patients, and all blebs in group 3 were considerably diminished (Fig 5). Complications included 1 transient pressure rise, 1 bleb failure, 6 pupillary retractions toward the bleb, 6 iatrogenic bleb leaks, and 1 cataract.

Conclusion.—Long-term follow-up indicates that the Nd:YAG laser is useful in repairing bleb-related problems while preserving the filtration function.

► Although not common, filtering blebs after cataract surgery can be a frustrating problem for the anterior segment surgeon. If they are small and

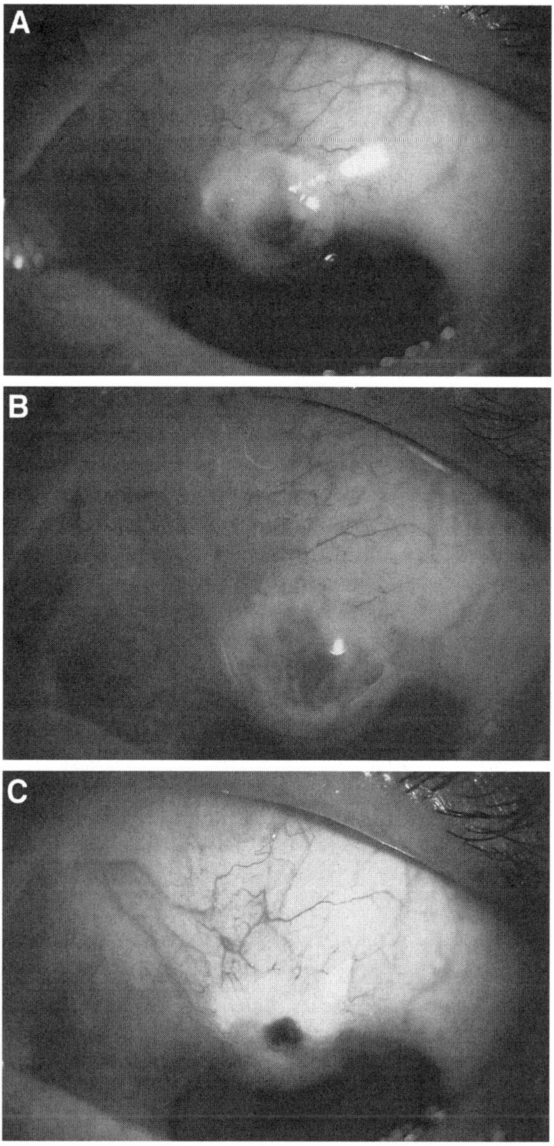

FIGURE 4.—Case 2. **A**, the eye of a 57-year-old woman before laser treatment. **B**, fluorescein staining of the filtering bleb showing leak. **C**, 2 years after Nd:YAG laser treatment. The leak had healed, the bleb was lower and thicker, and pigmentation was present along the treatment site. (Published courtesy of *Ophthalmology*, from Geyer O: Management of large, leaking, and inadvertent filtering blebs with the neodymium:YAG laser. *Ophthalmology* 105:983-987, 1998.)

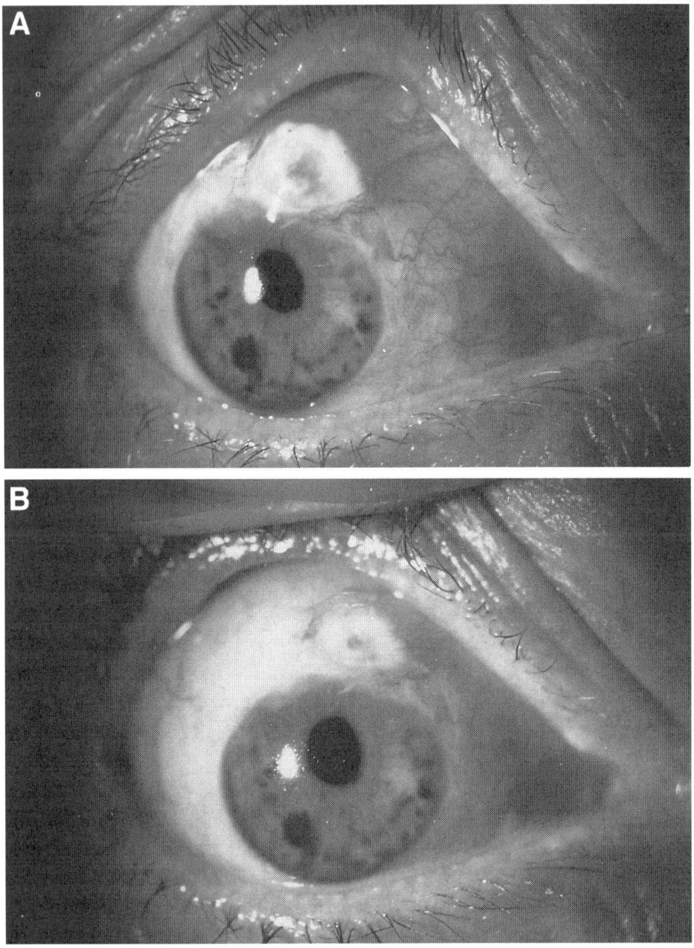

FIGURE 5.—Case 11. **A,** a-75-year-old woman with an inadvertent filtering bleb in the surgical wound of an otherwise uncomplicated cataract extraction. Surgical revision of the wound and cryotherapy to close the bleb had failed. The bleb induced an annoying foreign body sensation. **B,** at 2 years after laser treatment, the bleb had shrunk remarkably and symptoms were resolved. (Published courtesy of *Ophthalmology*, from Geyer O: Management of large, leaking, and inadvertent filtering blebs with the neodymium:YAG laser. *Ophthalmology* 105:983-987, 1998.)

not causing clinical symptoms, they can sometimes be simply observed. Ultimately, many will fail with time. There are, however, filtering blebs that cause local irritation and/or leak and need to be treated more aggressively.

In evaluating filtering blebs, it is important to determine where the leak is occurring. Sometimes gonioscopy can be helpful because a small internal cleft can be visible. If there is only a small gap in the sclera, procedures that induce inflammation will often cause the conjunctiva to scar and will seal the bleb. In these instances, I have found autologous blood injection to be very helpful.

In other cases, there is a large dehiscence of the incision, and autologous blood injections are usually not that helpful. Although direct surgical repair can be performed if the incision is closed, this will often induce an extreme amount of astigmatism. Another approach that I have found helpful in these situations is to tie silk sutures tightly through the area of the inadvertent bleb without completely closing the dehisced wound. This creates an extreme inflammatory response that causes the bleb to scar.

This article presents an interesting approach to treating large filtering blebs. Rather than having to go through a formal procedure, one can use the Nd:YAG laser to cause the bleb to scar. This obviously has an advantage in that it is less invasive and should not induce any additional astigmatism. As I see it, the downsides of this procedure include the need to administer retrobulbar or peribulbar anesthesia and localize patient discomfort afterwards.

When faced with a patient with a filtering bleb, I usually try to perform an autologous blood injection first if I think there is a chance that it may help. This is a relatively innocuous procedure and can be performed in the office without any supplemental anesthesia. If this fails, I consider Nd:YAG laser repair before going ahead with surgery.

R. Tipperman, M.D.

▶ This article was selected for inclusion in the YEAR BOOK because it represents a fairly standard type of article that is appearing more and more frequently. These articles deal with one of the major problems facing any glaucoma surgeon today—the management of problem filtering blebs. The author's contribution is a significant one, and it is good that his results were published. However, it would be a great disservice to patients to conclude that all or even most problem blebs should be treated with Nd:YAG laser.

Reviewing the list of references included with Geyer's article highlights the vast differences between different types of problem blebs. The first article, by Scheie and Guehl,[1] refers to a little-known technique that is highly useful in certain cases. When filtering blebs have been present for many years, some of them spread inferiorly over the cornea. Sometimes these spreading blebs overhang the limbus, reach as far as the visual axis, and interfere with sight. What seems to be amazingly unknown is how easy it is to treat such blebs. These were filtering cicatrices that originated in response to procedures done without antimetabolites, and in which evolution of the bleb occurred over many years. The blebs in such cases were inevitably loculated and were comprised of multiple tiny cysts. The blebs did not actually invade the cornea. All that is necessary to correct these problem blebs is to cut them off at the limbus. One needs nothing more than a Barraquer's sweep, a Vannas scissors, and a slit-lamp. The Barraquer's sweep is used to separate the overhanging bleb from the corneal surface, and then the bleb is simply amputated at the limbus. There may be some temporary leakage for a day or two, but this surgery is not associated with hypotony and has almost no complication rate. Surely one does not want to treat such a bleb with a Nd:YAG laser. Such blebs are functional, and they remain functional for the rest of the patient's life in most cases. Destroying the bleb is certainly not what is wanted.

The fourth reference in Geyer's bibliography, by Zalta and Wieder,[2] describes using cyanoacrylate tissue adhesive to close leaking filtering blebs. This method works very well in the immediate postoperative period if the surgeon has inadvertently caused a tear in the conjunctiva. In most cases in which it is possible to apply such glue promptly, the tissue will heal under the glue; when the glue comes off or is removed, the conjunctiva no longer leaks. Sometimes it is necessary to repeat such gluing, and it does not work in all cases. However, tissue glue in that type of bleb problem can work well. When blebs have evolved and have developed thinned areas that become so fragile they actually rupture (producing a hole in the surface), tissue glue may momentarily close the hole, but long-term results are poor. When the glue comes off, the hole is still present or, in almost every case, rapidly recurs.

Wilson and Kotas-Neumann refer to placing free conjunctival patch grafts over persistent late filtering bleb leaks.[3] Here the goal is to preserve the bleb but to prevent hypotonicity or the development of blebitis. This technique also has its downside, because the patch grafts do not always take, and in some cases they result in sufficient thickening of the bleb, causing the IOP to rise postoperatively. Additionally, if the basic problem is excessive filtration, the problem of an excessively filtering bleb usually occurs later.

Yannuzzi and Theodore describe closing filtering blebs that have occurred inadvertently following a cataract extraction.[4] Here, indeed, one wants to get rid of the bleb completely and in the least invasive way. That is certainly not the goal of treating blebs in patients who have glaucoma, in which one has gone to a great deal of difficulty to produce a filtering bleb. Thus, such patients are also not appropriately considered to be comparable with the type of group described in Geyer's report.

To summarize so far, then, patients in whom the goal is to eliminate a bleb because it should not have been present in the first place would probably not be good candidates for Nd:YAG laser treatment. Patients in whom there is an excessive bleb that dissects down over the cornea are best treated by amputating the bleb as described by Scheie and Guehl.[1] Patients with conjunctival leaks immediately following surgery may be best treated by applying tissue glue. And those in whom excessive filtration continues long-term postoperatively (because of excessive filtration through the sclera) usually need to have the scleral flap modified. There is yet another group of patients: specifically, those in whom filtering blebs have become excessively thin, usually in association with the use of an antimetabolite at the time of surgery. Such excessively thin blebs, however, can occur in association with full-thickness procedures or even occasionally following guarded filtration procedures. Here the goal is not to eliminate the blebs but to thicken the bleb so as to try to prevent the continuing leakage that is usually associated with hypotonicity and is often associated with blebitis. It is these cases which are the most problematic. If there is a frank hole in the bleb, the use of intra-bleb blood as described in the author's eighth reference usually does not work very well, whereas if the bleb simply needs thickening in the absence of a hole, such blood injections can be surprisingly effective.[5] Unfortunately, the blood can enter the anterior chamber, causing a temporary decrease in vision, and the blood injection can be associated with total failure of the blood. Irritating the tissue with an argon laser as suggested in the author's third reference may sometimes work, but it rarely achieves sufficient thickening of the bleb that has any lasting benefit.[6] The authors provide further cases using the technique initially described by Lynch et al.[7] However, this technique has 2 major drawbacks. The authors mention these but in my opinion do not stress their significance. First, when the technique works, it is usually associated with a rise in IOP because the bleb works less well following the treatment. Second, even in those cases in which it works, it is not unusual for the patient to again develop filtering bleb with excessive leakage, frank holes, and all the associated problems.

The reason this discussion has been so lengthy is that there appears to be a misunderstanding regarding the variety of basic causes for bleb problems. These separate and different causes need to be identified, and the treatment needs to be directed at the basic problem. When blebs dissect down the cornea over years of gradual evolution, they usually simply need to be amputated. When blebs become too thin because of excessive filtration through the sclera, the sclera usually needs to be repaired. Conjunctival holes occurring immediately after surgery can be helped to heal with tissue glue. When basically healthy conjunctiva becomes too thin because of years of filtration, such blebs can be thickened by irritating the tissue with a variety of techniques such as trichloroacetic acid, cryotherapy, blood, argon laser, or Nd:YAG laser. When tissue is basically necrotic because of the application of an antimetabolite at the time of surgery, it frequently needs to be excised and replaced with healthy, fresh tissue, either in the form of a sliding or patched graft.

G.L. Spaeth, M.D.

References

1. Scheie HG, Guehl JJ III: Surgical management of overhanging blebs after filtering procedures. *Arch Ophthalmol* 97:325-326, 1979.
2. Zalta AH, Wieder RH: Closure of leaking filtering blebs with cyanoacrylate tissue adhesive. *Br J Ophthalmol* 75:170-173, 1991.
3. Wilson MR, Kotas-Neumann R: Free conjunctival patch for repair of persistent late bleb leak. *Am J Ophthalmol* 117:569-574, 1994.
4. Yannuzzi LA, Theodore FH: Cryotherapy of post-cataract blebs. *Am J Ophthalmol* 76:217-222, 1973.
5. Smith MF, Magauran R, Doyle JW: Treatment of postfiltration bleb leak by bleb injection of autologous blood. *Ophthalmic Surg* 25:636-637, 1994.
6. Fink AJ, Boys-Smith JW, Brear R: Management of large filtering blebs with the argon laser. *Am J Ophthalmol* 101:695-699, 1986.
7. Lynch MG, Roesch M, Brown RH: Remodeling filtering blebs with the neodymium:YAG laser. *Ophthalmology* 103:1700-1705, 1996.

4 Cornea

Keratoconjunctivitis Sicca

by Peter R. Laibson, M.D.

Keratoconjunctivitis sicca—or "dry eye," as most patients refer to it—is characterized by a symptom complex that includes photophobia, burning, foreign body sensation, sandy or gritty feeling, and even a feeling of excessive tearing with some patients. Pathologic changes to the ocular surface (*drying of the superficial cells*) and lacrimal glands, including the accessory lacrimal glands (*lymphocytic infiltration*), are characteristic of this disease. Objective findings include superficial punctate staining of the cornea and conjunctiva, with fluorescein, rose bengal, or lissamine green in the exposed interpalpebral fissure area. Also, decreased aqueous tears in the pre-corneal tear film meniscus and increased mucus formation are found. Filamentary keratitis is also seen in the more severe cases.

The classification of the dry eye from the National Eye Institute/Industry Workshop Study by Lemp et al.[1] divides the dry eye into either a tear-deficient dry eye or an evaporative dry eye. The tear-deficient dry eye is further divided into the non-Sjögren's tear-deficient dry eye and the Sjögren's syndrome patient. The evaporative dry eye relates to lid problems, including blepharitis and obstructive meibomian gland disease and secondary changes caused by contact lenses and other lid-related problems. Also, conjunctival-destroying diseases, which damage the mucus-secreting goblet cells and meibomian glands, include cicatricial ocular pemphigoid and Stevens-Johnson disease.

The treatment of patients with keratoconjunctivitis sicca has not changed in many years.

The mainstay of treatment is tear-replacement drops. Non-preserved drops and tears with preservatives, which evaporate on exposure to air, are popular now. Solid bars of tear substitutes are useful for patients with the more severe keratitis sicca, but the manufacturers, particularly Merck & Company, have limited their supply.

Punctal closure on a temporary or permanent basis, depending on the severity of the dry eye, is common. In my experience, punctal plugs made of silicone are the most useful. The collagen plugs work less well, and I seldom use them. In the presence of filamentary keratitis, the use of acetylcysteine, 10% or 20%, can be very helpful.

There are new studies now to indicate that attacking the dry eye with anti-inflammatory and immunomodulatory drugs, such as cyclosporine, may be effective in ameliorating the disease and possibly altering its status significantly through their effects on the lacrimal and accessory lacrimal glands. Recent papers by Gao et al.[2] and Stern et al.[3] in the experimental animal and in man indicate that cyclosporine, in weak topical form, may prevent the production of inflammatory cytokines and eliminate the conjunctival and lacrimal gland lymphocytic infiltrates, thereby restoring function closer to normal. Allergan Pharmaceuticals has completed phase II of a prospective double-blind study testing cyclosporine and is into phase III studies now.[4]

New concepts concerning keratoconjunctivitis sicca now link the ocular surface, the corneal and conjunctival epithelium, as well as the main and accessory lacrimal glands and the mucus-secreting goblet cells of the conjunctiva and cornea. There very well may be interconnecting innervation among all of these tissues, so that they act as an integrated functional unit, rather than as individual units.[3] Sensory nerve impulses from the affected ocular surface cause stimulation of the higher centers. This stimulation then increases lacrimal gland production of tears and possibly increased mucin production and other protective mechanisms, such as blinking. This servomotor feedback may ameliorate symptoms.

Another recent interesting concept concerning the understanding of keratoconjunctivitis sicca is the influence of prolactin and the sex hormones, testosterone and estrogen, on human tear production.[5,6] Systemic androgens have been shown to decrease lymphocytic infiltration in the lacrimal gland in the mouse and also appear to reverse inflammation-induced changes of the acinar and ductal portion of lacrimal gland. When applied to the ocular surface of the canine with dry eye, androgens demonstrated a deapoptotic level in the lacrimal gland, as well as resolving lymphocytic infiltrates in the lacrimal acinar lobules.[4] These findings, which follow the work of Sullivan,[6] may provide a way to effectively treat the lacrimal gland dysfunction with androgen topically to increase tear production. These theoretical approaches to dry eye using cyclosporine, and possibly androgens, offer new hope to the patient with moderate or severe dry eye who does not do well with current therapy.

References

1. Lemp MA: Report of the National Eye Institute/Industry Workshop on Clinical Trials in Dry Eyes. *CLAO J* 21:221-232, 1995.
2. Gao J, Schwalb TA, Addeo JV, et al: The role of apoptosis in the pathogenesis of canine keratoconjunctivitis sicca: The effect of topical cyclosporin A therapy. *Cornea* 17:654-663, 1998.
3. Stern ME, Beuerman RW, Fox RI, et al: The pathology of dry eye: The interaction between the ocular surface and lacrimal glands. *Cornea* 17:584-589, 1998.
4. Tauber J (for the Cyclosporine Study Croup, Kansas City, Mo): Clinical efficacy and safety of cyclosporine ophthalmic emulsion in patients with keratoconjunctivitis sicca: A dose ranging study. Presented at SOE '97 XIth Congress of the European Society of Ophthalmology, Budapest, Hungary, June 1-5, 1997.

5. Mathers WD, Stoval D, Lane JA, et al: Menopause and tear function: The influence of prolactin and sex hormones on human tear production. *Cornea* 17:353-358, 1998.
6. Ariga H, Edwards J, Sullivan DA: Androgen control of autoimmune expression in lacrimal glands of MRL/Mp-Ipr/Ipr mice. *Clin Immunol Immunopathol* 53:499-508, 1989.

Acyclovir for the Prevention of Recurrent Herpes Simplex Virus Eye Disease

Beck RW, for The Herpetic Eye Disease Study Group (Jaeb Ctr for Health Research, Tampa, Fla)

N Engl J Med 339:300-306, 1998 4–1

Background.—Long-term treatment with antiviral agents can prevent recurrences of genital and orofacial herpes simplex virus (HSV) disease. Whether prophylactic therapy can prevent recurrences of ocular HSV disease is unknown.

Methods and Findings.—Seven hundred three immunocompetent patients experiencing ocular HSV disease within the preceding year were assigned randomly to oral acyclovir, 400 mg, or placebo twice a day. During the 12-month treatment period, 19% of acyclovir recipients and 32% of placebo recipients had a recurrence of any type of ocular HSV disease. The cumulative probability of recurrent stromal keratitis among 337 patients with a history of stromal keratitis was 14% in the acyclovir group and 28% in the placebo group. The cumulative probability of a recurrence of nonocular HSV disease was 19% in the acyclovir group and 36% in the placebo group. In the 6 months after acyclovir treatment cessation, no rebound was noted in the rate of HSV disease (Figure).

Conclusion.—One year of treatment with acyclovir after the resolution of ocular HSV disease decreases the rate of recurrent ocular HSV disease and orofacial HSV disease. Such treatment is especially important for patients with a history of HSV stromal keratitis, as it can prevent additional episodes and visual loss.

▶ For several years, ophthalmologists have used oral acyclovir to prevent recurrent herpetic disease in patients who have had corneal transplantation for herpes. This is the first study to prove, in a prospective, randomized study, that acyclovir can prevent recurrence of epithelial herpetic disease after an episode of ocular herpes. Although oral antiviral agents have prevented recurrence of genital and facial herpes, the prevention of ocular herpes has not been shown before with systemic antiviral medication.

The use of oral acyclovir, 400 mg twice a day, has the effect of reducing the incidence of recurrent herpes by about 50% in the first year. The oral acyclovir was well tolerated, and its use for 12 months is now recommended after an episode of active herpetic keratitis.

The big question is, Should this medication be used longer than 1 year? The question has not been answered in this study but, generally speaking,

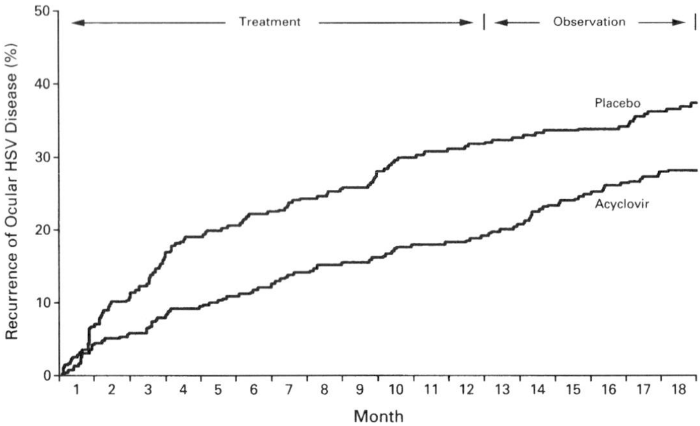

	1	2	3	4	5	6	7	8	9	10	11	12	13	14	15	16	17	18	Total
ACYCLOVIR GROUP																			
No. at risk	357	336	326	316	309	303	295	290	285	281	273	272	269	262	253	248	242	234	
Ocular HSV recurrence	15	6	8	4	5	6	5	5	2	6	1	3	5	9	5	5	5	1	96
Withdrawal or death	6	3	1	1	1	2				1						1	2		18
Loss to follow-up		1	1	2					2	1			2				1		10
PLACEBO GROUP																			
No. at risk	346	309	293	269	261	256	250	243	239	230	224	220	216	212	208	203	198	192	121
Ocular HSV recurrence	23	13	20	7	5	6	6	4	8	6	4	2	3	3	1	1	6	3	19
Withdrawal or death	10	2	2	1			1		1						2				17
Loss to follow-up	4	1	2									2	1	1	2	4			

FIGURE.—Kaplan-Meier estimates of the cumulative probability of a recurrence of ocular HSV disease, according to treatment. The cumulative probability of a recurrence of ocular herpes simplex virus (*HSV*) disease was 19% in the acyclovir group and 32% in the placebo group during the 12-month treatment period (*P* less than 0.001 by the Mantel log-rank test) and 28% and 38%, respectively, during the full 18 months of the study ($P = 0.005$ by the Mantel log-rank test). Two patients in the acyclovir group and 3 patients in the placebo group died; 11 and 8 patients, respectively, withdrew from the study; 3 and 8 patients, respectively, were withdrawn by their physicians; and 2 patients in the acyclovir group had their last study visit in month 17, rather than month 18. The numbers of patients at risk are the numbers who had not had a recurrence of ocular HSV disease at the beginning of each month. Data on patients who did not have a recurrence were censored at the time of the last study visit. (Reprinted by permission of *The New England Journal of Medicine*, from Beck RW, for The Herpetic Eye Disease Study Group: Acyclovir for the prevention of recurrent herpes simplex virus eye disease. *N Engl J Med* 339:300-306. Copyright 1998, Massachusetts Medical Society. All rights reserved.)

for patients who have multiple recurrences, we do use the medication longer than 1 year. For patients who have had genital herpes, oral acyclovir has been used longer than 1 year and it has been safe in that group. I believe that Valtrex or Famvir, 2 alternatives to acyclovir, could be used prophylactically also, although prospective placebo-controlled studies have not been done with these alternate drugs.

P.R. Laibson, M.D.

The Pathology of Dry Eye: The Interaction Between the Ocular Surface and Lacrimal Glands

Stern ME, Beuerman RW, Fox RI, et al (Allergan, Irvine, Calif; LSU Eye Ctr, New Orleans, La; Scripps Research Found, La Jolla, Calif; et al)

Cornea 17:584-589, 1998 4–2

Background.—Most dry-eye symptoms are associated with an abnormal, nonlubricative ocular surface that increases shear forces under the eyelids and reduces the ability of the ocular surface to respond to environmental challenges. Such dysfunction may result from systemic autoimmune diseases or may occur locally because of a reduction in systemic androgen support to the lacrimal gland that occurs in aging, most often in menopausal women.

Normal Physiology.—Normal ocular-surface maintenance requires appropriate concentrations of tear protein, including immunoglobulin A, lactoferrin, lysozyme, and growth factors, such as epidermal growth factor and transforming growth factor β. Mucins, which are produced by corneal epithelial cells and goblet cells in the conjunctival epithelium, serve as a major defense mechanism against various microtrauma. After wounding, the wing and basal cells of the corneal epithelium express mucins. Corneal sensation, which is very acute and processed centrally, is interpreted solely as pain. Research has shown that sex hormones significantly affect lacrimal gland function. Androgens exert essential, specific effects on the maintenance of normal glandular functions and suppress inflammation in normal and autoimmune animal models.

Changes in the Functional Unit.—The etiology of dry eye is thought to be multifactorial. It can be related to deficiencies in any of the 3 components of the tear film. Several studies have shown that the loss in systemic androgens that occurs in pre- and postmenopausal women results in less support for lacrimal secretory function and facilitates an inflammatory environment. This is still being investigated.

Authors' Hypothesis.—The current authors suggest that dry eye occurs when systemic androgen levels drop below the threshold needed to support secretory function and maintain an anti-inflammtory environment, and that this reduction causes lacrimal gland and ocular surface inflammation. Proinflammatory cytokine secretion would subsequently interfere with the normal connections driving the tearing reflex. Thus, the lacrimal gland is isolated, perhaps exacerbating atrophic changes of the glandular tissue. Such changes would promote antigen presentation at the surace of the lacrimal acinar cells and increase lymphocytic infiltration of the gland. Similar events may occur on the ocular surface.

Treatment for Dry-Eye Disease.—Cyclosporine, an immunomodulatory drug, and steroids decrease ocular-surface rose bengal staining. Topical ophthalmic cyclosporine A can eliminate both conjunctival and lacrimal gland lymphocytic infiltrates. Both epithelial cell apoptosis and lymphocytic apoptosis may be involved in the pathogenesis of autoimmune dry eye. Apoptosis appears to play an importan role in dry-eye mechanisms.

The apoptotic level appears to be reduced in the epithelial cells and increased in the lymphocytes after topical cyclosporine therapy, allowing elimination of follicular infiltrates. Androgens, both systemic and topical, may also be an important source of treatment for dry eye.

Conclusions.—The ocular surface, lacrimal gland, and interconnecting innervation serve as an integrated functional unit. After the lacrimal gland loses its androgen support, it is subject to immune-based inflammation, resulting in neurally mediated dysfunction. Anti-inflammatory agents can normalize the ocular surface and lacrimal neural reflex, improving the quality and quantity of the tear film. The ocular surface is an appropriate target for treatment.

▶ Our concepts of keratoconjunctivitis sicca are changing as we learn more about the ocular surface. The latest findings in keratoconjunctivitis sicca are outlined in this article, which presents the components of the ocular surface, cornea, conjunctiva, accessory lacrimal glands, and meibomian glands, as well as the main lacrimal gland, as all being interconnected and acting as a functional unit.

Restoration of lacrimal gland function may be possible using immunomodulating and anti-inflammatory drugs such a cyclosporine. Although cyclosporine is not yet available for general use in keratoconjunctivitis sicca, Allergan Pharmaceuticals has now finished phase II studies indicating its efficacy and is starting phase III studies. The article also mentions that lacrimal secretions may be controlled by circulating androgens. This is a new concept that is currently being explored and may lead to major findings in the future.

P.R. Laibson, M.D.

Ocular Trauma Following Penetrating Keratoplasty: Incidence, Outcome, and Postoperative Recommendations

Rehany U, Rumelt S (Western Galilee-Nahariya Med Ctr, Israel)

Arch Ophthalmol 116:1282-1286, 1998 4–3

Background.—The surgical wound created by penetrating keratoplasty has an increased vulnerability to contusive trauma. The incidence, causative factors, management, and visual outcome of ocular trauma after this procedure were determined.

Methods and Findings.—Five hundred fifty-nine patients undergoing penetrating keroplasty between 1986 and 1993 were included in the retrospective study. Surgical wound dehiscence caused by contusive ocular trauma occurred in 2.5% of the patients. These patients were significantly younger than the total group, mean ages being 30.6 and 49 years, respectively. The mean interval between transplantation and trauma was 6.7 months. In 11 of the 14 affected patients, the trauma occurred before the sutures were removed. In all patients, globe rupture occurred at the donor-recipient interface, accompanied by vitreous and lens loss in 57%. In 14%

of the patients trauma included retinal tissue disruption, resulting in poor visual outcome. Trauma usually occurred at home. After a mean follow-up of 29 months, the corrected visual acuity ranged from 0/120 to 20/20 in 86% of the patients.

Conclusions.—Ocular injury after penetrating keratoplasty is not rare, Patients should wear protective eyewear and should be told of the long-term vulnerability of the graft wound. Clinicians should repeatedly caution patients against high-risk environments and strenuous activity.

▶ Once a corneal transplant is performed, the weakest part of that eye, for the life of the patient, will be the junction between the donor tissue and the host cornea. This article documents 14 traumatic wound dehiscences in 559 patients over a 78-month period. The mean age of the patients was 30.6 years, indicating that younger patients were subject to this trauma. The mean age of corneal transplant recipients is much older.

These findings parallel our experience. In our experience, men are more likely to have wound dehiscence after keratoplasty than are women. It is critically important to warn everyone after corneal transplantation that the wound will be the weakest point of the eye for their lifetime. Men should avoid trauma by walking away from altercations and also by wearing safety glasses during participation in sporting events.

I feel the eye should be protected at all costs and at all times, and therefore safety glasses are necessary, particularly for children and young adults. The wound dehiscence may occur at any time after the corneal transplant, not just during the first year when the sutures are still in place. The sutures do not protect the cornea from wound dehiscence and suture removal certainly does not indicate a completely healed wound that is immune from trauma.

P.R. Laibson, M.D.

Ten-Year Postoperative Results of Penetrating Keratoplasty

Ing JJ, Ing HH, Nelson LR, et al (Mayo Clinic, Rochester, Minn)

Ophthalmology 105:1855-1865, 1998 4–4

Background.—The adult cornea typically loses 0.6% of endothelial cells per year. This rate of cell loss increases after intraocular surgery. Changes in central corneal endothelial cells and corneal thickness in transplanted corneas 5 to 10 years after grafting were studied, along with the development of glaucoma, graft rejection, and graft failure.

Methods.—Data on 500 consecutive penetrating keratoplasties performed by 1 surgeon were analyzed in this longitudinal cohort study. Patients were assessed at 2 months and at 1, 3, 5, and 10 years after grafting. Eyes regrafted during the study and the fellow eyes of patients bilaterally affected were excluded, leaving 394 grafts for analysis.

Findings.—By 10 years after keratoplasty, 80 patients had died and 68 grafts had failed. Among the 72 patients who returned for all scheduled

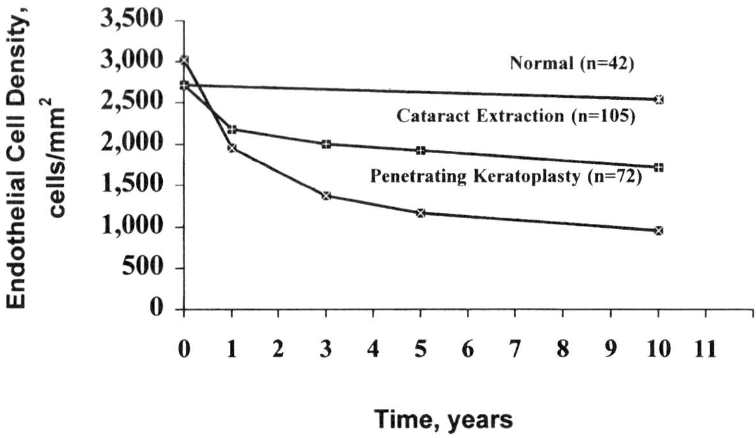

FIGURE 1.—Central endothelial cell density vs. time in normal adult participants and vs. postoperative time in patients after cataract extraction and after penetrating keratoplasty. The instantaneous exponential annual rate of endothelial cell loss was 0.6% per year in normal adults measured over a 10-year period, 2.5% per year in patients measured from 1 to 10 years after cataract extraction, and 4.2% per year in penetrating keratoplasties measured from 5 to 10 years after surgery. (Published courtesy of *Ophthalmology*, from Ing JJ, Ing HH, Nelson LR, et al: Ten-year postoperative results of penetrating keratoplasty. *Ophthalmology* 105:1855-1865, 1998.)

examinations, mean endothelial cell loss from preoperative donor levels at 10 years was 67%; mean endothelial cell density was 958 cells/mm^2; the coefficient of variation was 0.32; hexagonal cells were 56%; and corneal thickness was 0.58 mm. At 5 to 10 years, these changes were significant. Endothelial cell loss was greater in eyes with posterior chamber lenses (71%) than in eyes with anterior chamber lenses (51%). At 10 years, the cumulative risk of glaucoma was 21%; of rejection, 21%; and of failure, 22%. The primary cause for graft failure was late endothelial failure, accounting for 9 of 11 failures after postoperative year 5 (Fig 1; Table 4).

Conclusions.—In these patients, the annual rate of endothelial cell loss was 7 times the normal rate, at 5 to 10 years after penetrating keratoplasty.

TABLE 4.—Results for All Participants*

Examination	n	Endothelial Cell Density (Cells/mm^2)	Endothelial Cell Loss (%)	Coefficient of Variation of Cell Area	Hexagonal Cells (%)	Corneal Thickness (mm)
Preoperative	393*	2973 ± 550	—	0.26 ± 0.06	68 ± 11	—
Postoperative						
2 mos	355	2467 ± 675	17 ± 19	0.25 ± 0.06	60 ± 10	0.54 ± 0.05
1 yr	329†	1958 ± 718	34 ± 22	0.26 ± 0.06	62 ± 9	0.54 ± 0.05
3 yrs	231	1376 ± 586	53 ± 19	0.26 ± 0.07	64 ± 11	0.56 ± 0.05
5 yrs	187	1191 ± 523	59 ± 17	0.29 ± 0.09	61 ± 13	0.57 ± 0.05
10 yrs	119	960 ± 470‡	67 ± 17‡	0.33 ± 0.11‡	56 ± 12‡	0.58 ± 0.06‡

*Mean ± standard deviation

(Published courtesy of *Ophthalmology*, from Ing JJ, Ing HH, Nelson LR, et al: Ten-year postoperative results of penetrating keratoplasty. *Ophthalmology* 105:1855-1865, 1998.)

During this period, significant increases occurred in endothelial cell loss, pleomorphism, polymegethism, and corneal thickness; these indicated continued endothelial instability and dysfunction and resulted in a rising rate of late endothelial failure.

▶ The endothelium of a corneal transplant is critically important to the longevity of the transplant. This is one of the few studies that has looked at the endothelium 10 years after penetrating corneal transplant. Of 394 patients with transplants, 80 had died; 68 grafts had failed. Two hundred forty-six patients remained and of these, almost 50% returned for their 10-year examinations. So although 394 patients were operated on in this period, only 119 returned for their 10-year follow-up. Even so, this is an excellent follow-up, considering the time elapsed since the corneal transplant. The main finding in this study is that there is an endothelial cell loss that is 7 times the normal rate, and this loss continues to the 10-year mark at least. We must assume that the accelerated loss of endothelial cells will continue after that; therefore it is imperative to transplant the healthiest corneal tissue that we can obtain. By transplanting corneas with more endothelial cells, we can ameliorate loss so that corneal transplants can remain clear longer.

Eye Banks should realize that transplanting a bare minimum of 2,000 cells per square millimeter may mean that corneal transplants 20 to 30 years away will need repeat corneal transplants. For patients in their seventies or eighties, transplanting tissue with 2,000 cells per square millimeter is satisfactory, but for younger people the best tissue available must be used.

Another interesting finding in this study is that there was no statistical difference in failure rates between eyes with anterior chamber intraocular lenses (IOLs) and those with posterior chamber IOLs. Most people believe that posterior chamber IOLs cause less endothelial failure than anterior chamber IOLs do, but this was not borne out here.

This is further evidence supporting the use of an open loop anterior chamber lens, rather than a sutured-in posterior chamber lens, if there is to be an IOL exchange and the anterior chamber angle is healthy.

P.R. Laibson, M.D.

Combined Interrupted and Continuous Versus Single Continuous Adjustable Suturing in Penetrating Keratoplasty: A Prospective, Randomized Study of Induced Astigmatism During the First Postoperative Year

Karabatsas CH, Cook SD, Fiueiredo FC, et al (Bristol Eye Hosp, England)

Ophthalmology 105:1991-1998, 1998 4–5

Background.—Because extreme astigmatism may prevent or delay visual recovery after successful penetrating kerotoplasty (PKP), surgeons must try to keep postoperative astigmatism to a minimum. The postoperative astigmatism induced by 2 suturing techniques in PKP was compared.

Methods.—Ninety-two patients with 95 affected eyes were enrolled in the prospective, randomized, clinical trial. Fifty-one eyes were treated with

TABLE 2.—Preoperative Diagnosis of Recipient: No. (%)*

Diagnosis	ICS	SCAS	P†
Keratoconus	18 (35)	20 (45)	0.212
Fuch's endothelial dystrophy	10 (20)	4 (9)	0.124
Corneal decompensation	5 (10)	3 (7)	0.443
Pseudophakic bullous keratopathy	3 (6)	3 (7)	0.5888
Aphakic bullous keratopathy	—	1 (2)	0.463
Failed graft	6 (12)	4 (9)	0.467
Herpes simplex keratitis	3 (6)	3 (7)	0.588
Interstitial keratitis	2 (4)	2 (4)	0.633
Posterior keratoconus	1 (2)	—	0.563
Repeat PKP for high astigmatism	1 (2)	—	0.563
Corneal scarring (leukoma)	1 (2)	1 (2)	0.714
Reiss-Buckler dystrophy	1 (2)	—	0.563
Corneal melt	—	1 (2)	0.463
Acanthamoeba keratitis	—	2 (4)	0.211
Total	51	44	

*Percentages have been rounded off.
†Fisher's exact test.
Abbreviations: ICS, interrupted + continuous surgical technique; *SCAS*, single continuous adjustable suture; *PKP* penetrating keratoplasty.
(Published courtesy of *Ophthalmology*, from Karabastsas CH, Cook SD, Fiueiredo FC, et al: Combined interrupted and continuous versus single continuous adjustable suturing in penetrating keratoplasty: A prospective, randomized study of induced astigmatism during the first operative year. *Ophthalmology* 105:1991-1998, 1998.)

combined interrupted and continuous suturing (ICS) and 44 with single continuous adjustable suturing (SCAS). In the ICS group, combined suturing with 12 interrupted 10-0 nylon and 1 continuous 11-0 nylon sutures was performed. In the SCAS group, a single running 24-bite 10-0 nylon suture was used. Selective suture removal was begun at 10 weeks or later after surgery. Suture adjustment was done as soon as possible after surgery. Astigmatism was measured at 3, 6, 9, and 12 months postoperatively.

Findings.—Mean time to suture manipulation differed significantly between groups, being shorter in the SCAS group. Both interrupted-suture removal and suture adjustment significantly reduced astigmatism. However, the net astigmatic reduction in the 2 groups did not differ significantly. Mean vector changes in the SCAS and ICS groups were 7.4 and 6.3 diopters, respectively. Astigmatism did not differ significantly between groups at any point. At 1 year, refractive astigmatism was 2.66 in the ICS group and 3.12 in the SCAS, but no significant treatment effect occurred. Sixty-six percent of the ICS eyes and 58% of the SCAS eyes were within astigmatic target of the study (Table 2).

Conclusions.—Adjustment of a single running suture and selective removal of interrupted sutures can reduce postkeratoplasty astigmatism to comparable degrees. Neither SCAS nor ICS appears to have an advantage requiring fewer manipulations or producing less astigmatism, as has been suggested previously.

▶ This article compares, in a prospective fashion, 2 ways of suturing the corneal transplants. First, a combination of 12 interrupted 10-0 nylon sutures with a continuous 11-0 nylon suture compared with a single 24-bite 10-0 nylon running suture. The authors did not use interrupted sutures alone, which is a third valid technique. The authors found that suture adjustment varying from just a few days after surgery to up to 20 months after surgery showed no difference in the long run with these 2 suturing techniques. There was no advantage over ICS versus the adjustable suturing technique alone in either fewer manipulations or less astigmatism. Why would anyone do an adjustable running suture alone if this were the case. It is true that with an adjustable running suture, which is adjusted 1 or 2 weeks after the surgery, better vision is achieved early, but in the long run, visual acuity was the same in both groups. Is it safer to do an ICS versus an adjustable running suture with individual sutures? Surgeons must decide for themselves which technique they use, but I prefer z-belt and suspenders with the interrupted and running technique.

At Wills Eye Hospital, interrupted sutures alone are used on a large number of patients. Our guidelines are that interrupted sutures are used where the host cornea is unhealthy with thinning and/or vascularization and excessive edema. Where the host cornea is clear, interrupted and running sutures are used with suture removal starting months after the surgery. We try to tie the sutures looser, and we check the suture placement with a simple technique of either using the end of a safety pin or using one of the Avni plastic rings. Whether any of these suture techniques are used, the best visual acuity seems to be achieved by tying the sutures more loosely rather than more tightly to allow for a better ocular surface after the transplant.

P.R. Laibson, M.D.

Acanthamoeba Keratitis: Multicentre Survey in England 1992-1996

Radford CF, for the National Acanthamoeba Keratitis Study Group (Moorfields Eye Hosp, London; et al)

Br J Ophthalmol 82:1387-1392, 1998 4–6

Background.—Up to 92% of acanthamoeba keratitis (AK) cases have been associated with contact lens use. Changing trends in contact lens care and use appear to greatly influence the incidence of AK. The frequency, outcomes, and risk factors associated with AK in England in the past 4 years were reported.

Methods and Findings.—Two hundred forty-three patients with AK in 259 eyes were identified, for an annual incidence of 0.14 per 100,000 individuals. Between 1992 and 1996, 226 resident patients were diagnosed. Sufficient data for further analysis were available for 170 patients. Seventy-two percent of these patients were diagnosed within 30 days of initial assessment. Ninety percent were treated with polyhexamethyl biguanide or chlorhexidine, or both, and 16% underwent surgery. In 86% of the eyes, a visual acuity of 6/12 or better was achieved. Ninety-three percent of the patients wore contact lenses, and 84% wore soft contact lenses. Risk factors for AK among soft contact lens wearers included swimming with contact lenses, nonsterile contact lens rinsing, omitted disinfection, and chlorine release disinfection—all previously described risk factors. Non–contact lens users more often had delayed diagnosis, an increased need for surgery, and a worse visual outcome.

Conclusions.—For most patients, earlier diagnosis and better treatment have improved the prognosis of AK. This disease is highly preventable, as 91% of soft contact lens users could have avoided it by refraining from inadvisable practices. In addition, AK frequency dropped markedly after an intensive media campaign, possibly in conjunction with an increase in the use of new contact lens products.

▶ AK is seldom seen by the ophthalmologist in general practice and therefore is misdiagnosed frequently as either herpetic keratitis, fungal keratitis, atypical microbacterium, or bacterial keratitis. This large study of AK in the United Kingdom, of 259 eyes in 243 patients, tells us that the disease certainly has not been eradicated. The annualized incidence was 0.14 per 100,000 individuals. As previously noted, contact lens use was a high-risk factor for AK.

It is interesting to note that, in a large outbreak of AK seen in Iowa City, flooding in that region was felt to be responsible for the disease outbreak rather than contact lens use. In India, most cases of AK are not due to contact lens use. For the average ophthalmologist, where flooding and a high percentage of lower socioeconomic patients are not in the patient population, acanthamoeba must be suspected in order to treat it early and appropriately, which goes a long way to ensure a better visual outcome.

P.R. Laibson, M.D.

Baseline Findings in the Collaborative Longitudinal Evaluation of Keratoconus (CLEK) Study

Zadnik K, and the Collaborative Longitudinal Evaluation of Keratoconus (CLEK) Study Group (Ohio State Univ, Columbus; et al)

Invest Ophthalmol Vis Sci 39:2537-2546, 1998 4–7

Introduction.—A progressive, asymmetric, noninflammatory disease of the cornea, keratoconus is characterized by steepening and distortion, apical thinning, and central scarring of the cornea. A mild-to-marked decrease in vision secondary to high irregular astigmatism and frequently to central corneal scarring is caused by these corneal changes. As the disease progresses, more biomicroscopic corneal signs become more prevalent, such as inferiorly displaced, thinned protrusion of the cornea; corneal thinning over the apex of the cone; and Fleischer's ring, a full or partial ring of iron in the corneal epithelium at the base of the cone. Atopic disease, eye rubbing, genetics, and contact lens wearing have been associated with keratoconus. Changes in vision, corneal curvature, corneal status (such as corneal scarring), and quality of life in patients with keratoconus were evaluated.

Methods.—The Collaborative Longitudinal Evaluation of Keratoconus (CLEK) study included 1,209 patients with keratoconus who were evaluated for corneal scarring, visual acuity, keratometry, and quality of life. The factors associated with these changes across time were determined.

Results.—The patients had a mean age of 39.29 years with moderate-to-severe disease, as assessed by a keratometric-based criterion. Steep keratometric readings of at least 45 D were found in 95.4% of patients. Relatively good visual acuity was found in most patients, with 77.9% having had best corrected visual acuity of at least 20/40 in both eyes. Rigid gas-permeable contact lens were worn by 65% of patients, with 73% reporting that their lenses were comfortable. A family history of kerato conus was reported by 13.5% of patients. Serious systemic diseases that were previously reported to be associated with keratoconus were not reported by any of these patients. A history of atopy was reported by 53% of patients. Cornea scarring in 1 or both eyes was found in 53% of patients.

Conclusion.—Increased risk of connective tissue disease was not associated with keratoconus. Mild-to-moderate keratoconus was seen in this group. New information about the progression of keratoconus will be provided with an additional follow-up of at least 3 years, which will identify factors associated with progress and an assessment on its impact on the quality of life.

▶ The CLEK study, or the *C*ollaborative *L*ongitudinal *E*valuation of *K*eratoconus, is a National Eye Institute–funded study of keratoconus, primarily by optometrists. Optometrists see many keratoconus patients, and those that cannot be improved visually with contact lenses or glasses are then seen by an ophthalmologist, who may or may not recommend corneal transplantation. Since there are many patients with keratoconus who never see an ophthalmologist, this study should provide interesting information about the earlier phases of keratoconus. Many ophthalmologists do see such early patients, but a prospective organized study has not been done by ophthalmologists.

One previous paper by Zadnik et al.[1] also was an interesting study with information from this CLEK study. The baseline studies in this paper show that the great majority of 1,209 patients with keratoconus do not have other connective tissue diseases. About 13.5% of patients reported a family history with this disease in the study. Past reviews of keratoconus have pointed to a 10% family history of keratoconus, which is very similar. The CLEK study will follow patients longitudinally for at least the next 3 years trying to identify factors that may be associated with progression. I certainly will be watching for further CLEK reports to detail this interesting disease, whose etiology and course are not extremely well defined yet. Hopefully, this study will help us along those lines.

P.R. Laibson, M.D.

Reference

1. Zadnik K, Barr JT, Gordon MO, et al: Biomicroscopic signs and disease severity in keratoconus. Collaborative Longitudinal Evaluation of Keratoconus (CLEK) Study Group. *Cornea* 15:139-146, 1996.

Topical Treatment With Nerve Growth Factor for Corneal Neurotrophic Ulcers

Lambiase A, Rama P, Bonini S, et al (Univ of Rome; Hosp of Venice SS Giovanni e Paolo, Italy; Natl Research Council, Rome; et al)
N Engl J Med 338:1174-1180, 1998 4–8

Background.—Visual loss can result from corneal neurotrophic ulcers associated with impairment of corneal sensory innervation. No effective treatment currently exists for these ulcers. The efficacy of nerve growth factor was assessed.

Methods.—Twelve patients with severe corneal neurotrophic ulcers in 14 eyes were included in the study. The ulcers were associated with corneal anesthesia in all patients. Treatment consisted of topical nerve growth factor applied 10 times a day for 2 days, 6 times a day until healing, and for 2 weeks after healing. The patients were followed up for 15 months by slit-lamp examination, photography, fluorescein-dye testing, and tests of corneal sensitivity and best corrected visual acuity.

Findings.—Corneal healing started 2 to 14 days after nerve growth factor treatment was begun. Healing was complete in all patients within 10 days to 6 weeks. In 13 eyes, corneal sensitivity improved, returning to normal in 2 (15%). Corneal integrity and sensitivity were maintained during follow-up. In all patients, best corrected visual acuity progressively increased during treatment and follow-up. No adverse effects occurred.

Conclusions.—This preliminary, uncontrolled study suggests that treatment with nerve growth factor can induce prompt healing and restoration of corneal sensitivity in patients with corneal neurotrophic ulcers. This treatment also is apparently safe, causing no systemic or local side effects.

► Articles like this, even appearing in the prestigious *New England Journal of Medicine*, should be read very carefully. Corneal neurotrophic ulcers take a long time to heal and are treated in many different ways, including bandage contact lenses, lateral tarsorrhaphy, and conjunctival flaps. This is in addition to numerous medications that are used for these patients. In the past, epidermal growth factor and fibronectin have been extolled as very helpful in the treatment of neurotrophic ulcers, but when placebo-controlled prospective double-blind studies were done, neither compound was found to be effective. The same thing probably should be said about nerve growth factor for corneal neurotrophic ulcers.

The authors state that corneal healing began 2 to 14 days after initiation of treatment and the healing was completed from 10 to 42 days of treatment.

Many of these ulcers may well have gotten better in this extended period of time, even without nerve growth factor.

Certainly it is worthwhile to pursue uncontrolled studies but before we can be overly enthusiastic about exogenous nerve growth factor, a placebo-controlled prospective double-blind study is needed to determine the effectiveness of this drug.

P.R. Laibson, M.D.

Mutation Hot Spots in 5q31-linked Corneal Dystrophies

Korvatska E, Munier FL, Djemaï A, et al (Centre Hospitalier Universitaire Vaudois, Lausanne, Switzerland; Vanderbilt Univ, Nashville, Tenn; Augenklinik, Inselspital, Bern, Switzerland; et al)

Am J Hum Genet 62:320-324, 1998 4–9

Background.—There are 4 distinct bilaterally symmetrical disorders of the human cornea which are caused by mutations in the *BIGH3* gene on chromosome 5q31: granular (Groenouw type I), Reis-Bücklers, lattice type I, and Avellino corneal dystrophies. These disorders are marked by progressive accumulation of corneal deposits appearing in the first 10 or 20 years of life and can cause serious visual deficits. Phototherapeutic keratectomy or corneal transplantation is often required.

Patients.—Blood samples were analyzed from patients with 5q31-linked corneal dystrophy. The patients were from 10 different families. DNA was extracted from peripheral blood and analyzed. In these 10 families and 5 other families previously described, genotype analysis with microsatellite markers surrounding the *BIGH3* locus was performed.

Results.—A specific recurrent missense mutation was identified for each type of dystrophy. R555W, R124C, and R124H mutations were noted independently in several ethnic groups. These mutations do not represent a founder effect.

Conclusion.—These findings indicate that the R124 and R555 amino acids are important in the pathogenesis of 5q31-linked autosomal dominant corneal dystrophy. The phenotype appears to be perfectly correlated with these mutations.

► The relatively new field of molecular genetics has an important impact on corneal diseases. We now know that mutations on the *BIGH3* gene on chromosome 5q31 are responsible for the major corneal dystrophies, granular dystrophy, Reis-Bücklers' dystrophy (corneal dystrophy of Bowman's membrane 1 and 2), lattice dystrophy, and the Avellino corneal dystrophies, which are a combination of granular and lattice dystrophies. Molecular genetic techniques have localized these mutations, and a specific single amino acid mutation may be responsible for the autosomal dominant corneal dystrophies, which are linked to the 5q chromosome.

Unfortunately, the next step—preventing these changes—is much further away, but this is the beginning of a new era in diagnosing human diseases, and the ability to trace corneal dystrophies, as well as retinal dystrophies, to specific mutations of single amino acids is certainly major progress.

P.R. Laibson, M.D.

The Aetiology and Prevention of Peri-operative Corneal Abrasions

White E, Crosse MM (Southampton Gen Hosp, England)

Anaesthesia 53:157-161, 1998 4–10

Objective.—Corneal abrasions are a common complication of general anesthesia and may be responsible for significant pain and distress in the postoperative period. Although several different techniques of eye protection during general anesthesia have been proposed, few studies have been performed to compare these approaches. The causes and prevention of perioperative corneal abrasions were reviewed.

Perioperative Corneal Abrasions.—Most perioperative corneal abrasions result from lagophthalmos, i.e., failure of the eyelids to close properly, resulting in corneal drying. Direct trauma or chemical injury are possible as well. The cornea is very sensitive to lack of oxygen, which can result from pressure applied to the globe of the eye—e.g., from a poorly fitting face mask—causing reduced choroidal blood flow. Tracheal intubation, positive-pressure ventilation, or poor head positioning may lead to decreased venous return and increased intraocular pressure, and thus to corneal edema. General anesthesia reduces tear production and stability, and abolishes the protective Bell's phenomenon and blink reflex. The risk of corneal abrasions appears greatest for patients undergoing lengthy head-and-neck surgical procedures in the prone position.

Eye Protection Approaches.—Although many different methods for perioperative protection of the eyes have been proposed, few comparative studies have been done. Preventive measures include manual closure of the eyelids, taping the eyelids shut, instilling paraffin-based ointments into the conjunctival sac, and others. Ointments are commonly used because they are well retained in the eye. Studies using paraffin-based ointments have suggested that they are effective in preventing corneal abrasions; however, these ointments may be associated with increased morbidity. Aqueous solutions, viscous gels, and ointments do not appear to protect against abrasions. Aqueous solutions and viscous gels may be useful when applied regularly in patients whose eyes are opened during surgery to check pupillary dilation.

Discussion.—Perioperative corneal abrasions are a common problem for which preventive measures have been inadequately studied. Taping the eyes shut immediately after preoxygenation and IV induction of anesthesia is recommended. For operations with the patient in the prone position, the eyes should be taped shut and the head placed in neutral position to avoid pressure on the eyes. For patients in prone position, turning the head to one side may raise intraocular pressure in the lower eye, thus leading to corneal edema and abrasion. It is important to recognize the causes of corneal damage during operative procedures, and to take appropriate protective steps.

► Even though this article is in the anesthesia literature, it should be reviewed by all ophthalmologists. Corneal abrasions can be very embarrassing to the surgeon and the anesthesiologist if they occur while the patient is asleep, or during the perioperative period. Certainly the general ophthalmologist should be aware of this fact and instruct the anesthesiologist about ways to prevent corneal abrasions in the perioperative period.

The lids must be properly closed, and the anesthetic materials should not touch the cornea or conjunctiva. The use of antibiotic ointments or other nonpreserved paraffin-based ointments can be helpful if they are used judiciously and not in copious amounts. Even though the article states that ointments are associated with significant morbidity, ointments can be used effectively when used in small amounts to help protect the cornea. The ophthalmologist should be aware that general anesthesia reduces tear production, and the stability of the tear film is significantly affected if the eyelids are partially open. Taping the lids closed and using a small amount of lubricating ointment is helpful in addition to avoiding trauma to the eyes.

P.R. Laibson, M.D.

Iatrogenic Limbal Stem Cell Deficiency

Schwartz GS, Holland EJ (Associated Eye Care, Stillwater, Minn; Univ of Minnesota, Minneapolis)

Cornea 17:31-37, 1998 4–11

Background.—Deficiencies in the stem cells (SCs) that renew the corneal epithelium can lead to scarring, ulceration, and loss of vision. A limited number of specific diseases are associated with limbal SC deficiency. Some patients with SC deficiency do not have any of these diseases. A group of these patients were reviewed to characterize their SC deficiency, identify risk factors, and attempt to determine the cause.

Study Design.—The charts and operative records of all patients seen between 1987 and 1996 at the cornea clinic of the University of Minnesota who had SC deficiency without specific, known cause were reviewed. Risk factors, clinical findings, and sequelae were assessed.

Findings.—The study group consisted of 12 patients (14 eyes) with SC deficiency without a known cause. All the eyes had prior ocular surgery that involved the corneoscleral limbus, the location of SCs, and all had concurrent external disease. Of the 14 eyes, 11 had received long-term topical medication. The superior quadrants, the site of limbal surgery, were affected in all eyes. The disease sequelae included scarring and neovascularization, with 2 eyes having a visual acuity of no more than 20/150.

Conclusions.—A group of 14 eyes in 12 patients with SC deficiency without known cause was reviewed. All patients were affected at sites of prior limbal surgical incision, which suggests surgical trauma as the etiologic agent of SC deficiency in these patients. This damage probably made these cells more easily damaged by other factors, such as external disease and topical medication, which were present in many cases. Because SC deficiency in these patients is caused by ocular surgery trauma and toxicity from long-term topical medications, the term "iatrogenic limbal stem cell deficiency" is proposed for this condition.

▶ Limbal SCs are responsible for the renewal of corneal epithelium, and are located at the corneoscleral limbus. Aniridia, Stevens-Johnson disease, ocular cicatricial pemphigoid, and alkaline injuries are some of the entities that damage limbal SCs and cause a characteristic corneal opacity, which is difficult to treat. Recently, the limbal SC deficiency and the epitheliopathy produced by this deficiency has been better recognized. The pathology may occur anywhere around the limbus but generally occurs superiorly with these diseases.

Iatrogenic limbal SC deficiency now has been described after cataract surgery, but occasionally after other surgery. The pathology is only superior, where the limbal surgery has taken place. This points to the surgical trauma as a likely cause of this SC deficiency. In addition to the surgery, the long-term use of ocular medications with preservatives may damage the SCs and help lead to this disease.

Ophthalmologists should recognize that limbal SC deficiency may occur from ocular disease and also after surgery, and appropriate measures to limit the damage to the cornea should be taken. Removing the abnormal corneal epithelium to allow reepithelialization from the normal corneal epithelium, rather than from the abnormal limbal SC area, may hasten resolution of this problem.

P.R. Laibson, M.D.

Conjunctival Flaps

Alino AM, Perry HD, Kanellopoulos AJ, et al (Nassau County Med Ctr, East Meadow, NY; New York Eye and Ear Infirmary; Harvard Med School, Boston; et al)

Ophthalmology 105:1120-1123, 1998 4–12

Background.—The use of conjunctival flaps for numerous disparate corneal diseases with a persistently compromised ocular surface is a proven procedure. An experience with total conjunctival flaps (TCFs) and partial conjunctival flaps (PCFs) was reported.

Methods.—Sixty-one patients were treated in a 5-year period. Forty-eight had TCFs and 13 had PCFs. Indications for surgery were severe bullous keratopathy for chronic graft failure in 19 patients, herpes zoster ophthalmicus in 7, chronic ulcerative keratitis in 14, neurotrophic keratitis in 2, and herpes simplex keratitis in 9.

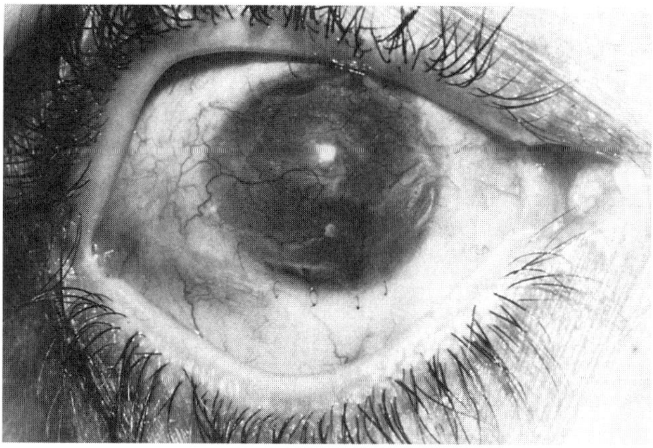

FIGURE 1.—Gundersen flap in a patient with severe Down's syndrome and persistent epithelial defect secondary to herpes simplex keratitis. (Published courtesy of *Ophthalmology*, from Alino AM, Perry HD, Kanellopoulos AJ, et al: Conjunctival flaps. *Ophthalmology* 105:1120-1123, 1998.)

Findings.—Seven complications occurred. Four flaps in the TCF group retracted, 2 of which needed resuturing. In the PCF group, 1 patient experienced 2 flap retractions and recurrent ulceration, necessitating tarsorrhaphy. One patient with a PCF had a perforation after flap retraction and needed penetrating keratoplasty (Fig 1; Table 1).

Conclusion.—Conjunctival flaps are currently underused. Clinicians should seriously consider the use of conjunctival flaps for bullous keratopathy, neurotrophic keratitis, recalcitrant keratitis, and persistent nonhealing epithelial defects.

▶ This paper reminds us that the conjunctival flap is a good alternative therapy for patients with chronic ocular surface disease, particularly that caused by herpes simplex virus, herpes zoster virus, and corneal ulcers. Ophthalmologists should not forget to include this in their thoughts about

TABLE 1.—Underlying Corneal Disease Preconjunctival Flap

Underlying Corneal Disease	No. (%) of Patients
HZV	7 (11)
HSV	9 (15)
Ulcer	12 (20)
Graft-associated	10 (16)
Bullous keratopathy	9 (15)
Neurotrophic	6 (10)
Neuroparalytic	3 (5)
Descemetocele	3 (5)
Band keratopathy	1 (2)

Abbreviations: HZV, herpes zoster virus; *HSV*, herpes simplex virus.
(Published courtesy of *Ophthalmology*, from Alino AM, Perry HD, Kanellopoulos AJ, et al: Conjunctival flaps. *Ophthalmology* 105:1120-1123, 1998.)

chronic nonhealing ulcers, whether from neurotrophic disease, viral disease, or other causes. The flap is not a difficult procedure to perform, although if the ophthalmologist has not performed a conjunctival flap recently, a review of the surgical technique is necessary.

I particularly like the Gunderson flap, which uses upper bulbar conjunctiva, leaving a bridge of tissue available nasally and temporally for a vascular supply. The flaps usually stay in place for at least 6 months and, in many cases, indefinitely if further surgery—such as corneal transplantation—is not contemplated.

P.R. Laibson, M.D.

Phototherapeutic Keratectomy for Map-Dot-Fingerprint Corneal Dystrophy

Örndahl MJF, Fagerholm PP (St Erik Eye Hosp, Stockholm; Karolinska Inst, Stockholm)

Cornea 17:595-599, 1998 4–13

Background.—Map-dot-fingerprint (MDF) dystrophy is the most common corneal dystrophy. A subgroup of patients with MDF dystrophy has a transient or more permanent reduction in visual acuity, sometimes combined with ghost images or subjective monocular diplopia. This results

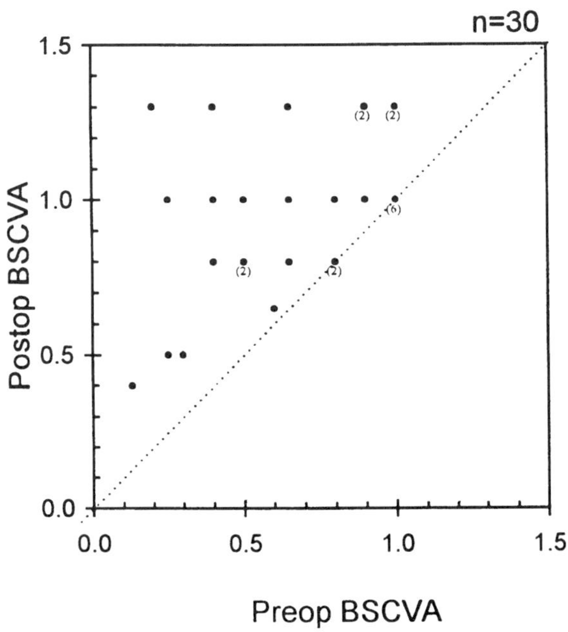

FIGURE 2.—Best spectacle-corrected Snellen visual activity (*BSCVA*) before and after phototherapeutic keratectomy at the final follow-up (mean, 30 months; range, 12-70 months.) (Courtesy of Örndahl MJF, Fagerholm PP: Phototherapeutic keratectomy for map-dot-fingerprint corneal dystrophy. *Cornea* 17:595-599, 1998.)

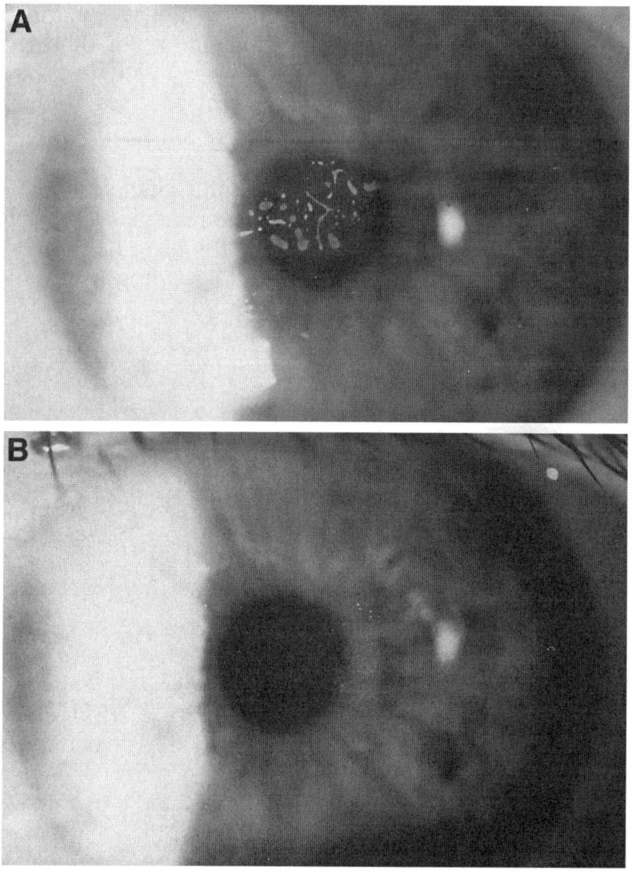

FIGURE 3.—Slit-lamp photographs of a 61-year-old man with map-dot-fingerprint dystrophy. **A**, preoperative appearance, spectacle-corrected visual acuity was 0.25. **B**, 3 months after 10 μm of stromal ablation, spectacle-corrected visual acuity was 1.0. There were no pathologic findings in the ablation zone. (Courtesy of Örndahl MJF, Fagerholm PP: Phototherapeutic keratectomy for map-dot-fingerprint corneal dystrophy. *Cornea* 17:595-599, 1998.)

from the irregular astigmatism and abnormal tear break-up that can occur in this disorder. In this subgroup, the clinical refraction often fluctuates, which may be at least partly responsible for the subjective decrease in vision. Though symptoms can sometimes lessen spontaneously, that may take months or years. The efficacy of the excimer laser in the treatment of MDF dystrophies is reported.

Methods.—Twenty-four patients with 30 affected eyes underwent phototherapeutic keratectomy (PTK). The treatment goal was to improve vision in 24 eyes and to resolve recurrent corneal lesions in 10. Symptoms included a long-standing decrease in visual acuity in 17 eyes, fluctuating visual acuity and clinical refraction in 12 eyes, and monocular diplopia in 8. Fourteen eyes had 2 or 3 symptoms, and 16 had only 1. Patients were studied for a mean of 30 months.

Findings.—Best spectacle-corrected Snellen visual acuity improved by 2 or more lines in 14 of 17 eyes that had long-standing reduction in visual acuity. By 1 to 3 months after PTK, all eyes with fluctuating visual acuity or clinical refraction were stabilized. The treatment resolved monocular diplopia or ghost images in all eyes. One recurrence in 1 of the 10 eyes with recurrent corneal erosions was documented during follow-up. All eyes healed shortly after PTK. No corneal dystrophic changes had recurred in the ablation zone at the last follow-up assessment. However, dystrophic changes were still noted outside the treatment zone in half the eyes. These changes were asymptomatic in all the eyes. The average refractive change was 0.34 diopters (Figs 2 and 3).

Conclusions.—Excimer laser photoablation appears to be effective, safe, and stable in eyes with MDF dystrophy. In some eyes, a refractive change, such as hyperopic shift, may occur.

▶ When anterior basement membrane dystrophy or MDF dystrophy is present in the visual axis, irregular astigmatism may cause blurred vision. There also may be recurrent corneal erosion resulting from this problem. This article documents the use of the excimer laser to remove epithelial pathology along with basement membrane complexes present with MDF dystrophy. If this treatment were inexpensive and readily available, it would be an excellent strategy for this problem. Unfortunately, it is expensive and not readily available to many ophthalmologists.

The use of the diamond burr following mechanical débridement can achieve a similar purpose and is far less expensive. PTK for anterior basement membrane dystrophy is probably a slightly better choice because of its control. However, an almost equally good and much less expensive way of treating this disease is with epithelial débridement and the use of a diamond burr, as described by Forstot almost 10 years ago.

P.R. Laibson, M.D.

Corneal Impression Test for the Diagnosis of Acute Rabies Encephalitis

Zaidman GW, Billingsley A (Westchester County Med Ctr, Valhalla, NY)

Ophthalmology 105:249-251, 1998 4–14

Background.—A young girl was described who had rabies diagnosed by the corneal cytologic impression test (CIT).

> *Case Report.*—Girl, 13 years, was examined at a local hospital for pain in her left arm and shoulder. She was given oral anti-inflammatory agents, but fever, neck stiffness, tremors, mood swings, difficulty swallowing, and parathesias in her left arm developed. She was transferred to Westchester County Medical Center, with a high fever, stiff neck, and left-sided numbness. Laboratory tests, CT scan of the brain, and chest x-ray showed normal

findings. The patient was admitted with a diagnosis of acute encephalitis of unknown origin. Lyme disease and tuberculosis test results were negative. During the next 72 hours, she became agitated and disoriented, and horizontal nystagmus and anisocoria developed. The possibility of rabies encephalitis was considered, although there was no known source. The ophthalmology department performed a CIT. Less than 24 hours later, the CIT was reported positive for rabies antigen. The patient became comatose and died 12 days after her symptoms began. The parents refused an autopsy.

Technique.—The CIT is performed under topical anesthetic. A clean, glass microscope slide is pressed firmly against the corneal epithelium and rocked to increase cell adherence. The slide is air dried, fixed in cold acetone, and stained with fluorescein-labeled mouse monoclonal antibody specific for rabies nucleocapsid protein. The slides are read with a microscope with immunofluorescent filters to detect intracytoplasmic inclusions of antigen.

Conclusions.—Ophthalmologists can assist in the diagnosis of rabies by using the CIT. Corneal smears should be part of the routine workup for suspected rabies to assist in early diagnosis.

▶ Most ophthalmologists probably do not realize that corneal impression cytology may help in diagnosing rabies. I had not realized myself that rabies can be diagnosed by corneal impression cytology using fluorescent antibody techniques to illuminate viral antigen in the conjunctival epithelial cells. This article, although referring to only 1 patient, led to the diagnosis of acute rabies encephalitis. The serum test would have also pointed to rabies as a cause of the encephalitis; however, the conjunctival cells are more easily removed and tested, thereby providing an answer within 24 hours.

The ophthalmologist who works in a general hospital and particularly the neuro-ophthalmologist should know of this important test for the diagnosis of rabies.

P.R. Laibson, M.D.

5 Retina

Alternative and Investigational Therapies in the Treatment of Age-related Macular Degeneration: A Cautionary Tale

by Joseph I. Maguire, M.D.

The word is out. Age-related macular degeneration is officially the "in" ocular disease. I've heard it called an "epidemic" by learned colleagues who should know better. I've watched prime-time news shows with a mixture of shock and bemusement as an elderly patient is brought before an eager press corps after undergoing ocular surgery with retinal cell transplantation, and we are cautioned that it may be several months before it is known if the surgery was successful in restoring vision in this series of one patient. P.T. Barnum is smiling somewhere, but I am not. The reason should be clear: Science should not be substituted for public relations, self-promotion, investment opportunities, or thin truths.

By design or accident, or both, our patients are increasingly exposed to reports of potential miraculous cures and benefits of formative and unproven treatments. The popular media is culpable in some of its reporting techniques; the Internet also accounts for dissemination of inaccurate data. But we, as physicians and scientists, are ultimately accountable. Recently, I searched online for a particular pharmaceutical with possible future application in choroidal neovascular disease. More than 30 references appeared. All but two were from business journals and periodicals. Of the two scientific articles, one was published in a peer-reviewed journal and the other was not yet in print.

So what is the truth regarding recent developments in unlocking the secrets of age-related macular disease (AMD)? The first truth is that, although we clearly know there is increased risk to contralateral eyes of individuals with unilateral exudative AMD, we still have little in the way of long-term natural history data regarding the risk of visual loss in eyes of individuals with no exudative disease.[1] Second, laser photocoagulation is still the only proven treatment for AMD, but this is woefully inadequate in over 90% of individuals seen with exudative maculopathy.[2] Third, any treatment or prophylactic regimen beyond that described above is unproved.

TABLE 1.

- A. Genetics and genetic engineering
- B. Prophylaxis
    - 1. Nutrition
    - 2. Laser
- C. Treatment
    - 1. Exudative
        - a. Photodynamic therapy
        - b. Submacular surgery
            - 1. Clot evacuation vitrectomy / retinotomy / t-pa pneumatic / t-pa
            - 2. Removal of choroidal neovascular membranes
        - c. Retinal translocation
        - d. Radiation
        - e. Antiangiogenesis medications
    - 2. Nonexudative
        - a. Nutrition
            - 1. Vitamins
            - 2. Antioxidants
        - b. Laser for drusen
    - 3. Exudative and nonexudative
        - a. Cell transplantation
        - b. Gene therapy

So what do we tell our patients regarding ongoing studies in the genetics, pathogenesis, epidemiology, prophylaxis, and treatment of AMD? I think first it helps to break down and outline different areas of current macular degeneration investigation and interest (Table 1). We can then logically discuss what is known and what is being studied. I emphasize to all macular degeneration patients under my care that AMD is without exact definition and describes a condition with protean presentations and degrees of severity. Like cancer, there will not be one cure, but different potential treatments that will evolve to benefit certain subsets of patients.

What do our patients want to know? If they have nonexudative AMD and reasonable visual acuity, or if they have close relatives with visual loss due to AMD, they want to know (a) What is my risk of visual loss? and (b) Is there any preventive treatment? To the former question, I emphasize that there is a dirth of prospective long-range longitudinal studies examining the risk of visual loss in eyes with nonexudative AMD and that the genetics of AMD is not Mendelian. Unlike hair and eye color, the heredity of macular disease in the aged population is certainly multifactorial. Recent studies have outlined genetic defects in juvenile forms of macular degeneration—for example, Best's disease, Stargardt's, Sorsby's—and some forms of dry AMD, but this is just the beginning, and there is no genetic test to assess risk let alone genetic engineering techniques to eliminate disease.[3,4] This is a fascinating but formative, area of investigation.

Prophylactic measures being evaluated involve nutrition, vitamins and antioxidants, and laser to drusen.[5] The AREDs study, an NIH-supported evaluation of the aging eye, is examining the impact of vitamins and antioxidants in AMD. Now nearly 10 years along, it evidently is to be extended an additional 5 years. The implication is that the current length of the trial was inadequate to assess any benefit between treatment and nontreatment groups. Studies evaluating laser for drusen have shown mixed results, with those individuals with unilateral exudative disease receiving laser for drusen to the contralateral eye actually having an increased risk of exudative disease.[6] Current focus is on whether laser to eyes of individuals with bilateral nonexudative maculopathy would create a decreased risk of exudative disease. Again, the premise of these papers suffers from the absence of good long-term longitudinal natural history studies that assess risk in elderly individuals with bilateral drusen alone.[1] Statistical models have been constructed, but are they reliable?

What about exudative macular degeneration treatment? Remember, our patients think in terms of "Does this treatment have the ability to let me be independent?" —specifically to read and to drive. They do not particularly care about "statistically significant" visual improvement; they want tangible benefit to their lifestyle. In my opinion, conventional laser for extrafoveal classic choroidal neovascularization is still the only treatment that affords this benefit. Unfortunately, only a minority of patients with exudative AMD (less than 10%) will derive any long-term benefit from such treatment.[2] This explains the multiple investigative protocols now being reviewed in the literature. These include submacular surgery (the submacular surgery trial, or SST), retinal translocation, photodynamic therapy, radiation, and anti-angiogenesis drugs.[7-11] Of all these, only photodynamic therapy is far down the investigative path. It has completed FDA-sanctioned phase I and II trials and moved onto phase III evaluation. Although its abilities show promise, its application is still limited and requires repetitive treatments because of recurrence within a dozen weeks of initial administration.

I believe all areas of potential investigation hold promise, but we have an obligation to our patients, and the public at large, to be meticulous in our presentation of the facts and to scrupulously avoid the tendency toward hyperbole that inevitably surrounds the popular reporting of medical research.

References

1. Klein R, Klein BE, Jensen SC, et al: The five-year incidence and progression of age-related maculopathy: The Beaver Dam eye study. *Ophthalmology* 104:7-21, 1997.
2. Moisseiev J, Alhalel A, Masuri R, et al: The impact of the macular photocoagulation study results on the treatment of exudative age-related macular degeneration. *Arch Ophthalmol* 113:185-189, 1995.
3. Felbor U, Doepner D, Schneider U, et al: Evaluation of the gene encoding the tissue inhibitor of metalloproteinase-3 in various maculopathies. *Invest Ophthalmol Vis Sci* 38:1054-1059, 1997.
4. Dryja TP, Briggs CE, Berson EL, et al: ABCR gene and age-related macular degeneration. *Science* 279:1107, 1998.
5. Bressler NM, Bressler SB: Preventative ophthalmology: Age-related macular degeneration. *Ophthalmology* 102:1206-1211, 1995.

6. The Choroidal Neovascularization Prevention Trial Research Group: Laser treatment in eyes with large drusen: Short-term effects seen in a pilot randomized clinical trial. *Ophthalmology* 105:11-23, 1998.
7. Anand-Apte B, Pepper MS, Voest E, et al: Inhibition of angiogenesis by tissue inhibitor of metalloproteinase-3. *Invest Ophthalmol Vis Sci* 38:817-823, 1997.
8. Guyer DR, and the Pharmacological Therapy for Macular Degeneration Study Group: Interferon Alfa-2a is ineffective for patients with choroidal neovascularization secondary to age-related macular degeneration: Results of a prospective randomized placebo-controlled clinical trial. *Arch Ophthalmol* 115:865-872, 1997.
9. Ibanez HE, Williams DF, Thomas MA, et al: Surgical management of submacular hemorrhage: A series of 47 consecutive cases. *Arch Ophthalmol* 113:6269, 1995.
10. Little CW, Castillo B, DiLoreto DA, et al: Transplantation of human fetal pigment epithelium rescues photoreceptor cells from degeneration in the Royal College of Surgeons rat. *Invest Ophthalmol Vis Sci* 37:204-211, 1996.
11. Kramer M, Miller JW, Michaud N, et al: Liposomal benzoporphyrin derivative verteporfin photodynamic therapy: Selective treatment of choroidal neovascularization in monkeys. *Ophthalmology* 103:427-438,1996.

Age-related Macular Degeneration: Clinical Features in a Large Family and Linkage to Chromosome 1q

Klein ML, Schultz DW, Edwards A, et al (Oregon Health Sciences Univ, Portland; The Rockefeller Univ, New York)
Arch Ophthalmol 116:1082-1088, 1998 5–1

Background.—Although the pathogenesis of age-related macular degeneration (AMD) remains uncertain, evidence suggests that genetic influences are important. The chromosomal location of a disease-causing gene was sought in this study, and the clinical characteristics of a large family with AMD were described.

Methods.—Twenty-one members of a family with an AMD pedigree participated in the study. To identify the chromosomal regions likely to be involved, the authors used a genome-wide screen at about 6-centimorgan spacing with a DNA-pooling strategy combined with shared-segment analysis.

Findings.—Ten family members were found to be affected. AMD was characterized by large, soft, confluent drusen and varying degrees of retinal pigment epithelial degeneration and/or geographic atrophy. The disease segregated as an autosomal-dominant trait. The disease locus mapped to chromosome 1q25-q31 between markers *D1S466* and *D1S413*, with a multipoint lod score of 3.00.

Conclusion.—In this large family with a predominantly dry phenotype, AMD localized to chromosome 1q25-q31. Identifying AMD genes can facilitate early diagnosis and improve understanding of the molecular pathophysiologic mechanisms of AMD.

► The development of our genetic disease database continues to grow throughout medicine and particularly in ophthalmology. The eye with its amitotic component of sensory cells (i.e., the retina and retinal pigment epithelium) present the perfect medium for genetic engineering and repair. As with all endeavors, preparation is 90% of the effort and it is time-consuming, with a host of dead ends and disappointments. Genetic disease of the retina has a habit of exhibiting less than perfect mendelian genetics and often gives very similar phenotypes with vastly different genotypes.

This report by Klein and colleagues is exciting in that a pedigree of autosomal-dominant non-exudative AMD has been discovered, evaluated, and described. Like retinitis pigmentosa, however, 1 locus is not the all-encompassing answer. It is, however, a fascinating start on a long journey of discovery which will eventually give insight to macular degeneration's pathophysiology and treatment(s).

J.I. Maguire, M.D.

High-risk Characteristics of Fellow Eyes of Patients With Unilateral Neovascular Age-related Macular Degeneration

Sandberg MA, Weiner A, Miller S, et al (Harvard Med School, Boston; Massachusetts Eye and Ear Infirmary, Boston)
Ophthalmology 105:441-447, 1998 5–2

Background.—The leading cause of legal blindness among persons aged 50 years and older in the United States is age-related macular degeneration (AMD). In about 10% of the patients, visual loss is related to a choroidal neovascular membrane (CNVM). More severe visual loss results from subretinal exudation, bleeding, and scarring. In 4% to 12% of patients with a CNVM in 1 eye, a CNVM will develop in the fellow eye within 1 year. Whether clinical tests of ocular function and macular appearance can independently predict which patients with unilateral neovascular AMD will have CNVM development in the fellow eye was determined.

Methods.—One hundred twenty-seven patients with unilateral neovascular AMD were monitored for up to 4.5 years. Visual acuity, macular visual field, glare recovery time, and foveal electroretinogram amplitude and implicit time were assessed.

Findings.—A CNVM developed in an average of 8.8% of patients each year. In a Cox proportional hazards model, independent risk factors for CNVM development in the fellow eye were glare recovery time in minutes and the extent of visible macular abnormalities on a 4-point scale. In affected eyes, the interval to CNVM development was correlated inversely with the foveal electroretinogram implicit time.

Conclusions.—In patients with unilateral neovascular AMD, independent risk factors for CNVM development in the fellow eye include a slower recovery from glare and more extensive funduscopic changes. A slower foveal electroretinogram implicit time may be a sign of early-stage development of a CNVM.

▶ My patients with unilateral exudative AMD always want to know their chances for bilateral disease. Clearly, previous papers have analyzed the importance of clinical factors such as drusen and retinal pigment epithelial changes in predicting risk of choroidal neovascularization (CNV) in uninvolved eyes when the contralateral eye has exudative disease. This prospective study differs in that it attempts to determine whether macular appearance and ocular function tests (foveal electroretinogram, macular visual field, and glare recovery time) independently predict risk of CNV.

Sandberg and associates found an annual risk of 8.8% for CNV. In addition, increased presence of drusen and retinal pigment epithelial changes conferred higher risk as found in previous work. However one other independent predictor was found—an increased glare recovery time. Glare recovery time is easily tested in an office setting with normally available equipment, i.e., a transilluminator and a watch! Among study eyes whose glare recovery spanned periods of less than 1 minute to greater than 10 minutes, the increased risk of CNV proliferation was 10 times greater!

J.I. Maguire, M.D.

Pneumatic Displacement of Subretinal Hemorrhage Without Tissue Plasminogen Activator

Ohji M, Saito Y, Hayashi A, et al (Osaka Univ, Japan; Retinal Diagnostic Ctr, Campbell, Calif)

Arch Ophthalmol 116:1326-1332, 1998 5–3

Introduction.—Poor visual outcome has been associated with the natural course of subfoveal hemorrhage caused by age-related macular degeneration or macroaneurysms. A potential treatment for subfoveal hemorrhage is vitreous surgery, but final visual outcomes have generally been disappointing because of the trauma on the sensory retina and retinal pigment epithelium. To improve foveal function, it is necessary to clear the subretinal hemorrhage from the fovea; however, it has not been determined whether actual evacuation of subretinal hemorrhage from the subretinal space is necessary. Foveal function would be expected to be restored if clearance of subretinal hemorrage from the fovea could be achieved with an intervention less traumatic to the sensory retina and retinal pigment epithelium. The question of whether subretinal hemorrhage could be moved by gas injection into the vitreous cavity after face-down positioning without the use of intravitreal tissue-type plasminogen activator was determined in a small case study.

Methods.—The study included 5 patients with subretinal hemorrhage involving the fovea because of age-related macular degeneration (4 eyes) or ruptured retinal arterial macroaneurysm (1 eye). Pure perfluoropropane gas at 0.4 to 0.5 mL was injected into the vitreous cavity while the patients were in a prone position.

Results.—Before gas injection, visual acuity ranged from 20/300 to 20/2000. In 3 eyes, subretinal hemorrhage was dramatically displaced on the day after surgery, and slightly displaced with a reduction in the thickness of subfoveal hemorrhage in the remaining 2 eyes. In all eyes, final visual acuity improved, ranging from 20/15 to 20/220. A final visual acuity of 20/50 or better was seen in 3 eyes. Two complications occurred. In 1 eye, vitreous hemorrhage caused by migration of subretinal hemorrhage into the vitreous cacity occurred. In another eye retinal detachment occurred. Vitrectomy resolved both complications.

Conclusion.—In some patients, gas injected into the vitreous cavity can displace subretinal hemorrhage without the use of tissue plasminogen. An improvement of visual acuity after gas injection can occur, making this treatment an alternative to evacuation of subretinal hemorrhage with vitrectomy.

▶ As our professional community scrambles to evaluate new forms of management, macular degeneration continues to taunt us. Like cancer, age-related macular degeneration is not generic, but protean in its clinical presentation. As such, 1 treatment will probably never fit all cases and a final "cure" will be elusive and involve multiple regimens.

The patient presenting with thick subfoveal hemorrhage is difficult. Usually these patients are asymptomatic until an acute event occurs, and then evaluation is hampered by the presence of blood that obscures underlying choroidal detail even with the use of indocyanine green videoangiography techniques. Reports of surgical removal with vitreoretinal techniques, even modified with the use of clot-lysing tissue plasminogen activator (t-PA) are disappointing visually. Mechanical manipulation has the unfortunate ability to disturb and damage sensory retina and retinal pigment epithelium above and beyond the clot already present.

A recent report by Heriot[1]—using t-PA and intraocular expansile gas with head-down positioning in acute macular bleeds—sparked interest due to its ability to move macular hemorrhage peripherally without the expense and trauma of mechanical manipulation in the subretinal space. Simple is usually safer, and in this small consecutive case series Ohji and colleagues have successfully reproduced Heriot's results, but without the use of t-PA. As in all nonrandomized small-case series, treatment benefit requires a more critical assessment and long-term follow-up. However, pneumatic retinopexy, with or without t-PA, should be considered in eyes with macular hemorrhage when not a candidate for standard therapy.

J.I. Maguire, M.D.

Reference

1. Heriot WJ: Further experience in management of submacular hemorrhage with intravitreal TPA, in *Program and Abstracts of Vitreoretinal Update 1997*. San Francisco, Oct 24-25, 1997.

External Beam Radiation Therapy for Choroidal Neovascularization

Spaide RF, Guyer DR, McCormick B, et al (Manhattan Eye, Ear, and Throat Hosp, NY; Mem Sloan Kettering Cancer Ctr, New York)

Ophthalmology 105:24-30, 1998 5–4

Background.—Radiation therapy has been suggested for treating choroidal neovascularization (CNV). The effect of external beam radiation treatment on CNV caused by age-related macular degeneration (AMD) was studied.

Methods.—Ninety-one patients treated with external beam radiation were compared with 119 control patients retrospectively. Patients with subfoveal CNV not meeting the Macular Photocoagulation Study Group criteria for laser therapy or who did not want laser therapy were considered for radiation treatment in a nonrandomized, prospective clinical study. All had visual acuity of 20/320 or better and a lesion of less than 12 disc areas in size. Radiation treatment consisted of 5 fractions of 200 cGy 6 MV external beam photons. Baseline visual acuity was compared with visual acuity at 1 year.

Findings.—At baseline, the mean visual acuity of patients undergoing radiation therapy was 20/80. At 1 year, the mean visual acuity of the 83 patients (91.2%) completing follow-up was 20/200. In the control group, mean baseline visual acuity was 20/80 and, at 1 year, 20/125. Thirty-eight percent of the control group and 49.4% of those treated with radiation therapy lost 3 or more lines of visual acuity by the 1-year assessment.

Conclusions.—External beam radiation consisting of 1,000 cGy in 5 fractions is not effective in patients with CNV caused by AMD. This dose, which has been used in previous studies, should not be given in an attempt to treat such patients.

► The current list of ongoing studies investigating therapeutic options—other than laser—for AMD is growing. Most have responsibly progressed from pilot studies to prospective randomized trials. These include thalidomide, laser treatment for drusen, submacular surgery, and photodynamic therapy. However, most published reports on external beam radiation in the treatment of exudative AMD have suffered from short follow-up and lack of randomization.

In Spaide and colleagues' current report, treated patients are evaluated in a prospective manner using a historical control group of matched demographics and entry visual acuities. In addition, this analysis benefits from a 1-year follow-up and more than 90% retention of study patients. Results show no benefit to vision in eyes with foveal choroidal neovascularization from AMD when compared with historical controls treated with 5 Gy of fractionated external beam radiation. In our study at Wills Eye, initial data support a nominal to nonexistent effect on vision. Any additional treatment of exudative AMD with radiation therapy should be through hospital internal review board oversight and performed in a randomized fashion at higher than current dosages.

J.I. Maguire, M.D.

The Prognosis of Idiopathic Choroidal Neovascularization in Persons Younger Than 50 Years of Age

Lindblom B, Anderson T (Göteborg, Sweden)

Ophthalmology 105:1816-1820, 1998 5–5

Introduction.—An uncommon disorder affecting primarily individuals aged 50 years or less, idiopathic or juvenile choroidal neovascularization (CNV) is not accompanied by other ocular pathology. A previous study suggested that age was important for the prognosis of idiopathic CNV, and that the outcome was more favorable in younger patients. For many years, there was a reluctance to treat extrafoveal membranes in patients aged less than 50 years. The prognosis of idiopathic choroidal neovascular membranes (CNVMs) in patients younger than 50 years at the time of diagnosis was reported in a retrospective series.

Methods.—The study included 18 patients who had 20 eyes with idiopathic CNV in the macular area. They were followed up for a mean of 55 months that ranged from 5 months to 187 months. Patients were treated conservatively. They were informed about argon laser photocoagulation, but most were not encouraged to have the treatment. Computerized image analysis was used to determine the dimensions of the CNVM and its distance to the foveola. The correlation of these two variables with final visual acuity was determined.

Results.—A visual acuity of 20/60 or better was retained in 15 (75%) of the 20 eyes. The acuity was 20/25 or better in 10 eyes (50%). Laser photocoagulation was performed on 6 eyes. Only 1 had a membrane located 200 μm or more from the foveola at the time of treatment. The outcome for treated and untreated eyes was the same, although the 2 groups were not directly comparable. No initially juxtafoveal or extrafoveal membrane grew under the foveola in any of the eyes.

Conclusion.—For eyes with choroidal membranes associated with age-related macular degeneration, the prognosis of idiopathic CNV was much better than previously reported. Consideration should be given to a conservative treatment regimen. The belief that laser photocoagulation would have improved the outcome in the nontreated eyes could not be supported.

▶ The benefits of laser in the treatment of discrete CNVMs associated with age-related macular degeneration (AMD) and ocular histoplamosis is well documented by the Macular Photocoagulation Study (MPS). Laser treatment benefit for CNVM in idiopathic cases is also documented by the MPS, but involves a heterogeneous grouping of eyes and included patients who were in the AMD age group.

Recent reports have shown the ability of subfoveal idiopathic CNVMs to do well with observation alone. Lindblom and associates have demonstrated that juxta and extrafoveal lesions also have a strong tendency to do well with conservative observation in the 50 and younger age grouping. Although this report is retrospective in nature, taken along with other reports on the natural history of foveal idiopathic CNVM, it clearly indicates the option for less aggressive management. Current tendency is to lump CNVM visual prognosis from a multitude of conditions into 1 grouping, that is, the poor outcome associated with AMD. Therefore we see aggressive management, such as submacular surgical techniques, for eyes which apparently may do very well on their own.

J.I. Maguire, M.D.

Cystoid Macular Edema and Anterior Uveitis Associated With Latanoprost Use: Experience and Incidence in a Retrospective Review of 94 Patients

Warwar RE, Bullock JD, Ballal D (Wright State Univ, Dayton, Ohio)

Ophthalmology 105:263-268, 1998 5–6

Background.—Latanoprost, a prostaglandin analogue, is the first of a new class of drugs developed to reduce intraocular pressure. This drug has been reported to be effective and safe in studies following up patients for 6-12 months. The incidence of cystoid macular edema (CME) and anterior uveitis associated with the use of latanoprost was examined retrospectively.

Methods and Findings.—Data on 94 patients and a total of 163 eyes were reviewed. Signs and symptoms of ocular inflammation during latanoprost treatment were documented. The extent of anterior uveitis and CME were measured. Anterior uveitis developed in 6.4% of the patients and in 4.9% of all eyes during latanoprost treatment. CME occurred in 2.1% of patients and in 1.2% of all eyes.

Conclusions.—Although latanoprost is an effective ocular-hypotensive agent, the incidences of anterior uveitis and CME are significant. Clinicians need to be aware of these possible complications when using latanoprost therapy.

▶ The effect of latanoprost in the treatment of open angle glaucoma has been a boon to our patients. However, no therapy is without potential risk. This current retrospective report cites the development of CME and anterior uveitis as associations with the use of latanoprost. As a prostaglandin analogue, it should not be surprising that an association with iritis has been made. This is made more believable by the redevelopment of iritis in eyes rechallenged with latanoprost after their iritis was quiescent and the medication removed.

The claim of CME is less supportable, especially given the retrospective nature of this report and the ocular history of the 2 eyes (1.2% of treated eyes) deemed to have developed CME through the use of latanoprost. Each of these patients had undergone previous cataract extraction. One had an anterior chamber lens with previously documented CME from cataract surgery complications, and the other eye had a very recent history of iritis before the start of latanoprost. Both eyes had minimal follow-up.

Although these results should be taken with appropriate skepticism, the increasing use of this effective medication should lead us to consider its involvement in cases of iritis and CME.

J.I. Maguire, M.D.

Incidence of Idiopathic Full-thickness Macular Holes in Fellow Eyes: A 5-Year Prospective Natural History Study

Ezra E, Wells JA, Gray RH, et al (Moorfields Eye Hosp, London; Univ of South Carolina, Columbia)

Ophthalmology 105:353-359, 1998 5–7

Background.—Idiopathic full-thickness macular hole (FTMH), a major cause of central visual loss, affects 3.3 per 1,000 persons, about 70% of whom are female. The incidence of idiopathic FTMH in normal fellow eyes was determined, and the role of electrodiagnostic and psychophysical tests in identifying eyes at risk was assessed.

Methods.—One hundred fourteen patients were initially enrolled in a prospective, longitudinal study. All patients had unilateral holes and normal, asymptomatic fellow eyes without posterior vitreous detachment. Baseline examination included pattern reversal electroretinography, electro-oculography, and color contrast sensitivity (CCS) testing for protan, deutan, and tritan thresholds. Eighty patients were available for follow-up assessment at 18 months, and 74 patients at 5 years.

Findings.—At 18 months, 6 of 80 patients had full-thickness macular holes in the fellow eye. At 5 years, an additional 5 patients had holes in the

TABLE 1.—Mean Values of Test at Baseline for Affected Eyes and Fellow Eyes

Objective Test	Normal Value (Age Adjusted)	Affected Eye	Fellow Eye	P
Electro-oculogram (EOG) (%)	180	197	203	0.86
Pattern electroretinogram (PERG) (P50)* (μV)	1.5	1.50 (0.37)	1.63 (0.41)	0.82
Color contrast sensitivity (CCS) (%)				
Protan	7.5	23.0 (17.0)	8.97 (7.0)	0.0001
Deutan	7.5	26.7 (21.0)	15.4 (9.9)	0.0001
Tritan	8.5	42.2 (27.0)	11.2 (9.2)	0.0001

Values in parentheses indicate SD. A value of $P = 0.05$ or less was taken as indicating statistical significance.
*P50 indicates the initial corneal positive response.
(Published courtesy of *Ophthalmology*, from Ezra E, Wells JA, Gray RH, et al: Incidence of idiopathic full-thickness macular holes in fellow eyes: A 5-year prospective natural history study. *Ophthalmology* 105:353-359, 1998.)

fellow eye. At baseline, mean CCS protan, deutan, and tritan thresholds were increased significantly in affected eyes (Table 1).

Conclusions.—Patients with idiopathic FTMH have a 15.6% 5-year estimated risk of fellow eye involvement. Although electrodiagnostic and psychophysical assessment did not predict fellow eye involvement, baseline tritan CCS loss in apparently normal fellow eyes may indicate subclinical foveal dysfunction. The nature of this is unclear.

▶ Since the application of vitrectomy techniques to idiopathic macular holes by Kelly and Wendel, this surgery has enjoyed enormous popularity and increasing success rates of 80% or greater in properly selected eyes. In addition, greater morbidity is described, with the incidence of retinal tear, retinal detachment, and visual field loss seemingly greater in this procedure than other conditions requiring vitrectomy. As always it is important when advising patients of their therapeutic options to communicate surgical risk and risk to the contralateral eye. Ezra and associates' prospective study clearly shows a substantial risk—about 16%—to the contralateral eye developing a FTMH within 5 years of the initial eye *if* there was no evidence of posterior vitreous detachment. Presence of posterior vitreous detachment in unaffected eyes conferred almost no risk of macular hole development. These are the things our patients want to know to make an informed decision when contemplating surgery.

J.I. Maguire, M.D.

Reopening of Macular Holes After Initially Successful Repair

Christmas NJ, Smiddy WE, Flynn HW Jr (Univ of Miami, Fla)

Ophthalmology 105:1835-1838, 1998 5–8

Introduction.—The anatomical success rate of vitreous surgery for a macular hole is more than 90%, with about half of the patients recovering at least 20/40 visual acuity. Reopening of the macular hole has been reported in about 5% of patients, despite the fact that visual acuity usually continues to improve after successful macular hole surgery. Little is known about the patients who require reoperation. The frequency and prognosis of reopened macular holes after initially successful surgery was evaluated in a retrospective review.

Methods.—The study included 17 patients with reopened macular holes among 390 who had idiopathic macular holes that previously involved macular hole surgery. An evaluation was conducted of the patients' demographics and visual acuity, both preoperatively and postoperatively, after reopening of macular hole and after reoperation.

Results.—After initial successful surgical closure, 17 (4.8%) of 353 patients had a reopened macular hole. Initial success was defined as resolution of the cuff of surrounding subretinal fluid, usually with complete disappearance of the invisible edges of the macular hole at the 3-month postoperative visit. Before reopening, the mean visual acuity was

TABLE 1.—Reopened Macular Holes

	Mean Visual Acuity	≥20/40 (%)
Before MHS (N = 17)	20/109	6
Before reopening (N = 17)	20/48	35
After reopening (N = 17)	20/133	0
After reoperation (N = 11)	20/54	36

Abbreviation: MHS, macular hole surgery.
(Published courtesy of *Ophthalmology*, from Christmas NJ, Smiddy WE, Flynn HW, Jr: Reopening of macular holes after initially successful repair. *Ophthalmology* 105:1835-1838, 1998.)

20/58, and after reopening, it was 20/133 (Table 1). Reoperation was performed on 12 eyes, resulting in improvement to a mean visual acuity of 20/54. A mean visual acuity of 20/200 was found in the 5 eyes that did not require reoperation. Cataract surgery was performed on 10 of the eyes between macular hole surgeries, but only 1 of the eyes appeared to show an association with cataract surgery. Cataract surgery was performed on 269 (80%) of the 335 eyes whose macular holes did not reopen.

Conclusion.—A previously successfully operated macular hole rarely reopens and seems to be a spontaneous event. Results similar to those present before the reopening usually occur with reoperation. It is rare to see reopening of a macular hole associated with cataract surgery. The exact mechanism by which the macular hole reopens is still not known, but possibly relates to mechanical or inflammatory factors.

▶ Macular hole repair via pars plana vitrectomy, membrane peeling, intraocular gas infusion, and postoperative positioning has evolved rapidly to an efficient procedure with an impressive success rate in both hole closure and visual improvement. Of interest is a subgroup of macular hole patients who, despite initial successful repair, redevelop foveal defects. In this retrospective, consecutive, noncomparative case series, Christmas and colleagues confirm that reopening of macular holes after initial closure is uncommon, occurring in less than 5% of cases. In addition, previous reports that this event is related to cataract surgery or YAG capsulotomy is not supported. The mechanism by which macular holes reopen is still unclear, but a standard repeat surgical repair has a high rate of both anatomical and visual success.

J.I. Maguire, M.D.

Intraocular Lens Changes After Short- and Long-term Exposure to Intraocular Silicone Oil: An In Vivo Study

Khawly JA, Lambert RJ, Jaffe GJ (Duke Univ, Durham, NC; Alcon Labs, Ft Worth, Tex)

Ophthalmology 105:1227-1233, 1998 5–9

Background.—The use of silicone as a vitreous substitute after complex vitreoretinal procedures is common. The effects of short-term and long-term exposure to silicone oil on polymethylmethacrylate (PMMA), silicone, and soft acrylic intraocular lenses (IOLs) were studied.

Methods.—In this experimental animal study, 41 New Zealand white rabbits were subjected to lensectomy, vitrectomy, capsulotomy, and placement of 1 of 3 IOL types into the ciliary sulcus. The short-term study involved fluid-air exchange followed by a coating of silicone oil applied to the posterior lens surface, immediately after which an air-fluid exchange was done. The remaining silicone on the posterior lens surface was aspirated and/or wiped for 1 minute using a soft-tipped extrusion cannula. In the long-term study, all rabbits, at 3 months, underwent silicone-fluid exchange, an attempt to manually remove any remaining silicone oil, and lens explantation.

Findings.—In the short-term study, none of the rabbits with PMMA or acrylic IOLs had silicone oil remaining after manual wiping or aspiration. In the rabbits with silicone IOLs, a significant amount of silicone oil remained on the posterior lens surfaces. In the long-term study, 6 of 9 PMMA IOLs and all 10 silicone IOLs showed aqueous droplet formation on the posterior lens surface at 3 months. The group with acrylic IOLs showed no opacities. Adherent silicone oil was noted in 2 of 9 PMMA IOLs and in none of the 10 acrylic IOLs. In addition, lens weights were significantly increased before and after implantation in the silicone IOL group but not in the PMMA or acrylic group.

Conclusions.—Removing the remaining silicone oil from the posterior surface of a silicone IOL after short-term or long-term exposure to silicone oil is extremely difficult, if not impossible. Such oil can interfere with the surgeon's view of the retina and can reduce the patient's visual acuity. By contrast, removing oil from the posterior surface of an acrylic IOL is easy. Thus, a soft acrylic or PMMA IOL should be used instead of a silicone IOL for lens implantation in patients who may need vitreoretinal procedures with silicone oil tamponade.

▶ This excellent comparative study by Khawly and associates should highlight the clear advantages of acrylic foldable IOLs over silicone IOLs in cataract surgeries involving patients at higher risk for future vitreoretinal procedures. Such patients include high myopes, diabetics, younger individuals, and patients with previous retinal detachments in the contralateral eye.

If an anterior segment surgeon asks me my preference of IOL types, I voice my preference for PMMA, or—if a foldable—acrylic lenses. All of my retinal colleagues have probably by now experienced the need to use silicone oil in an eye with a silicone IOL. My experience is that these IOLs always require removal and exchange when silicone oil is likewise removed or exchanged due to the oil's adhesion to the silicone IOL's surface. This phenomenon impedes both the surgeon's and patient's view alike.

J.I. Maguire, M.D.

Visual Recovery in Macula-Off Rhegmatogenous Retinal Detachments

Ross WH, Kozy DW (Univ of British Columbia, Vancouver)

Ophthalmology 105:2149-2153, 1998 5–10

Introduction.—It has been known that there is a progressive decline in visual recovery of macula-off retinal detachments during a 1- to 79-day period. After 4 weeks of macular detachment, approximately 1 line of vision is lost for each additional 10 to 11 days until 71 days. However, it is not known whether there is a difference in visual acuity within the first week. It was determined whether delay in surgical repair correlates with visual acuity outcome within the first week after development of macula-off retinal detachment. The visual results of macula-off detachments operated on within the first 7 days of macular involvement were reviewed.

Methods.—The study included 104 patients with macula-off detachments of 7 days or less. The time of the macular detachment was determined within the first 7 days. A primary scleral buckling procedure was used to repair all 104 detachments. Patients were operated on between 1 and 2 days (group 1) 3 and 4 days (group 2) or 5 and 7 days (group 3) after macular involvement. To compare the visual results of the 3 groups of patients, statistical methods were used.

Results.—After surgery, the mean visual acuity was 20/60. A visual accuity of 20/50 or better was attained by 59% of patients; a visual acuity between 20/60 and 20/200 was attained by 35% of patients; and a visual acuity of less than 20/200 was achieved by 5% of patients, regardless of their grouping. No statistical difference in visual recovery (Fig 4) was observed among the 3 groups.

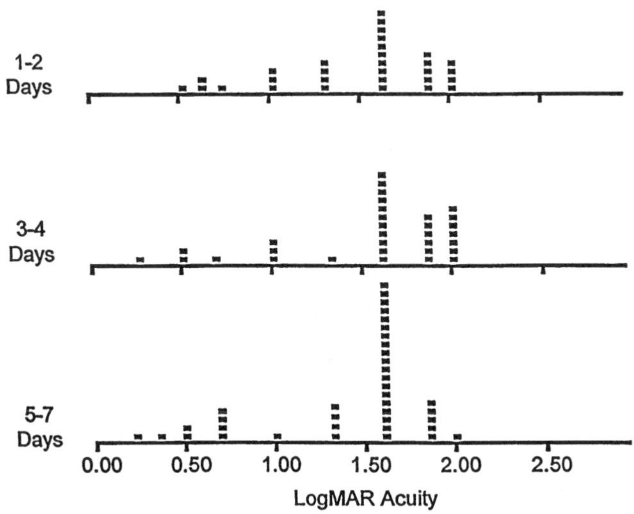

FIGURE 4.—Dot-plot of preoperative logMAR acuities. *Abbreviation: logMAR*, logarithm of the minimal angle of resolution. (Published courtesy of *Ophthalmology*, from Ross WH, Kozy DW: Visual recovery in macula-off rhegmatogenous retinal detachments. *Ophthalmology* 105: 2149-2153, 1998.)

Conclusion.—Delay in surgical repair does not adversely affect visual outcome within the first week after development of macula-off retinal detachment. This data supports the contention that good preoperative vision portends a better postoperative result. Macula-off detachments are not emergent and can wait for the next scheduled available operating room.

► In my practice, referring physicians routinely inquire about the emergent timing of evaluation and repair of their patients with retinal detachment. This, of course, depends on many factors, but certainly the first 2 questions I ask are (1) is the macula off and for how long?; and (2) what is the visual acuity?

Previous reports in the literature have nicely demonstrated the progressive degenerative changes to the sensory retina with increased chronicity of retinal detachment. This prospective study by Ross and associates offers convincing data that the length of macular detachment within the first week does not influence the final postoperative visual acuity. This information allows a certain comfort level in the more efficient and cost-effective timing of surgical repair in such patients.

Additional findings of this report include the tendency for more shallow macular detachments to experience better final visual acuity over their bullous counterparts and the observation that nondrainage procedures also achieve better final postoperative visions over their drainage counterparts.

J.I. Maguire, M.D.

What Happens to Untreated Asymptomatic Retinal Breaks, and Are They Affected by Posterior Vitreous Detachment?

Byer NE (Univ of California, Los Angeles)
Ophthalmology 105:1045-1050, 1998 5–11

Purpose.—Clinical reports have suggested that asymptomatic, unsuspected retinal breaks are common. There have been few studies of the natural history of these retinal breaks, or of the effects of posterior vitreous detachment (PVD) on pre-existing retinal breaks. This prospective study evaluated the long-term outcomes of asymptomatic retinal breaks, and the effects of PVD.

Patients.—The study included 235 eyes with asymptomatic retinal breaks, in 196 patients. All patients received clinical follow-up, including binocular indirect ophthalmoscopy with scleral indentation. Fifty eyes underwent posterior vitreous examination as well. The patients were studied, without treatment, for an average of 11 years.

Outcomes.—Subclinical retinal detachment—defined as a detachment containing subretinal fluid that extended at least 1 DD from the retinal break, but no more than 2 DD posterior to the equator—developed in 8% of eyes. Though remaining asymptomatic, 2 of these were treated because they were associated with moderate extension. One patient had a small peripheral clinical retinal detachment develop from a subclinical detachment over a 14-year period. Posterior vitreous detachment was found in 24% of eyes undergoing examination with a Goldmann lens and slit lamp.

Conclusions.—Clinical retinal detachment appears to be rare in phakic, nonfellow eyes with asymptomatic retinal breaks. In this prospective, 11-year follow-up series, the combined risk of retinal detachment requiring treatment was only 1% to 2%. The results suggest that PVD has no adverse effect on the outcomes of pre-existing retinal breaks. Thus, prophylactic treatment of retinal breaks is not required before or after the development of PVD.

► One of the 10 most common queries I receive, from residents and general ophthalmologists alike, involves the management of incidental retinal tears found on routine examination. We are indebted to Dr. Byer, who over the years—and indeed decades—has painstakingly recorded the findings of not only in retinal tears but in lattice degeneration and subclinical retinal detachments. In this cohort study of consecutive patients, we find significant evidence that retinal tears without associated presenting symptoms, in phakic eyes without a history of contralateral retinal detachment, do not require treatment, even in the face of age-indeterminate posterior vitreous detachment. This was found to be true not only for operculated holes, but also for flap tears.

J.I. Maguire, M.D.

Proliferative Vitreoretinopathy: A Natural History of the Fellow Eye
Schwartz SD, Kreiger AE (Jules Stein Eye Inst, Los Angeles, Calif)
Ophthalmology 105:785-788, 1998 5–12

Background.—Proliferative vitreoretinopathy (PVR) is the most frequent cause of failure in retinal reattachment surgery, with an estimated postoperative incidence of 5% to 10%. There is little information about the risk of vision-threatening conditions in the contralateral eye of patients with PVR. The decision to proceed with multiple PVR operations can be difficult. This retrospective study of individuals with PVR investigated the incidence of vision-threatening disorders in the contralateral eye at first diagnosis, the incidence of development of a vision-threatening condition in the contralateral eye, and the incidence of loss of vision in the contralateral eye.

Methods.—A search of the diagnostic database of one of the authors identified 249 patients with PVR. Patients with less than grade C-3 PVR, giant retinal tears, trauma, inherited vitreoretinopathy, or diabetic retinopathy were excluded.

Results.—The main outcome measure was the presence of vision-threatening conditions in the contralateral eye of patients with PVR. Reliable follow-up information was available for 205 patients. Bilateral PVR was initially present or developed later in 11 of the 205 patients. Of the 205

TABLE 2.—Fellow Eye: Vision-Threatening Pathology

Pathology	No.
Proliferative vitreoretinopathy	11
Previous retinal detachment repair	18
Acute retinal detachment (present on referral or during follow-up)	18
Previous retinal break repair	12
Acute retinal break (present on referral or during follow-up)	22
Rhegmatogenous events (total	81 (74.3%)
Age-related macular degeneration	11
Myopic degeneration	4
Macular hole	2
Cataract (patient too apprehensive for surgery)	2
Corneal disease (requiring keratoplasty)	2
Amblyopia	1
Anophthalmos (malignant melanoma)	1
Phthisis bulbi (etiology unknown)	1
Central retinal vein occlusion	1
Optic atrophy (meningioma)	1
Diabetic retinopathy	1
Glaucomatous field loss	1
Total	109

(Published courtesy of *Ophthalmology*, from Schwartz SD, Kreiger AE: Proliferative vitreoretinopathy: A natural history of the fellow eye. *Ophthalmology* 105:785-788, 1998.)

patients, a total of 109 had a vision-threatening disorder in the contralateral eye; 64 had vision-threatening disorders in the contralateral eye at the time of initial diagnosis, and in 45 patients, vision-threatening disorders developed in the contralateral eye during follow-up. A variety of vision-threatening conditions was seen, including a high prevalence of rhegmatogenous events (Table 2). The mean follow-up period was 9.5 years for patients who had vision-threatening disorders in the contralateral eye and 5.4 years for patients who did not. This suggests that the rate of vision-threatening disorders in the contralateral eye may be even greater over longer periods of time. Regarding final visual acuity, 10 of 205 fellow eyes finished with no light perception. In contralateral eyes in which vision-threatening disorders developed, 51 of 109 ended with visual acuity of 20/50 or worse.

Discussion.—Patients with PVR in one eye are at significant risk of vision-threatening disorders or vision-damaging conditions in the contralateral eye. The high rate of rhegmatogenous events in the contralateral eye seen in these patients indicates that the contralateral eye should be carefully scrutinized during initial examination and also during follow-up. This information should be carefully considered before decisions about surgery are made.

▶ The bane of vitreoretinal surgeons is the development of PVR repair after retinal detachment. Recurrent retinal detachment secondary to PVR carries a poorer visual prognosis and a greater risk of redetachment from reproliferation and additional retinal hole formation. Although the advent of modem vitreoretinal techniques and the use of silicone oil, intraocular gas, and perfluorocarbon liquid has made the overall rate of anatomic reattachment high, poor final visual results may not always warrant multiple aggressive and expensive surgical procedures, especially in the managed care era.

The current study may give sufficient ammunition to those who advocate an aggressive posture toward recurrent detachment from PVR. This interesting retrospective analysis points out the high degree of vision-threatening disorders in the contralateral eye. More than half of the contralateral eyes demonstrated potentially vision-threatening changes; one third had these changes at the time of the initial eyes' presentation! Almost 75% of these events were of a rhegmatogenous nature, including retinal breaks and retinal detachment. The incidence of bilateral PVR was also high (5.4%). This study outlines the need for aggressive management of eyes with retinal detachment and PVR and the need for careful evaluation of the contralateral eye at the time of presentation.

J.I. Maguire, M.D.

A Comparison of Laser Photocoagulation With Trans-scleral Cryotherapy in the Treatment of Threshold Retinopathy of Prematurity

Connolly BP, McNamara JA, Sharma S, et al (Jefferson Med College, Philadelphia)

Ophthalmology 105:1628-1631, 1998 5–13

Background.—Laser photocoagulation has largely replaced cryotherapy in the treatment of retinopathy of prematurity (ROP). The visual outcomes of eyes with threshold ROP treated by transscleral cryotherapy and by laser photocoagulation were compared.

Methods.—Fifty-two patients with bilateral threshold ROP were randomly assigned to cryotherapy in 1 eye and laser photocoagulation in the other. Follow-up data on 25 patients were available for analysis.

Findings.—At a mean follow-up of 5.8 years, the odds of a good clinical outcome were 6.91 times greater in eyes treated with laser than for eyes treated with cryotherapy. The laser-treated eyes were also less myopic, with a mean spherical equivalent of −3.05 D, compared with −5.08 D in cryotherapy-treated eyes (Fig 1; Table 2).

Conclusions.—Laser photocoagulation appears to be superior to transscleral cryotherapy for the treatment of threshold ROP. In this series, visual acuity was better and myopia was less after photocoagulation than after cryotherapy.

► Anyone who has experience using cryotherapy in the treatment of ROP will understand the positive reception with which previous reports demonstrating the efficacy of laser for threshold ROP were greeted. Laser is more portable, more easily applied without excessive manipulation of the premature infant, and, in my experience, better tolerated by far. Connolly and associates' report is thus "sauce for the goose." Although half of their initial

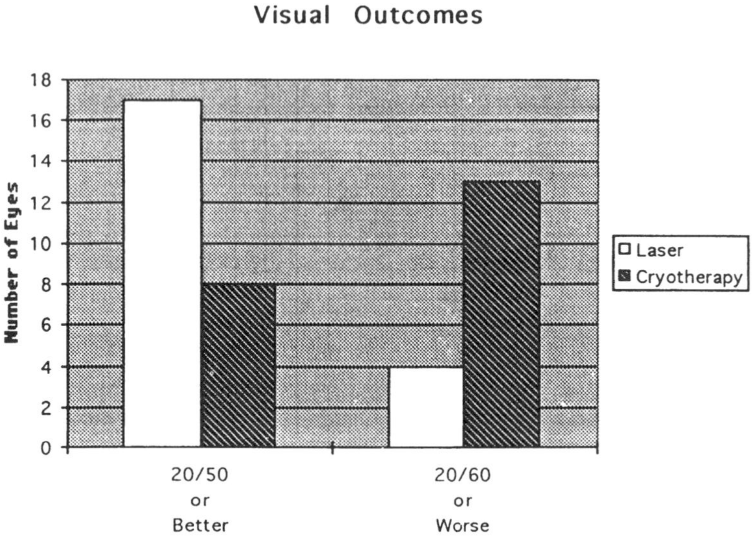

FIGURE 1.—Laser-treated eyes were 6.91 times more likely to have a good visual outcome than cryotherapy-treated eyes. (Published courtesy of *Ophthalmology*, from Connolly BP, McNamara JA, Sharma S, et al: A comparison of laser photocoagulation with trans-scleral cryotherapy in the treatment of threshold retinopathy of prematurity. *Ophthalmology* 105:1628-1631, 1998.)

treatment study population (with bilateral threshold disease treated in 1 eye with cryopexy and in the other with laser) were unable to be evaluated for this report, the results are still impressive.

The laser-treated group had an almost 7-fold greater chance of achieving a favorable visual result (20/50 or better) and had far less myopia than their matched cryopexy-treated eyes. The reasons for this difference are unknown but may be related to the finer placement abilities of laser with less insult to the sclera. Whatever the reasons, laser should be considered equal

TABLE 2.—Refractive Outcomes

Laser Used	Laser Treated Eyes (Mean Spherical Equivalent) (D)	Cryotherapy Treated Eyes (Mean Spherical Equivalent) (D)	Difference of Means (D) (95% Confidence Interval)	*P*
All (n = 23)	−3.05	−5.08	2.02 (0.63 to 3.41)	0.0072
Argon (n = 10)	−3.25	−6.08	2.83 (0.55 to 5.10)	0.020
Diode (n = 13)	−2.90	−4.31	1.40 (−0.61 to 3.42)	0.155

(Published courtesy of *Ophthalmology*, from Connolly BP, McNamara JA, Sharma S, et al: A comparison of laser photocoagulation with trans-scleral cryotherapy in the treatment of threshold retinopathy of prematurity. *Ophthalmology* 105:1628-1631, 1998.)

if not superior to cryotherapy and should be used with impunity in the treatment of threshold ROP.

J.I. Maguire, M.D.

Can Convulsions Alone Cause Retinal Haemorrhages in Infants?

Tyagi AK, Scotcher S, Kozeis N, et al (Birmingham and Midland Eye Centre, England; Birmingham Children's Hosp, England)

Br J Ophthalmol 82:659-660, 1998 5–14

Background.—Retinal hemorrhages in infants are a classic sign of nonaccidental injury that can result from direct head trauma, severe chest compression, or severe shaking of the head. Retinal hemorrhages are seen in up to 89% of infants with nonaccidental injury. Before retinal hemorrhages in young children are attributed to nonaccidental injury, other potential causes, such as birth trauma, blood dyscrasias, infections, cardiopulmonary resuscitation, and seizures, must be excluded. Because it is believed that the vascular systems of infants are vulnerable to sudden changes in central venous pressure, the likelihood of convulsions that alone may cause retinal hemorrhage in children younger than 2 years was investigated.

Methods.—In a prospective study, 32 consecutive children less than 2 years of age who were admitted to the hospital after convulsions underwent a detailed ocular examination within 48 hours of admission. Convulsions were categorized according to the international classification of epileptic seizures, which would exclude children with associated head trauma or children who underwent cardiopulmonary resuscitation. Statistical analysis was performed with the use of Hanley's rule of 3.

Results.—Of the 32 children, 10 were admitted after epileptic seizures and 22 were admitted after febrile convulsions. None of the children had direct head trauma or needed cardiopulmonary resuscitation. None of the 32 children had retinal hemorrhages. Hanley's rule of 3 demonstrated that the chance of retinal hemorrhages resulting from convulsions alone in children younger than 2 years was at most 10% (95% confidence interval). In a previous study of 32 children younger than 14 years, the same authors found no retinal hemorrhages resulting from convulsions alone. When the results of the present and previous studies are combined, the chance of retinal hemorrhages resulting from convulsions alone in children younger than 14 years is less than 5% (95% confidence interval).

Discussion.—These findings suggest that convulsions alone are unlikely to cause retinal hemorrhages in children younger than 2 years. When retinal hemorrhages are detected in very young children admitted after convulsions, it is important to search for other causes for the hemorrhages, especially nonaccidental injury.

Nonaccidental Head Injury in Infants: The "Shaken-Baby Syndrome"

Duhaime A-C, Christian CW, Rorke LB, et al (Univ of Pennsylvania, Philadelphia)

N Engl J Med 338:1822-1829, 1998 5–15

Introduction.—Inflicted head injuries are the major cause of traumatic death in infants. Research has established the diagnostic characteristics of nonaccidental head injuries in infants and toddlers. The mechanisms, findings, diagnosis, and management of "shaken-baby syndrome," the most common type of inflicted head injury in infants, are reviewed.

Shaken-Baby Syndrome.—Most severe inflicted brain injuries are thought to result from sudden deceleration resulting from striking the head against a surface. The attending physician must understand the biomechanics of these injuries to make the diagnosis in a situation where the history is often vague or unreliable. Diffuse brain injuries result from forces causing the brain to rotate about its center of gravity; these types of forces are highly unlikely to result from household falls in infants and young children. Patients with "whiplash shaken-baby syndrome" have subdural and subarachnoid hemorrhage, traction-type metaphyseal fractures, and retinal hemorrhage, related to rotational deceleration. The magnitude of the deceleration forces is much greater when the head strikes a surface; the injury results not from the contact forces applied to the head, but from the deceleration forces placed on the brain and blood vessels. The term "shaking-impact syndrome" might be a more accurate description, though it remains unclear whether shaking alone can cause the typical constellation of findings. In any case, the forces causing these injuries are clearly greater than those involved in normal child care activities.

Most cases of shaking-impact syndrome occur during the first year of life, and almost all in children less than 3 years old. Many victims show evidence of previous abuse. Risk factors include young parents, unstable families, low socioeconomic status, and child disability or prematurity. Fathers, boyfriends, and babysitters are more often perpetrators than mothers.

Patient Findings.—The reported history usually involves a minor blunt impact to the head. The history may be vague, inconsistent, or incompatible with the child's developmental status. The infants may show lethargy, irritability, seizures, increased or decreased tone, impaired consciousness, vomiting, poor feeding, or breathing abnormalities. About half of patients are severely impaired to moribund. Up to 95% of patients have retinal hemorrhage, which is best appreciated with mydriatic agents. The biomechanics leading to the development of retinal hemorrhage are unknown. Though they are strongly associated with inflicted head injury, they are not a specific finding, and may also occur after accidental trauma. However, severe bilateral retinal hemorrhage accompanied by retinal folds or detachments strongly suggests nonaccidental injury. The available evidence suggests that the injury is followed immediately by a decrease in the level of consciousness, with no interval of lucidity before the onset of symptoms.

Differential Diagnosis.—No other condition shares all the same features as shaking-impact syndrome. The definitive findings are a history of trivial or no trauma in an infant with acute subdural hemorrhage and unexplained extracranial bony injuries or inflicted soft tissue injuries; or a definite history of no trauma in the presence of clear evidence of head impact with subdural hemorrhage. Retinal hemorrhage and multiple fractures in various stages of healing support the diagnosis. In some cases, there are insufficient findings to make a definite diagnosis. Accidental injuries may cause small epidural hemorrhages or traumatic subarachnoid hemorrhages; MRI scanning can help to rule out subdural hematoma.

Discussion.—"Shaking-impact syndrome" is caused by major mechanical forces. If this diagnosis is suspected, the child should be hospitalized and child-welfare and law-enforcement agencies notified. Careful attention is needed to documentation for medicolegal reasons. To protect its young victims, physicians must be able to recognize the features of this common inflicted head injury.

▶ Domestic and childhood abuse has become an epidemic of heartwrenching proportions. Trauma is certainly the most common cause of death in children, and in the under 3 age group nonaccidental head injury, including the "shaken-baby syndrome," may be responsible for nearly one fourth of pediatric admissions for head injury in some urban areas. The presence of a neurologically impaired, convulsing or obtunded infant with subdural and subarachnoid hemorrhage, traction-type metaphyseal fractures, and retinal hemorrhages implies significant rotational and deceleration-type brain trauma. The role of the ophthalmologist is to document the presence of retinal pathology, specifically the presence of retinal hemorrhages. Although the presence of retinal hemorrhages is not pathognomic of nonaccidental head injury it is present in between 65% and 95% of cases. Hemorrhage can be bilateral or unilateral and if associated with retinal folds and detachment strongly suggests abuse. In Tyagi and associates' prospective series (Abstract 5–14) of 32 consecutive children admitted for convulsions, none had associated retinal hemorrhages! These data, combined with a previous report (Abstract 5–15) placed the statistical likelihood of retinal hemorrhages due to seizures in children younger than 14 years of age at no more than 5%. As physicians, we shoulder a grave responsibility and have a strong moral imperative to protect innocent lives from life-threatening abuse. Recognizing the symptoms and signs of the "shaken baby syndrome," doing the appropriate examination, and meticulously documenting and reporting suspicious findings helps protect those with whom we are entrusted.

J.I. Maguire, M.D.

Discontinuation of Maintenance Therapy in Patients With Quiescent Cytomegalovirus Retinitis and Elevated CD4+ Counts

Vrabec TR, Baldassano VF, Whitcup SM (Thomas Jefferson Univ, Philadelphia; Temple Univ, Philadelphia; Natl Eye Inst, Bethesda, Md)

Ophthalmology 105:1259-1264, 1998 5–16

Background.—Up to one fourth of patients with AIDS have cytomegalovirus (CMV) retinitis (CMVR). Highly active antiretroviral therapy (HAART), which includes proteinase inhibitors combined with nucleoside analog antiretroviral agents, has been reported to increase CD4+ T-lymphocyte counts and to reduce HIV load in some patients. Whether maintenance treatment can be discontinued safely in patients with quiescent CMVR and increased CD4+ counts after HAART was investigated.

Methods.—Eight HIV-positive patients with quiescent CMVR treated by HAART were studied. All had CD4+ counts exceeding 100 cells/μL and elected to stop anti-CMV maintenance therapy. Twelve previously affected eyes in the 8 patients were assessed repeatedly for recurrent retinitis. Biweekly to monthly indirect ophthalmoscopy and fundus photography were done, along with monthly to quarterly CD4+ counts and quarterly HIV viral load testing.

Findings.—During a mean follow-up of 11.4 months, none of the patients had retinitis reactivation or progression. No CMVR developed in any of the previously unaffected eyes. In all patients, CD4+ levels remained increased. Viral load ranged from undetectable to 139,000 copies.

Conclusions.—Patients may consider discontinuing maintenance treatment if they have (1) HAART-induced increased CD4+ counts exceeding 100 cells/μL, (2) prolonged relapse-free intervals during reconstitution before CD4+ counts rise to more than 100 cells/μL, and (3) completely quiescent retinitis characterized by retinal pigment epithelial scarring only. Potential benefits include a decrease in the risks of drug toxicity and drug-resistant organisms. Close surveillance for evidence of recurrent retinitis is warranted.

▶ Ten years ago the diagnosis of CMVR visited on the afflicted patient certain death within several months, independent of the catastrophic visual loss it also created. Much has changed in the treatment of AIDS-related infections and HIV in general over the last decade. Aggressive systemic therapies aimed at controlling viral load have become popular. This entails the use of combination drugs with different modes of action to combat HIV. HAART combines the use of protease inhibitors with nucleoside antiretrovirals. One consequence of this treatment has been the elevation of CD4+ counts in many individuals above levels where opportunistic infections such as CMVR occur. The question is whether these T cells are functional.

This report by Vrabec and colleagues gives us hope that indeed they are, at least in some patients. However, this enthusiasm needs to be tempered by caution. Patients should have CD4+ counts greater than 100 cells/μL, prolonged CMVR-free periods during the time T-cell counts are rising on

HAART, and quiescent retinitis on detailed funduscopic examination prior to cessation of CMV therapy.

The benefits to patient lifestyle, cost, and increasing drug resistance, as well as the avoidance of significant systemic side effects, make this an important and exciting development.

J.I. Maguire, M.D.

Laser Chorioretinal Venous Anastomosis for Nonischemic Central Retinal Vein Occlusion

Browning DJ, Antoszyk AN (Charlotte Eye, Ear, Nose, and Throat Associates, NC; Uniformed Services Health Sciences Univ, Bethesda, Md)

Ophthalmology 105:670-679, 1998 5–17

Objective.—Patients with central retinal vein occlusion (CRVO) sometimes have severe visual loss. None of the many proposed treatment approaches has been effective. The exception is a laser-induced chorioretinal venous anastomotic technique, reported to be effective in one third of cases in 1 study. This technique was tried in 8 patients to see whether the results could be replicated by another group of surgeons.

Methods.—The authors attempted laser chorioretinal anastomosis in 8 eyes of 8 consecutive patients with CRVO. All patients had nonischemic but progressively worsening CRVO, with none having afferent pupillary defect or perfusion defects in the midperiphery on fluorescein angiography. All had decreased vision as a result of macular edema. All eyes were treated using the argon laser, according to the technique of McAllister and Constable. The patients were studied for a median of 11 months.

Results.—Two of twenty attempted anastomoses were successful, but neither of these produced a therapeutic response. There were 3 patients with rubeosis, retinal neovascularization at the laser treatment site, and vitreous hemorrhage. There were 2 cases of traction retinal detachment and 1 of neovascular glaucoma. Three patients underwent secondary panretinal photocoagulation, 1 had pars plana vitrectomy, and 1 had glaucoma seton. Two patients had improvements in visual acuity, despite the lack of successful anastomosis. The remaining 6 patients—including both of those with successful anastomoses—all had unchanged or worsening vision.

Conclusions.—This experience does not replicate the initial report of good responses to laser chorioretinal anastomosis for CRVO. Even when anastomosis is successfully carried out, vision may not improve, and successful anastomosis may be followed by conversion to ischemic CRVO, leading to an elevated risk of ocular neovascularization. Laser chorioretinal anastomosis may be a high-risk, low-efficacy procedure.

► In 1995, McAllister and Constable reported a technique for the treatment of nonischemic CRVO with chorioretinal anastomosis created by high energy focused laser delivery. This involved the rupture of Bruch's membrane with the penetration of both retinal and choroidal veins. The technique has been shown to be successful in reversing the vision-robbing effects of progressive cystoid macular edema in selected individuals with progressive nonischemic CRVO. However, for Browning and colleagues these results were not reproducible, and treatment was associated with significant side effects. Three major points are emphasized regarding effects of laser anastomosis: (1) even successfully developed anastomosis did not lead to visual improvement; (2) eyes with CRVO and successfully developed anastomosis may still develop ischemic CRVO; and (3) the rate of anterior segment neovascularization development is higher in nonischemic CRVOs subjected to laser anastomosis attempts. Such observations, and other well-recognized complications like vitreous hemorrhage, proliferative retinopathy, and retinal detachment, should lead one to employ such a technique judiciously. As always, exacting informed consent is mandatory.

J.I. Maguire, M.D.

6 Oculoplastic Surgery

Evolving Trends in Oculoplastics

by Robert B. Penne, M.D.

Keeping up with the latest trends in a field involves continuous evaluation of new products and techniques. Meetings, exhibits, and journals all allow for the evaluation of new trends, but each does so in a different way. Exhibitors show the latest and newest, but the quality of this information can be highly variable. Information presented at a meeting is more likely to be of high quality. A well-referred journal should offer the highest quality, but the speed of passing on new ideas may suffer.

Evaluating trends continues to be one of my aims in this chapter. I find one of the best ways to evaluate what is working, and what is not, is through informal discussions with colleagues at the hospital, during meetings, or over the phone. One-to-one discussions give me the real story on a product. This type of frank evaluation may not be given if 300 people are listening to a formal lecture. Although this introduction is not a one-to-one discussion, I will try to outline the trends that have changed in oculoplastics this past year.

The new products at oculoplastics meetings seem to be new materials used to rebuild lids and orbits, and to cover implants. The trend is away from using banked human tissue. New ways of processing human dermis have been developed that leave a collagen and extracellular protein matrix as a graft. This works well in place of fascia, sclera, hard palate, or buccal mucosal grafts. It saves the patients significant postoperative oral discomfort. Amniotic membrane is another tissue material that has been introduced. Its potential uses for corneal reconstruction have become well known. The potential for reconstruction of scarring diseases of the lids may be just beginning. Time will tell the usefulness of these products.

Some concepts and ideas that were popular continue to see their use on the decline. Laser dacryocystorhinostomy (DCR) surgery is being used less and less. Studies continue to show a much lower success rate with this than with traditional external DCR. There are still some indications for this, especially associated with DCR failure, but these are few.

While still commonly used, skin resurfacing is no longer seen as the perfect way to resurface skin. There are significant potential side effects and complications. This will remain a valuable tool for the cosmetic surgeon, but it will find its place next to the various facial peels, lifts, and implants. The initial swell of enthusiasm that often accompanies the hype of a new product is gone. This was evidenced at a recent oculoplastics meeting. Two years ago, the crowd around the laser resurfacing booths was huge. This year, the booths were much smaller; you could walk right up to the lasers.

Some trends that were new in the last few years have become accepted standard procedures. The balloon dacryoplasty for partial nasolacrimal obstruction appears to have a success rate as high as 80%. Recent investigation suggests that the procedure without placement of a silicone tube may be as successful as with silicone intubation. Porous polypropylene implants continue to be popular and are now available in different shapes.

One disease entity that has undergone significant changes in its management is thyroid-related ophthalmopathy (TRO).[1] The usefulness of orbital irradiation has been suggested for years but only recently has it's use become widespread. In my practice, orbital irradiation has made a large improvement in the management of TRO. The severity of disease is less, and thus the rehabilitative surgery is less. No large prospective study has been completed to prove this, but they are underway. Partially because of the need for smaller decompression in TRO, decompression surgery itself is changing.

The selected articles that follow attempt to give a glimpse at the changing ideas, technologies, and procedures presented in the literature over the past year. Which of these prove valuable, only time will tell.

Reference

1. Bartalena L, Marcocci C, Bogazzi F, et al: Relation between therapy for hyperthyroidism and the course of Graves' ophthalmopathy. *N Engl J Med* 338:73-78, 1998.

Relation Between Therapy for Hyperthyroidism and the Course of Graves' Ophthalmopathy

Bartalena L, Marcocci C, Bogazzi F, et al (Univ of Pisa, Italy; Natl Research Council, Pisa, Italy)

N Engl J Med 338:73-78, 1998 6–1

Objective.—The effects of radioiodine therapy for treatment of hyperthyroidism in Graves' ophthalmopathy are unknown. Results of a prospective, randomized study of the effects of the treatment of Graves' hyperthyroidism with methimazole or radioiodine therapy, and the effects of corticosteroids in patients with mild or moderate Graves' ophthalmopathy or none at all, are presented.

Methods.—After 3 or 4 months of treatment with methimazole, 443 patients with Graves' disease were randomly allocated to receive radioiodine therapy (120-150 μCi) for 18 months, radioiodine therapy plus prednisone (0.4-0.5 mg/kg) for 3 months, or continuing methimazole.

Ocular examinations were performed every 2 months. Thyroid function was assessed every 1 or 2 months for 1 year. Hypothyroidism or persistent hyperthyroidism was corrected.

Results.—Within 6 months, ophthalmopathy developed or worsened in 23 (15%) of 150 patients treated with radioiodine alone. Smokers were significantly more likely than nonsmokers to have ophthalmopathy or worsened ophthalmopathy (83% vs 50%). In the 145 patients treated with radioiodine plus prednisone, 50 of 75 patients (66.7%) with ophthalmopathy at baseline had regression, and those without ophthalmopathy at baseline did not change. Of the 148 patients receiving methimazole, 3 (2%) with ophthalmopathy improved, 4 (3%) had new or worsened ophthalmopathy, and 141 (95%) had no change. The frequency of development or progression in the radioiodine group was significantly higher than in either the radioiodine-prednisone group or the methimazole group.

Conclusion.—Patients with Graves' hyperthyroidism, treated with radioiodine only, may show new or worsened ophthalmopathy to a greater extent than patients treated with methimazole. The ophthalmopathy is transient and regresses or can be prevented with prednisone therapy.

▶ This is an important study for anyone involved in the treatment of thyroid-related ophthalmopathy (TRO). This was a prospective, randomized study looking at the effect of various treatments of hyperthyroidism on the eye disease. The study compared the results of using for radioactive iodine vs. medical treatment of hyperthyroidism with those using methimazole. This debate has raged for years. Some studies have shown there is no difference in the type of treatment for hyperthyroidism and how it affects TRO. A few studies have shown worsening of TRO with use of radioiodine. This study is by no means the last word on this subject, but it is a good study and certainly puts weight on the side of radioiodine alone worsening TRO.

There are a lot of details to consider in this study. One theme that is recurrent from other studies is that smokers have more frequent and more severe TRO. This once again emphasizes the need to get these patients to stop smoking. Patients who received radioiodine had a 15% incidence of worsening of their disease. This was only 3% in the methimazole-treated patients. However, if patients received systemic prednisone with radioiodine, none worsened and 67% improved. Only 3% of methimazole patients improved. It is not surprising that systemic prednisone improved TRO or was protective from worsening. The difference between 15% worsening with radioiodine and 3% with methimazole is the real significant finding.

We still lack a huge amount of knowledge concerning systemic thyroid abnormalities and TRO. This will be refined as research continues. For now, any patient receiving radioiodine with TRO needs to be aware of the increased risk of worsening their disease. The option of systemic steroids needs to be considered as it appears protective in these patients and particularly in those patients with other risk factors, such as smoking. The total treatment of 3 months with steroid is fairly long for some people and may evoke some adverse effects. We still lack the knowledge on why these patients get a worsening of their TRO. How radiation to the orbits, which is now used often, may affect this worsening is another of many questions that needs to be answered.

R.B. Penne, M.D.

Prospective Randomized Comparison of External Dacryocystorhinostomy and Endonasal Laser Dacryocystorhinostomy

Hartikainen J, Grenman R, Puukka P, et al (Univ of Turku, Finland; Social Insurance Institution, Turku, Finland)
Ophthalmology 105:1106-1113, 1998 6–2

Background.—Endonasal laser dacryocystorhinostomy (ENL-DCR), introduced in the early 1990s, showed promise as a minimally invasive procedure. The efficacy and safety of this treatment were compared with that of traditional external dacryocystorhinostomy (EXT-DCR).

Methods.—Sixty-one patients with primary acquired nasolacrimal sac or duct obstruction in a total of 64 eyes were first classified by symptoms (simple epiphora or chronic dacryocystitis), then randomly assigned within symptom groups to EXT-DCR or ENL-DCR. Silicone tubes were removed 6 months after surgery. Patients were followed up for 1 year. Lacrimal passage patency was investigated by irrigation.

Findings.—At 1 year after surgery, success rates were 91% for EXT-DCR and 63% for ENL-DCR after primary surgery, a significant difference. Duration of the ENL-DCR procedure was 3 times shorter than that of EXT-DCR, with means of 23 and 78 minutes, respectively (Table 4).

Conclusions.—Currently, EXT-DCR is more successful than ENL-DCR for patients with primary-acquired nasolacrimal sac or duct obstruction. In addition, more frequent postoperative visits are needed after ENL-DCR to clean mucus and debris intranasally at the site of the rhinostomy. However, many patients prefer ENL-DCR because it avoids cutaneous wounding. The efficacy of ENL-DCR will increase as new techniques are developed and more experience is gained.

TABLE 4.—Symptoms at 12 Months Postoperatively by Questionnaire With Reference to Patency to Irrigation

	External Dacryocystorhinostomy			Endonasal Laser Dacryocystorhinostomy		
	No.	(%)	Patent to Irrigation	No.	(%)	Patent to Irrigation
Asymptomatic	27/32	(84)	25/27	19/32	(59)	19/19
Watering indoors	2/32	(6)	1/2	11/32	(34)	1/11
Watering outdoors	5/32	(16)	4/5	13/32	(41)	1/13
Discharge	1/32	(3)	0/1	7/32	(22)	0/7

Abbreviation: No., number of patients.

(Published courtesy of *Ophthalmology*, from Hartikainen J, Grenman R, Puukka P, et al: Prospective randomized comparison of external dacryocystorhinostomy and endonasal laser dacryocystorhinostomy. *Ophthalmology* 105:1106-1113, 1998.)

▶ There has been ongoing debate between external and internasal-laser DCR surgery for years. Despite many papers touting the success of ENL-DCR surgery, this is the first prospective, randomized study comparing these approaches. Proponents of EXT-DCR will hail this as proof that ENL-DCR is much less successful, and indeed, that is what this study says. The flip side is there are many variations in approaches to laser DCR surgery, and whether this study used the best laser techniques is debatable.

The success rate of 91% for EXT-DCR versus 63% for ENL-DCR is a huge difference. This is the reason that many surgeons have moved away from the ENL-DCR as their primary choice. I feel it is tough to justify an internal approach when the success rate is so much worse. Another difference between the 2 procedures that was surprising to me was the operating time. The EXT-DCR took 78 minutes with the laser taking 23 minutes. One disadvantage to ENL-DCR in my mind was that it always took longer. All my experience has been with oculoplastic surgeons doing the endoscopic surgery, so I could understand that a more experienced endoscopic surgeon could take less time. I am surprised at the very long time for the EXT-DCR. I would think 30 to 40 minutes would be an average.

ENL-DCR also required a higher number of follow-up visits to clean out the nasal ostium or for other problems. My experience is similar, and I find laser surgery requires more postoperative care.

This study certainly suggests that EXT-DCR is superior to ENL-DCR. Whether this holds true for other laser approaches such as a transcanalicular approach remains to be shown. For now this certainly suggests that EXT-DCR should be chosen over ENL-DCR for routine cases of complete dacryostenosis.

R.B. Penne, M.D.

Intervention Within Days for Some Orbital Floor Fractures: The White-eyed Blowout

Jordan DR, Allen LH, White J, et al (Univ of Ottawa Eye Inst, Ont; Univ of Western Ontario, London; Univ of Saskatchewan, Saskatoon; et al)

Ophthal Plast Reconstr Surg 14:379-390, 1998 6–3

Background.—Management of orbital blowout fractures is controversial. Treatment varies from conservative treatment for 4 to 6 months to a waiting period of 2 weeks before beginning treatment. The authors have encountered a group of patients younger than 16 years old who have sustained blows to the periocular area but who have little or no evidence of soft tissue trauma (i.e., a white eye, diplopia with restricted vertical gaze, no enophthalmos, and minimal or no radiologic signs of bone displacement). These patients sometimes have signs of tissue herniation into the maxillary sinus. The authors have termed these cases "white-eyed blowouts."

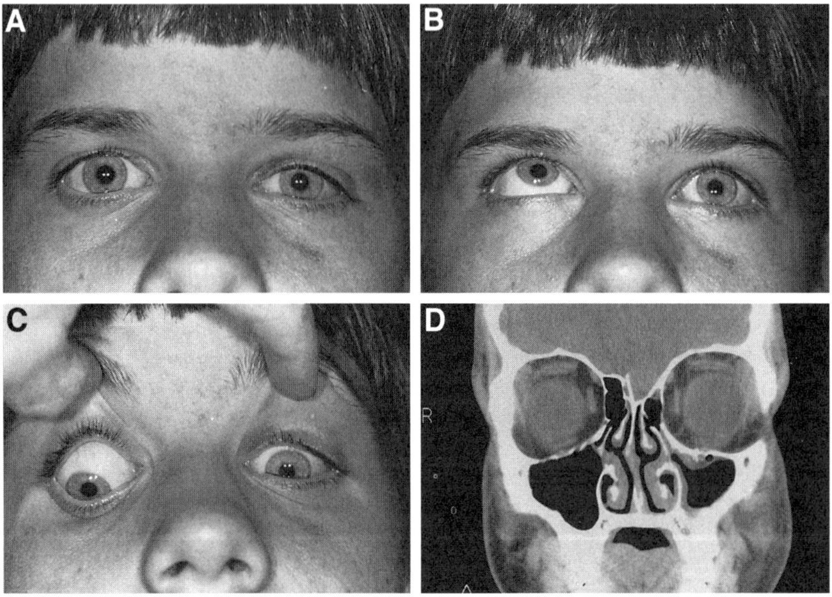

FIGURE 1.—A, a 14-year-old after a fist blow with minimal sign of injury; B, upgaze restriction; C, downgaze restriction; D, CT scan results reveal a small crack on the floor with a small teardrop sign. (Courtesy of Jordan DR, Allen LH, White J, et al: Intervention within days for some orbital floor fractures: The white-eyed blowout. *Ophthal Plast Reconstr Surg* 14:379-390, 1998. Copyright American Society of Ophthalmic Plastic & Reconstructive Surgery.)

Methods.—In a retrospective study, the medical records of patients with floor fractures with minimal signs of soft tissue trauma, diplopia with restriction of gaze, and lack of enophthalmos were reviewed. Patient age, nature of injury, clinical examination, results of CT scan, timing of surgery, reoperation necessitated, and postoperative course were recorded.

Results.—The review identified 20 patients with the "white-eyed blowout." All patients were between 4 and 18 years old. The nature of the injury included a blow from a fist, elbow, knee, or head; falls; and motor vehicle accidents. Clinical examination results showed few signs of soft tissue trauma, even in cases of significant blows to the periocular area. All patients reported diplopia with restriction in up-and-down gaze, and some patients reported pain when attempting vertical gaze. There was no enophthalmos. In most patients, CT results showed a small crack on the floor or a "trap door" type of defect with little bone displacement (Fig 1). Some patients had slight tissue herniation. Surgery was performed from 48 hours to 40 days after injury. Of the 20 patients, 6 had surgery within 4 days of injury, and 5 of these had resolution of symptoms between 3 and 6 weeks after surgery. None of these patients had permanent restriction. Among the other 14 patients, surgery was performed between 5 and 40 days after injury. Three of these patients had resolution of symptoms within 4 weeks. Of the other 11 patients, 8 patients had slow resolution of signs and symptoms from 4 to 10 months, and 3 patients had continued restriction at 12 months. The patients who had surgery at 2 to 3 weeks after injury had slower resolution of symptoms, and some of them had permanent restriction. Reoperation was performed in 4 of 20 patients at 2 to 4 weeks. Two of these patients still had impaired extraocular motility at 12 months, 1 patient had resolution of restriction by 12 months, and 1 patient had almost complete recovery at 8 months.

Discussion.—Early treatment of "white-eyed blowouts" is recommended because there is little benefit to a 2-week waiting period and because such a waiting period may harm the patient's motility. Surgery is recommended within a few days of injury to help prevent permanent motility restriction.

▶ The timing of surgery for repair of orbital fractures remains a controversial subject. The search for a single approach to all fractures has lead to this problem. Not all fractures are the same nor can they be treated the same. By separating orbital floor fractures into subsets, the timing of treatment makes more sense and is more effective.

The authors have chosen an important subset of orbital fractures to look at and discuss treatment. These are small fractures with minimal swelling and significant restriction. The muscle is tightly trapped in this small "trapdoor" fracture. The restriction in this case will not get better, and delay in repair may result in permanent ischemia or additional scarring of the muscle. Early repair of this subset of fractures is important. I do not believe repair within 2 to 4 days is an absolute requirement, but treatment within a week is more desirable than waiting 2 weeks.

A second theme that comes from this paper is the need to individually evaluate and treat all fractures. Most fractures do not require this "early surgery," and many will not need surgical repair at all. Small fractures only need repair if there is diplopia. If there is a lot of swelling and diplopia, then observation for improvement in the diplopia as the swelling resolves is indicated. The time should be at least 2 weeks but sometimes longer if there is continuing improvement and little CT evidence of entrapment and the swelling is still present.

Larger fractures are less likely to have entrapment but may need to be repaired to prevent development of enophthalmos. Observation for up to 2 to 3 weeks as the swelling improves, especially if the diplopia is minimal, is warranted. Entrapment without improvement needs repair within 2 weeks. If the development of enophthalmos is not definite with moderately large fractures and there is no entrapment, observation with late repair is reasonable.

Education about various types of orbital floor fractures is important, and this paper does a good job. Becoming aware of the need to get patients seen for potential repair as soon as possible is the greatest educational goal this paper provides.

R.B. Penne, M.D.

Involutional Lower Lid Entropion: To Shorten or Not to Shorten?

Danks JJ, Rose GE (Moorfields Eye Hosp, London)

Ophthalmology 105:2065-2067, 1998 6–4

Background.—In older adults, involutional entropion of the lower eyelid, often with manifest horizontal laxity, is common. There are several etiologic factors, including horizontal lid laxity, vertical lid laxity with attenuation or disinsertion of lower lid retractors, and overriding of preseptal orbicularis muscle. Although a low recurrence rate is seen after surgical procedures that address all of these factors, the effect of horizontal eyelid laxity is unknown. The cure rate of involutional lower lid entropion with or without horizontal eyelid shortening was examined.

Methods.—In a retrospective study, 583 cases of entropion surgery were identified. The cases of patients with involutional entropion and sufficient follow-up information were evaluated.

Results.—Of 313 primary procedures, 180 included horizontal shortening. Of these 180 patients, cure was achieved in 178 (99%). Of the 133 patients who did not have horizontal shortening, cure was achieved in 104 (78%). Of 47 reoperations for recurrent entropion or consecutive ectropion, 28 included horizontal shortening. Of these 28 patients, cure was achieved in 28 (100%). Of the other 19 patients who did not have horizontal shortening, cure was achieved in 12 (63%) (Table 1).

Discussion.—In these patients, the incidence rate of recurrent malposition of the eyelid was significantly higher in patients who did not have horizontal eyelid shortening at the time of primary operation or reoperation for recurrence or overcorrection. Surgical correction without horizontal eyelid shortening probably does not have a role in the treatment of age-related entropion because horizontal laxity may be the primary pathogenic factor of this condition.

▶ There are many different approaches to entropion surgery. Most of these techniques include some form of horizontal shortening. Simpler techniques, such as Quickert sutures, can easily be done in the office, but do not address

TABLE 1.—Surgical Success for Involutional Lower Lid Entropion, With Respect to Horizontal Shortening at Primary or Re-do Surgery

	Type of Surgery			
	Primary Surgery		Reoperation	
Outcome	Not Shortened (133 Cases)	Shortened (180 Cases)	Not Shortened (19 Cases)	Shortened (28 Cases)
Success	104 (78%)	178 (99%)	12 (63%)	28 (100%)
Failure				
Recurrence	11 (8%)	1 (<1%)	4 (21%)	0
Overcorrection	18 (14%)	1 (<1%)	3 (16%)	0
Fisher's exact test	$P < 0.001$		$P < 0.001$	

(Published courtesy of *Ophthalmology*, from Danks JJ, Rose GE: Involutional lower lid endotropion. *Ophthalmology* 105:2065-2067, 1998.)

horizontal laxity. It is generally accepted that procedures without horizontal shortening are less effective. This simple, retrospective study confirms that procedures that include horizontal shortening have a much lower rate of recurrence of the entropion when compared with procedures that do not shorten the lid.

I rarely do a procedure for a noncicatricial entropion that does not include horizontal shortening. On occasion, I will treat a patient in the hospital or office with an entropion and I will place Quickert sutures (this involves no horizontal shortening and is not the "Quickert" procedure referred to in the paper) as a temporary treatment. For some of these patients, this form of repair may be long lasting. Because it is so simple, I sometimes wonder if it should be used more. This study shows the much higher failure rate if eyelids are not horizontally shortened. Because lid laxity is probably the main factor in the development of the entropion, it follows that not addressing this factor would result in a higher failure rate.

There are many different procedures to choose from in repairing entropions. Many of the older and "simpler" procedures do not shorten the eyelid. From this study, any procedure that does not shorten a lax lid that is entropic must be viewed as less than optimal and should only be done as a potentially temporizing procedure when horizontal shortening is unable to be done safely.

R.B. Penne, M.D.

Modified Levator Aponeurotic Advancement With Delayed Postoperative Office Revision

Mauriello JA Jr, Abdelsalam A (UMD-New Jersey Med School, Newark)

Ophthal Plast Reconstr Surg 14:266-270, 1998 6–5

Objective.—The optimum timing for early revision of aponeurotic repair is controversial, with recommendations varying from 3 days to 2 weeks. Results of 8- to 14-day delayed office revision are retrospectively reviewed.

Methods.—Between February 1989 and November 1994, modified levator advancement was performed on 122 eyelids in 110 patients.

> *Technique.*—After a lid crease incision and mobilization of the skin-orbicularis muscle flap, the orbital septum is incised, and a cotton-tip applicator is introduced into the space occupied by the preaponeurotic fat pad between the orbital septum and the levator aponeurosis. A strip of orbicularis oculi muscle just above the upper tarsal border is excised with a hand-held cautery. The underlying Müller muscle is exposed, and the edge of the levator is advanced. The edge of the levator is stitched with three 6-0 silk sutures to adjust the position of the upper eyelid.

Results.—Of 110 patients who had modified levator advancement surgery, 5 required revision of undercorrection that varied from 2.0 to 2.5 mm. Four underwent revision between 8 and 14 days after surgery. Patients were followed for an average of 31 months, and all had excellent results. Two patients had a transient granuloma at the site of a suture.

Conclusion.—Delaying revision of aponeurotic repair for 8 to 14 days allows time for resolution of postoperative edema and leads to excellent results.

▶ There are many different approaches to ptosis surgery. The small details such as type of suture, placement of suture, and type of local used vary greatly among surgeons. Most ptosis surgeons have developed a technique that works well for them. The technical aspect of the surgery is the easy part. The judgment on where exactly to set the lid is the difficult part. Swelling, bleeding, levator function, and healing—among other factors—make each case different. No matter how hard we try to make rigid rules for levator surgery, including how much to lift the lid, they do not hold. There will always be judgment and uncertainty involved.

Every surgeon will have a certain number of cases that will require postoperative adjustment. How and when that is done is also variable, depending on the surgeon. I prefer to see my patients with ptosis 5 to 7 days after surgery. At that time, any needed adjustment can often be made without anesthesia as the lid still has some postoperative anesthesia, especially the lid skin. There is some healing, but the tissues can usually be separated with a cotton-tip applicator. This makes revision of overcorrection very simple. Undercorrection still will require sutures and, likely, some local anesthesia. My experience has been that at 14 days after surgery, the wounds are much better healed, and the dissection is difficult and produces more bleeding.

I have also tried the procedure with and without epinephrine for my local block. I found that the increased bleeding produced when not using epinephrine made the case much more difficult. As my own technique, I have adjusted where I set the final lid height to compensate for the use of epinephrine. I cannot really say how much more I lift the lid, but my approach works for me. Use of the needle bovie or CO_2 laser may make the bleeding less, but I still use epinephrine in my block.

R.B. Penne, M.D.

Changes in Astigmatism After Ptosis Surgery Measured by Corneal Topography

Holck DEE, Dutton JJ, Wehrly SR (Wilford Hall Med Ctr, San Antonio, Tex; Duke Univ, Durham, NC; MacDill AFB Hosp, Tampa, Fla)

Ophthal Plast Reconstr Surg 14:151-158, 1998 6–6

Background.—Changes in astigmatism after ptosis surgery have been reported. The current study used a computerized topographic analysis system to determine the effects of ptosis surgery on corneal topography.

Methods.—Corneal astigmatic changes were assessed after blepharoptosis surgery on 29 eyelids in 22 patients. Fifteen untreated eyelids undergoing unilateral ptosis repair made up a control group. All patients were assessed before and 6 weeks after surgery. In addition, 15 surgically treated eyelids and 5 control lids were evaluated 12 months after treatment to determine the stability of these measurements.

Findings.—At 6 weeks after surgery, corneal topography showed increased with-the-rule astigmatism in 72.4% of surgically treated eyes, increased against-the-rule astigmatism in 13.8% of treated eyes, and no change in 13.8% of treated eyes. None of the control eyes showed changes in corneal astigmatic axis or significant change in central corneal power. By 12 months after surgery, all surgically treated eyes showed a regression toward the amount and pattern of preoperative astigmatism. Only 2 of 15 eyes maintained a difference of more than 0.3 D of central corneal power greater than their preoperative measurement at 1 year.

Conclusions.—Steepening of the superior cornea can occur after ptosis repair, which is probably a cause of the blurred vision commonly reported after such surgery. However, these changes tend to regress over time. Few patients will require permanent changes in refractive correction.

▶ The message of this article is that corneal astigmatic changes are common after ptosis surgery. This was a simple study, which measured corneal topography before ptosis surgery, 6 weeks after surgery, and (in 5 patients) 1 year after surgery. The astigmatic changes are shown, however, how these changes affected visual acuity is not mentioned. This is a major omission, because the amount of astigmatic change does not always correlate with changes in vision. Snellen's visual acuity test would have been helpful, but even mention of subjective change in vision would have added valuable information. This study could have been improved from that aspect and with longer follow-up of these patients after ptosis surgery.

This article does make everyone aware of the astigmatic changes that can occur with ptosis surgery. It is well recognized that ptosis and ptosis surgery can change the astigmatism in children, but this is less well recognized in adults. Most of these changes have resolved by 6 weeks after surgery. Often when we see patients in the first week after ptosis surgery and they complain of blurring, we blame this on tear film changes or the use of ointment. We now have another cause of this blurring but, except in very unusual cases, the cure is the same:*observation*.

A study of the effect of other upper or lower eyelid surgery on corneal astigmatism and how it effects vision may show similar changes. Much of the blurred vision that we routinely blame on tear film changes could actually be astigmatic changes.

R.B. Penne, M.D.

Blepharospasm: Past, Present, and Future

Anderson RL, Patel BCK, Holds JB, et al (Univ of Utah, Salt Lake City; Anheuser-Busch Eye Inst, St Louis; Ottawa Gen Hosp, Ont)

Ophthal Plast Reconstr Surg 14:305-317, 1998 6–7

Objective.—Blepharospasm encompasses a variety of eyelid and facial spasms, but the greatest disability occurs to patients with eyelid spasms (Fig 2). A history and causes of blepharospasm were presented, and the efficacy of full myectomy, botulinum-A toxin, oral drugs, and help from the Benign Essential Blepharospasm Research Foundation (BEBRF) were evaluated retrospectively by patient questionnaire.

Methods.—Questionnaires were mailed to 4,000 patients with blepharospasm treated before 1988, and 41% (1,653) responded.

Results.—Causes are varied. Eyelid malpositioning as a result of chronic forceful squeezing tends to exacerbate the problem. Subjective improvement remains the best indicator of treatment efficacy. Help from the BEBRF benefitted 90% of patients, and the patient acceptance rate was 96%. Full myectomy benefitted 88%, with an acceptance rate of 82%. Botulinum-A toxin benefitted 86%, with an acceptance rate of 95%. Drug therapy benefitted 43%, with an acceptance rate of 57%. Treatment must be tailored to the patient; it is also important to treat the stress created by the condition and to provide familial and psychological support. Full myectomy is usually reserved for patients who fail botulinum A toxin and drug therapy. Limited myectomy can improve results in patients who also respond to botulinum A toxin.

Conclusion.—There appear to be multiple causes of blepharospasm. The condition is frequently misdiagnosed. Of the 4 main treatments available—drug therapy, botulinum A toxin, myectomy, and support from the BEBRF—the last has proven to be the most beneficial and has the highest level of patient satisfaction.

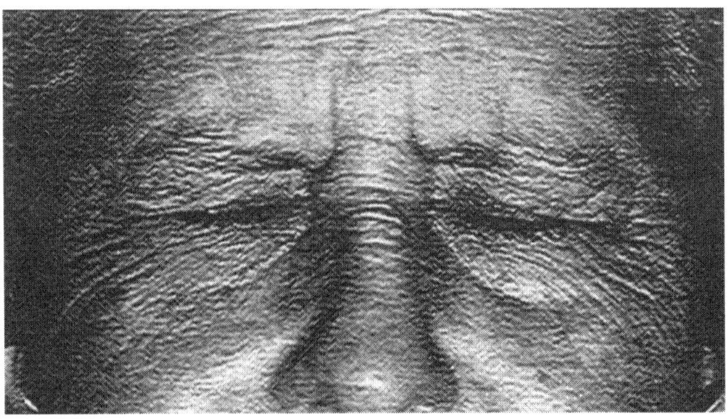

FIGURE 2.—Blepharospasm. Spasm only in eyelids. (Courtesy of Anderson RL, Patel PCK, Holds JB, et al: Blepharospasm: Past, present, and future. *Ophthal Plast Reconstr Surg* 14:305-317, 1998. Copyright American Society of Ophthalmic Plastic & Reconstructive Surgery.)

► This article provides a very good overview of the history of blepharospasm as well as the current thought on etiology and treatment. Anyone dealing with these patients will find this article worth reviewing. Blepharospasm and its treatment are very subjective. It is appropriate that the evaluation of treatments and their value for blepharospasm patients were done subjectively through a survey. This approach may not have as much scientific merit as prospective, masked studies, but this disease would not lend itself to any evaluation that did not have significant subjectivity.

The most valuable treatment for these patients was the resources of the BEBRF. The BEBRF provides patient education and support to help them understand and cope with this disease, which is often poorly understood by the public and very frustrating to the patient. The foundation is an important resource for all providers to be aware of.

Botulinum-A toxin injection was highly accepted but was not perfect and did not work for all patients. Myectomy was the most "permanent" of the treatments. It is especially helpful for patients who are not responsive to botulinum-A toxin. Drug therapy provided help to some patients but was not nearly as helpful as the above 3 approaches. The general feeling is that the spasm improvement was similar to the amount of generalized sedation, which is not well tolerated. Blepharospasm remains a poorly understood disease. It is evident that education and patient support must be a primary part of any successful treatment. This article makes an excellent attempt to summarize a disease process that remains extremely puzzling.

R.B. Penne, M.D.

Basal Cell Carcinoma of the Eyelids and Solar Ultraviolet Radiation Exposure

Lindgren G, Diffey BL, Larkö O (Sahlgrenska Univ Hosp, Gothenberg, Sweden; Newcastle Gen Hosp, England)

Br J Ophthalmol 82:1412-1415, 1998 6–8

Background.—Because the highest incidence of basal cell carcinoma is seen in countries with intense sunlight exposure, solar ultraviolet radiation exposure is believed to be an important factor in the cause of basal cell carcinoma. The risk of basal cell carcinoma is related to the length and pattern of exposure to ultraviolet radiation. The distribution of eyelid basal cell carcinoma was compared with the relative exposure to ultraviolet radiation at different sites on the eyelids.

Methods.—The location of basal cell carcinoma on the eyelids was evaluated in 319 patients with 329 tumors. There were 140 men, 189 women, and the median patient age was 73 years. The eyelid area was divided into 7 sites. Sunlight exposure was recorded with a polymer film attached to the eyelids in a manikin and in the human subjects.

Results.—Of the 329 tumors, 225 were on the lower eyelids and 87 were on the medial canthal regions. No association between doses of ultraviolet radiation at the 7 sites on the eyelids and location of basal cell carcinoma

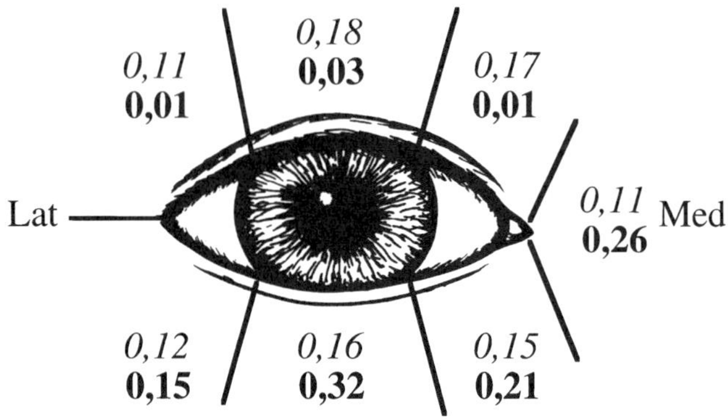

FIGURE 4.—Fraction of the total number of basal cell carcinomas (*bold*) and fraction of the total ultraviolet radiation (*italic*) at the 7 different sites of the eyelids (assuming that the areas are approximately the same size). The right and left eyes are combined. (Courtesy of Lindgren G, Diffey BL, Larkö O: Basal cell carcinoma of the eyelids and solar ultraviolet radiation exposure. *Br J Ophthalmol* 82:1412-1415, 1998. By permission of the B.J. Publishing Group.)

was found. The number of tumors on the lower eyelids outnumbered the number of tumors on the upper eyelids by a factor of 13, although measurements of ultraviolet radiation exposure showed that exposure to sunlight was similar on both the upper and lower eyelids (Fig 4).

Discussion.—Although basal cell carcinoma can develop in skin not exposed to ultraviolet radiation, there is strong evidence that ultraviolet radiation does have a role in this disease. The large difference between the number of tumors on the upper and lower eyelids is difficult to explain. These findings indicate that the cause of periorbital basal cell carcinoma is only partially explained by solar ultraviolet radiation exposure.

▶ This study attempts to correlate the location of periocular basal cell carcinoma with the amount of ultraviolet light each area receives. The results do not show good correlation in either the human or the manikin models.

The poor correlation may be because of the way the the ultraviolet light exposure was analyzed or because there are other unidentified factors that influence the development and location of basal cell carcinoma. The ultraviolet light exposure in manikins and humans showed some differences, but they achieved similar exposures to ultraviolet light. Thus, it is most likely that ultraviolet light plays a major role in the development of basal cell carcinoma but is not the only factor. Many unknown factors inherent to the skin and each individual may modulate the risk of development of basal cell carcinoma.

Clinically, there are many patients with significant sun exposure who never develop basal cell carcinoma. Likewise, patients with little sun exposure may develop basal cell carcinoma. These observations mirror the study results in that the amount of ultraviolet exposure is not the only factor in developing basal cell carcinoma.

This was an interesting study, but it does not give us any direct knowledge to help our patients. The study emphasizes how little we really do understand about this very common skin malignancy. We know that basal cells rarely occur on non–sun exposed areas, so avoiding ultraviolet exposure is still the best advice for prevention of basal cell carcinoma. Early detection and treatment are the second line of treatment.

R.B. Penne, M.D.

► Various lesions have a predilection for different parts of the eyelid. Xanthelasmas typically affect the skin of the inner canthi. Sebaceous carcinoma involves the upper eyelid in two thirds of cases, presumably reflecting the much greater mass of meibomian gland tissue in the upper lid. Basal cell carcinoma, which accounts for 80% to 90% of all eyelid malignancies, affects the lower eyelid.

Exposure to ultraviolet light is thought to play a major role in the pathogenesis of basal cell carcinoma. This study suggests that other factors must be involved. Although the incidence of basal cell carcinoma was 13 times greater in the lower lid than the upper lid, dosimetry studies showed that the upper lid actually received slightly more ultraviolet radiation.

R.C. Eagle, Jr., M.D.

Multiple Aesthetic Unit Flaps for Medial Canthal Reconstruction

Harris GJ, Logani SC (Med College of Wisconsin, Milwaukee)

Ophthal Plast Reconstr Surg 14:352-359, 1998 6–9

Objective.—Correction of defects involving the medial canthal region is aesthetically complicated because of the various anatomical units present. An approach is described that combines flaps from each of the aesthetic units anchored to the medial canthal tendon or associated deep fibrous tissue. This helps to maintain the normal concavity and minimize web formation.

Technique.—Aesthetic units are identified and component flaps are designed. These include an inverted V-Y flap for the glabellar component, a bilobed flap for the nasal sidewall component, advancement flaps in the upper and lower eyelids with relaxing incisions in the natural creases, advancement cheek flaps with relaxed skin tension-line incisions, and direct closure of brow defects. Flaps are anchored to the anterior limb of the medial canthal tendon or to the fibrous tissue above or below it.

Results.—This technique has been used in 58 patients to repair a variety of defects. Defects of the nasal sidewall and lower eyelid or cheek have been repaired with medially advanced cheek flaps and nasal skin (Fig 3). A small glabellar flap and a small V-Y or bilobed flap from the nasal sidewall

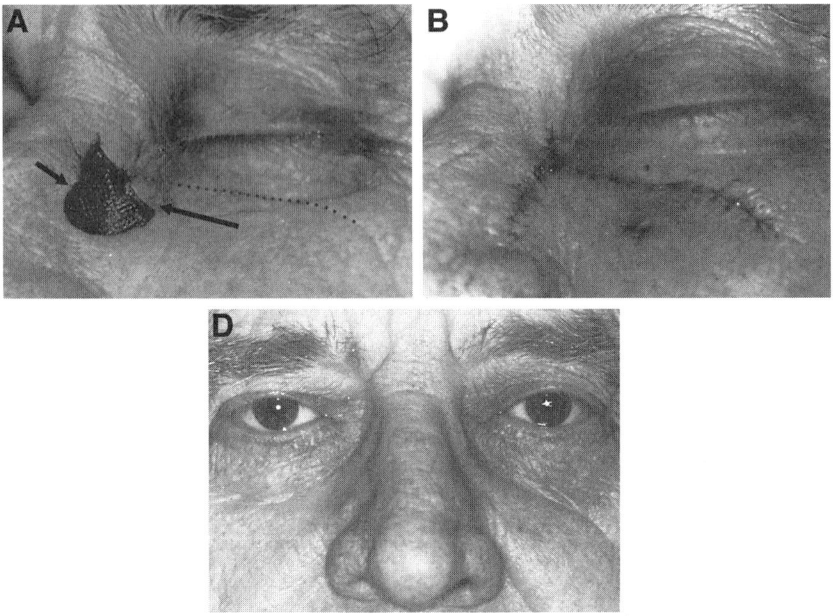

FIGURE 3.—A, the defect includes the nasal sidewall and lower eyelid/cheek. The nasal and cheek skin will each be advanced centrally (*arrows*) and anchored in deep fibrous tissue. B, flaps advanced. D, 4 months after surgery. (Courtesy of Harris GJ, Logani SC: Multiple aesthetic unit flaps for medial canthal reconstruction. *Ophthal Plast Reconstr Surg* 14:352-359, 1998. Copyright American Society of Ophthalmic Plastic & Reconstructive Surgery.)

is useful for reconstructing large medial canthal defects associated with recurrent tumors that have been treated by various methods (Fig 11).

Conclusion.—Flaps of various kinds individually designed to cover a specific component area and anchored to the medial canthal tendon or deep fibrous tissue above or below it minimize web formation and maintains normal concavity.

▶ The medial canthus is the second most common area for skin malignancies to occur around the eye. This area offers special challenges for reconstruction because of its concave contour. The approach separates the medial canthus into multiple areas to utilize multiple flaps. The fact that there are so many areas contributing to the medial canthus adds to the complexity of reconstruction. The article presents a unified approach to medial canthal defects and utilization of these multiple potential flaps. Having knowledge of the multiple flaps and the different approaches allows reconstruction of many varied defects. The defect size cannot always be accurately estimated before surgery. The knowledge of different approaches is valuable in reconstructing these defects.

I recommend reading this article in its entirety because of all the pictures. The techniques described are simple in themselves, but combining them in the appropriate manner is the challenge, but also the fun. Although I am not sure that these flaps are entirely unique, they do help contribute a solid

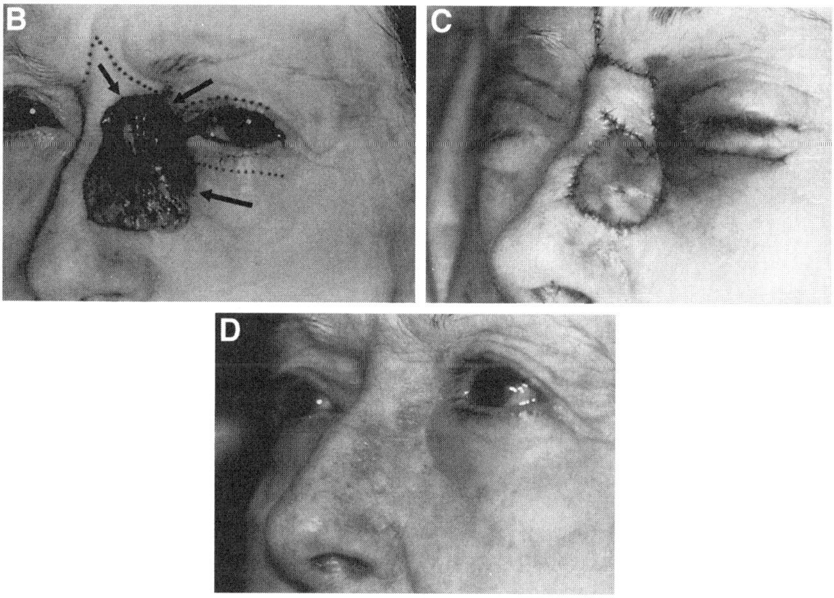

FIGURE 11.—B, The tumor-free defect involves all components of medial canthal region. The reconstructive plan includes upper eyelid flap, lower eyelid/cheek flap, glabellar flap, and full-thickness graft (*white arrow*). C, flaps transposed and graft placed. D, 8 months after surgery. (Courtesy of Harris GJ, Logani SC: Multiple aesthetic unit flaps for medial canthal reconstruction. *Ophthal Plast Reconstr Surg* 14:352-359, 1998. Copyright American Society of Ophthalmic Plastic & Reconstructive Surgery.)

approach to medial canthal reconstruction. I, for one, am always interested in any new ideas for reconstructing that unusual defect that I may see tomorrow.

R.B. Penne, M.D.

Long-term Results of Frontalis Suspension Using Irradiated, Banked Fascia Lata

Esmaeli B, Chung H, Pashby RC (Univ of Toronto)
Ophthal Plast Reconstr Surg 14:159-163, 1998 6–10

Background.—Frontalis suspension is the surgical treatment of choice in patients with blepharoptosis with poor or absent levator function. The long-term rate of recurrence of ptosis and other postoperative complications after frontalis suspension with banked irradiated fascia lata was determined.

Methods.—Seventy-two patients with a total of 132 affected lids underwent frontalis suspension between 1980 and 1989. Preoperative diagnoses were severe congenital ptosis in 83%, blepharophimosis in 10%, third nerve palsy in 4%, and chronic progressive external ophthalmoplegia in 3%. Mean age at the time of surgery was 3 years 5 months, with a range of 5 months to 19 years. Sixty-four percent of the patients underwent surgery before the age of 3 years. Mean follow-up was 10 years.

Findings.—In all but 3 patients, lid height was good to excellent immediately after surgery. Ptosis recurred in 21% of the eyelids. Mean time to reoperation was 3 years. Eighty percent of the patients with recurrence were younger than 3 years. Only 3% of the patients had reactions to donor fascia lata. One patient had excessive exposure keratopathy, necessitating sling revision.

Conclusions.—Banked fascia lata should be considered an alternative suspensory material for the treatment of congenital ptosis in children younger than 3 years. In the current series, the long-term reoperation rate was greater than that associated with autogenous fascia but lower than that associated with banked fascia lata.

► Correction of congenital ptosis with banked fascia has become a commonly performed procedure. The success of autogenous fascia vs. that of banked fascia has been debated for years. Banked fascia is much easier to obtain; however, it must be remembered that it is a banked tissue and, despite radiation treatment, there may be unknown risks. Most surgeons I know prefer banked fascia for congenital ptosis for most routine cases.

This study finds a 28% reoperation rate after correction of congenital ptosis with banked fascia in patients followed up for 10 years. There is a large variation in rates of reoperation when various studies are compared. These variations have multiple potential reasons, and one should not just assume it is the material used to correct the ptosis that accounts solely for this variation. Variables include surgical technique, the child's age, variability in fascia quality, and subjective variation in when and why to redo surgery. Parents may be happy to have their child's eyelid just above the pupil at age 1; however, when the child starts to school and is teased about the droopy lids, the decision may be made to operate again, even if very little has changed with respect to the lid position. There is no mention of the amount of correction of ptosis achieved with surgery or how far the lid fell before repeat surgery was performed. Without objective numbers in this study, it is difficult to compare studies of banked fascia vs. autogenous fascia.

What is needed is a study of congenital ptosis in which banked fascia is used in one lid and autogenous fascia in the other lid. Since congenital ptosis is often bilateral, this is a perfect setup. It makes sense that, with time, in a growing child there will be some failures of ptosis surgery. I think we need to be cautious about the exact cause of these failures and not make changes in our surgical technique until better proof is shown.

R.B. Penne, M.D.

Enhancement of the Cosmetic and Functional Outcome of Enucleation With the Conical Orbital Implant

Rubin PAD, Popham J, Rumelt S, et al (Massachusetts Eye and Ear Infirmary, Boston; Colorado Oculoplastics, Denver; Wills Eye Hosp, Philadelphia; et al)
Ophthalmology 105:919-925, 1998 6–11

Background.—Many attempts have been made over the years to improve the shape and composition of enucleation implants. A new design of a conical-shaped enucleation implant is discussed that helps to minimize the occurrence of superior sulcus defects and maximize prosthesis motility. (Figs 1 and 2).

Methods.—Forty-five patients, aged 13 to 75 years, were implanted with the new prosthesis. Thirty-nine had primary enucleations and 6, secondary implants. The implant, in the shape of a modified sphere, has a posterior conical projection that parallels the orbital walls, a superior projection supporting the soft tissues of the upper eyelid sulcus, a flattened anterior surface, and channels for each rectus muscle. In all primary and in 2 of the secondary placements, the anterior part of the implant was covered with autologous fascia. The remaining secondary implants were covered with a pseudocapsule harvested from the explanted primary implant. The prostheses were fit 6 to 10 weeks postoperatively.

Outcomes.—Forty-three patients had minimal or no superior sulcus defect. The other 2 patients had moderate defects. No severe sulcus defects

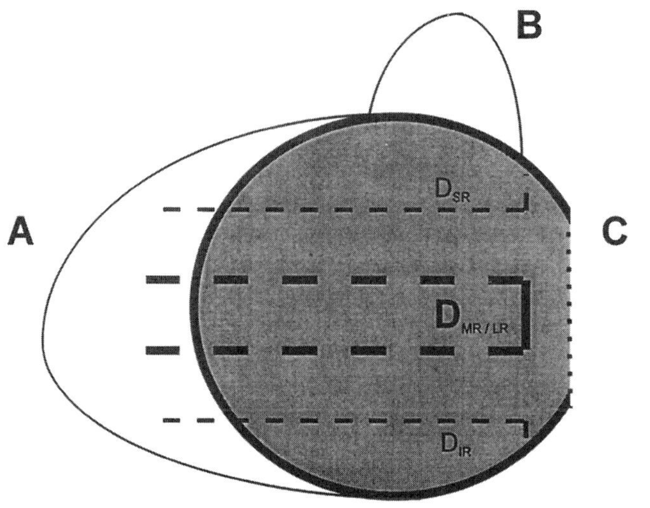

FIGURE 1.—Schematic of enucleation implant, sagittal view. The implant is a modification of a sphere. A posterior projection *A* parallels the orbital walls. A superior projection *B* provides support for the soft tissues of the superior sulcus. The front end of the implant is flattened *C* to ease conjunctival closure and to provide a broad area of contact with the overlying prosthesis. Channels for each rectus muscle *D* permit positioning of the extraocular muscles closer to the core of the implant. (Published courtesy of *Ophthalmology*, from Rubin PAD, Popham J, Rumelt S, et al: Enhancement of the cosmetic and functional outcome of enucleation with the conical orbital implant. *Ophthalmology* 105:919-925, 1998.)

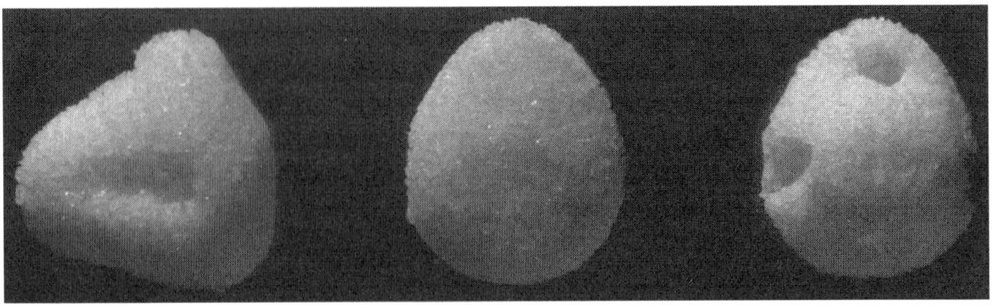

FIGURE 2.—Final prototype of implant. Lateral (*left*), anterior (*center*), and posterior (*right*) views. (Published courtesy of *Ophthalmology*, from Rubin PAD, Popham J, Rumelt S, et al: Enhancement of the cosmetic and functional outcome of enucleation with the conical orbital implant. *Ophthalmology* 105:919-925, 1998.)

occurred. All patients were satisfied with their appearance and did not seek further corrective procedures. In all patients, good prosthetic motility was achieved, with small-angle ductions and saccades. Two cases of conjunctival wound dehiscence occurred, both within 4 weeks of surgery. One required suturing, and the other healed spontaneously. No implant extrusions, migrations, or infections occurred.

Conclusions.—This conical orbital implant allows appropriate reconstitution of orbital volume. Superior sulcus defects are minimized, and prosthetic motility is adequate.

► During the past 8 to 10 years there have been a number of new porous implants introduced, and many are now in common usage. The advantages of porous implants are many. The spherical shape of these implants is a constant that has not changed. This is the first nonspherical implant introduced in the recent past.

The conical implant seeks to improve motility, improve the time of vascularization of the implant, and decrease the superior sulcus deformity. This is done by modification of the spherical shape of the implant. This can be seen in Figure 2.

The improved motility will be hard to prove. The actual documentation of motility of the prostheses is difficult to standardize. That along with the fact that only about 10% to 15% of patients have their implant drilled in the average practice make the need for more motility over what we have questionable. The real potential for advantage will be if there is less superior sulcus deformity. Superior sulcus deformities occur years after the enucleation so proof of effectiveness may take many years.

There are disadvantages to this implant. I do not cover my medpor implants nor do I directly suture the muscle to the implant. Both these steps are required with this implant and are added steps. The importance of orientation with this implant can also lead to potential problems.

Any change from the standard is at first perceived with skepticism. That is my reaction to this new implant. However, I think it is important to keep the idea of modification of the shape of the implant in mind as further evaluation is done. Years from now we may wonder why anyone would have ever used a spherical implant.

R.B. Penne, M.D.

Efficacy of Probing as Treatment of Epiphora in Adults With Blocked Nasolacrimal Ducts

Guinot-Saera A, Koay P (Darlington Mem Hosp, Darlington, England)

Br J Ophthalmol 82:389-391, 1998 6–12

Background.—Idiopathic or primary acquired nasolacrimal duct obstruction (NLDO), a syndrome of unknown origin, accounts for most NLDO in adults. Although probing is known to be an effective treatment for NLDO in young children, the risk of failure increases with age, doubling every 6 months. The efficacy of probing in the initial treatment of epiphora in adults with NLDO was investigated.

Methods.—Eighty-five eyes in 65 patients, aged 19-89, were treated. The probe was advanced to the point of obstruction and gently pushed through. Patency was confirmed by syringing. Mean follow-up was 7.4 months. Outcomes were determined by a patient questionnaire and interview.

Findings.—In 35% of the eyes, there was no watering after probing. Seventeen percent had mild watering; 35% had moderate watering; and 11% had severe watering. Eighty-two percent of the patients were satisfied with the results. The mean symptom-free period was 11.3 months in eyes with no watering, 8.2 months in eyes with mild watering, 5.4 months in eyes with moderate watering, and 1 month in eyes with severe watering. The symptom-free period between eyes with no watering and those with severe watering was significant.

Conclusions.—Probing can be recommended as the initial treatment for NLDO in adults. This procedure has a relatively good efficacy and a high level of patient satisfaction. If unsuccessful, it does not compromise subsequent surgical treatment.

► Simple probing of the lacrimal system offers an interesting alternative approach to NLDO that most ophthalmologists would rarely consider. Unfortunately, this study is not well designed and serves to offer probing as a consideration but gives little proof of its effectiveness.

The study uses a questionnaire about severity of tearing in a retrospective manner to obtain results rather than evaluation with irrigation of the lacrimal system to prove lacrimal system patency. Although relief of symptoms of tearing is the ultimate desired result, evaluation of the system with irrigation gives the most accurate assessment of surgical success. There are multiple other factors that may result in improvement in tearing symptoms other than the lacrimal system being open. We really have no idea how many of the patients have patent lacrimal systems.

Use of a control group treated only with drops would have eliminated the improvement due to factors other than the probing. The 82% improvement rate is deceptive. Thirty-five percent had no tearing, and 17% had mild watering, thus, 52% of patients had no or mild tearing. Clearly, the success rate is different if you look at those patients with improvement and at those left with no or only mild symptoms of tearing. There is no mention of whether these patients had partial or complete obstructions. The success rate in these two very different groups is very different, and the groups should be separated. A group of patients with partial obstructions would have a higher success rate than those with complete blocks.

The use of probing is rarely considered for treatment of adult complete NLDO in the United States, but probing is useful in congenital NLDO. Over the past few years, the use of a balloon catheter for treatment of partial NLDO has become more popular, with success rates said to approach 90%. This rate is much better than the rates reported in this study. If balloon dacryoplasty is successful as an office procedure, then this will be the procedure of choice for partial obstruction. Probing of complete lacrimal obstructions in the office has some merit in elderly patients who are unable to have a dacryocystorhinostomy with the understanding that the success rate is lower and the long-term results are questionable.

R.B. Penne, M.D.

The Endoscopic Forehead Lift

Steinsapir KD, Shorr N, Hoenig J, et al (Univ of California, Los Angeles)

Ophthal Plast Reconstr Surg 14:107-118, 1998 6–13

Background.—Eyebrow elevation is traditionally done by coronal and pretrichial forehead elevation, midforehead elevation, direct brow lift, and browpexy through a blepharoplasty incision. Endoscopic forehead techniques provide the opportunity to manage brow ptosis and glabellar wrinkles without significant scarring and postoperative anesthesia or dysesthesia. The indications, anatomy, surgical techniques, potential complications, and outcomes of endoscopic forehead lift were discussed.

Discussion.—Endoscopic techniques in patients with eyebrow and forehead ptosis depend on extensive subperiosteal and subgaleal release of the forehead and scalp flap, permitting soft tissue elevation. Skin folding in the glabellar region can be managed by ablation of the depressor supercilli and procerus. The mobilized frontotemporal flap is elevated, fixated with microscrews to the outer table of the skull and laterally to the deep temporalis fascia. Surgeons need a good knowledge of regional anatomy and the use of specialized instruments currently available to dissecting under the flap. The outcomes of the endoscopic forehead lift are comparable with those obtained by the open coronal forehead lift. With the endoscopic procedure, the incidence and extent of postoperative cutaneous anesthesia and telogenic hair loss that often follow coronal forehead surgery are minimized. Also, the endoscopic technique will not cause scarring in balding men with eyebrow ptosis.

Conclusions.—Endoscopic forehead lifting should be considered by surgeons now performing coronal petrichial, midforehead, and direct eyebrow lifting procedures. The learning curve for mastering this technique is especially steep for surgeons who have not performed open forehead elevating procedures.

▶ Forehead and brow lifts are an important aspect of cosmetic rehabilitation of the periorbital area. Many patients who present with ptosis or upper eyelid dermatochalasis have a significant component of eyebrow droop contributing to the excess skin. This paper completely describes the endoscopic approach to lifting the forehead and brow. Although most ophthalmologists will not be doing this surgery the method and advantages are worth understanding.

The most difficult aspect of this procedure is the visualization and anatomy. Good training is essential because the physician learning curve can be steep. This is especially true for someone less familiar with the use of endoscopy. The procedure when done initially often takes hours but with experience the time is less.

Indications for brow lifts are very subjective. When a patient presents with a complaint of excess skin on the upper lids careful evaluation of the brows will be required. There are some patients who have no brow ptosis and some whose brows are the entire problem. For the remaining patients, which is the majority, they have some brow ptosis and some true dermatochalasis. For these patients deciding on simple blepharoplasty versus brow lift and blepharoplasty can be difficult. Many of these patients do very well with a blepharoplasty but the brow and its position must be discussed. Often keeping the surgery simple is the best approach. Those patients requiring a brow lift the endoscopic approach offers many advantages which are touched on in the paper.

R.B. Penne, M.D.

Meibomian Gland Dysfunction in Patients With Sjögren Syndrome

Shimazaki J, Goto E, Ono M, et al (Tokyo Dental College)

Ophthalmology 105:1485-1488, 1998 6–14

Objective.—Patients with meibomian gland dysfunction experience ocular surface abnormalities and discomfort as a result of excessive evaporation of tears. Patients with Sjögren syndrome (SS) often have more severe changes in the ocular surface than patients with dry eye who do not have SS. Patients with SS and age- and sex-matched non-SS dry eye patients were compared in this prospective clinical study.

Methods.—Twenty-seven consecutive patients with SS were age- and sex-matched with 29 non-SS patients with dry eye. Ocular surface tests were performed and tear evaporation rate, tear function, and meibomian glands were examined.

Results.—The SS group had significantly higher fluorescein and rose bengal staining scores than did the non-SS group. Tear break-up time and rate of tear production were similar for the 2 groups, but tear evaporation rate was significantly faster in the SS group than in the non-SS group under normal and forced blinking. The incidence of meibomian gland dropout was significantly higher in the SS group (16/19) than in the non-SS group (15/27). Whereas most eyes revealed orifice obstruction, the incidence was significantly higher in the SS group (n = 7) than in the non-SS group (n = 3).

Conclusion.—Meibomian gland dysfunction is involved in ocular surface changes in patients with SS.

▶ This study investigated meibomian gland dysfunction in patients with SS and found that 57.9% of them had loss of meibomian glands compared with 18.5% of controls. This indicates that the surface problem in patients with SS is not just a problem with the aqueous layer; there is a lipid problem as well. These findings may explain poor response to artificial tear treatment. The study also presents the new problem of how to treat lipid layer deficiencies. Our ability to treat lipid layer problems is less effective than our ability to treat aqueous problems.

A potential broader use for this evidence is the fact that these patients may provide a model for treating combined aqueous/lipid layer problems in patients other than those with SS. One of the most common ocular disorders is blepharitis. Blepharitis is a poorly understood disease and a disease that has few universally successful treatments. Whether the abnormality of the meibomian glands in blepharitis acts like the loss of meibomian glands in SS is unknown. It is clear clinically that some of the most difficult dry eye patients to treat are those that also have significant blepharitis. If this information leads to improvements in the treatment and study of blepharitis, many patients and physicians will be grateful.

R.B. Penne, M.D.

Ritleng Intubation System for Treatment of Congenital Nasolacrimal Duct Obstruction

Pe MRL, Langford JD, Linberg JV, et al (West Virginia Univ, Morgantown; Midwest Eye Inst, Indianapolis, Ind)

Arch Ophthalmol 116:387-391, 1998 6–15

Background.—The Ritleng lacrimal intubation system allows bicanalicular silicone intubation without the need to retrieve metal probes from the inferior meatus. One experience with this system was described.

Equipment.—The Ritleng probe is a rigid, hollow, polished stainless steel tube 105 mm long. Its diameter is 1 mm, comparable to that of a Bowman 0 probe. The superior end of the probe has a funnel-shaped opening to facilitate Prolene monofilament leader insertion. The clinician holds and orients the probe using a disk attached to the superior end. On the blunt inferior end, a lateral opening 5 mm above the tip serves as an exit for the Prolene probe that prevents impaling the mucosa on the nasal fossa floor. There is a narrow slit running the length of the probe. The lacrimal intubation set consists of silicone tubing attached firmly to a Prolene monofilament leader at each end. The silicone tubing is 300 mm long, with an outer diameter of 0.64 mm. The 2 Prolene leaders, consist of a thicker dark blue initial portion 0.4 mm in diameter and a thinner, light blue portion 0.2 mm in diameter. Only the thinner part can pass through the probe's slit. A Ritleng hook or small muscle hook is needed occasionally to engage the Prolene under the inferior turbinate.

Application.—The Ritleng lacrimal intubation system was used in 28 patients with 34 eyes affected by congenital nasolacrimal duct obstruction. A Prolene monofilament guide thread, fastened securely to the silicone tubing, was introduced into a tubular metal probe that opened into the inferior meatus. Ninety-four percent of the lacrimal systems were intubated successfully. In 2 eyes (6%), passing the Prolene thread through the probe and out the tip was difficult, necessitating conversion to a Crawford intubation system. In 75% of 32 eyes, the prolene emerged spontaneously from the nose, making retrieval simple and uncomplicated. Signs and symptoms of obstruction were relieved in 97% of the eyes treated by the Ritleng system. Both eyes treated by the Crawford system showed symptomatic relief.

Conclusion.—Bicanalicular silicone intubation using the Ritleng intubation system is an effective, easy method for treating congenital nasolacrimal duct obstruction. The Prolene suture is soft and atraumatic and is retrieved from the nasal cavity more easily than traditional rigid metal probes. In most cases, the Prolene emerges spontaneously from the nose.

► Retrieval of the lacrimal probe from the nasal cavity can sometimes be the most difficult part of intubation of the lacrimal system. This difficulty results in intranasal trauma, prolonged operation times, and postoperative nasal congestion. The use of a nasal endoscope may simplify probe retrieval. However, endoscopes are not always available nor are all ophthalmologists familiar with their use. For all of these reasons, the potential for a system that provides simpler tube retrieval from the nose is desirable.

The paper describes the successful treatment of congenital nasolacrimal duct obstruction with the Ritleng system. The system and its unique design are completely described by the author. The ease of retrieval of the tubes is what is emphasized in the study.

My experience with this system has been only recent, but it appears to work very well. The system provides an overall easier tube retrieval, which is a great advantage for those surgeons less experienced with this type of surgery. For my practice, there is even a greater potential advantage: In adults, the attempt to pass and retrieve tubes from the nose is uncomfortable and requires significant sedation or even general anesthesia. This system offers a much less traumatic approach. Together with the recent interest in performing balloon dacryoplasty in the office setting, this technique may provide an approach to intubation that can also be done in the office without sedation.

R.B. Penne, M.D.

Prediction of Late Enophthalmos by Volumetric Analysis of Orbital Fractures

Raskin EM, Millman AL, Lubkin V, et al (New York Eye and Ear Infirmary; Manhattan Eye, Ear and Throat Hosp, New York)

Ophthal Plast Reconstr Surg 14:19-26, 1998 6–16

Background.—Traumatic enophthalmos results from atrophy and prolapse of orbital fat, displacement of orbital walls with a significant increase in orbital volume, and cicatricial contraction of orbital tissue. Whether CT assessment of orbital volume provides additional information for the examination and treatment of orbital blowout fractures was investigated.

Methods.—The records of 30 patients with orbital blowout fractures treated surgically or conservatively were reviewed. Orbital volumetric analysis was assessed by digitized CT scans.

Findings.—Fracture-related volume expansion (compared with the unaffected fellow eye) was associated with motility defects and enophthalmos location and degree. Hertel measurements obtained within 4 weeks of injury, available in 21 patients, were uncorrelated with the computer volumetric values or subsequent late enophthalmos. Hertel measures obtained after 4 weeks in 13 of 15 conservatively treated eyes and in 5 of 15 surgically treated eyes showed that 92% of patients with 13% or more orbital volume expansion had significant enophthalmos, compared with 17% of patients with less than 13% orbital expansion. Eyes with enophthalmos on initial assessment had extensive medial wall involvement along with the floor fracture (Fig 4).

Conclusion.—Assessment of orbital volume on CT can be used for predicting the final extent of late enophthalmos, possibly facilitating the planning of surgical treatment. The current data confirm that enophthalmos after orbital blowout fractures is correlated linearly with the volumetric expansion of the fractured orbits.

▶ Predicting which patients will have enophthalmos after orbital fracture is a valuable tool in the management of orbital fractures. Currently, the general rule is that a fracture of greater than 50% for the floor has a significant risk of enophthalmos development, and repair should be considered for preventing enophthalmos. Within the 50%, there can be great variability in the amount of displacement of bone. This study defines a more precise limit of increased orbital volume at which the risk of enophthalmos becomes significant.

Patients with orbital fractures who have significant diplopia and muscle restriction will go on to surgery within 2 weeks no matter what the orbital

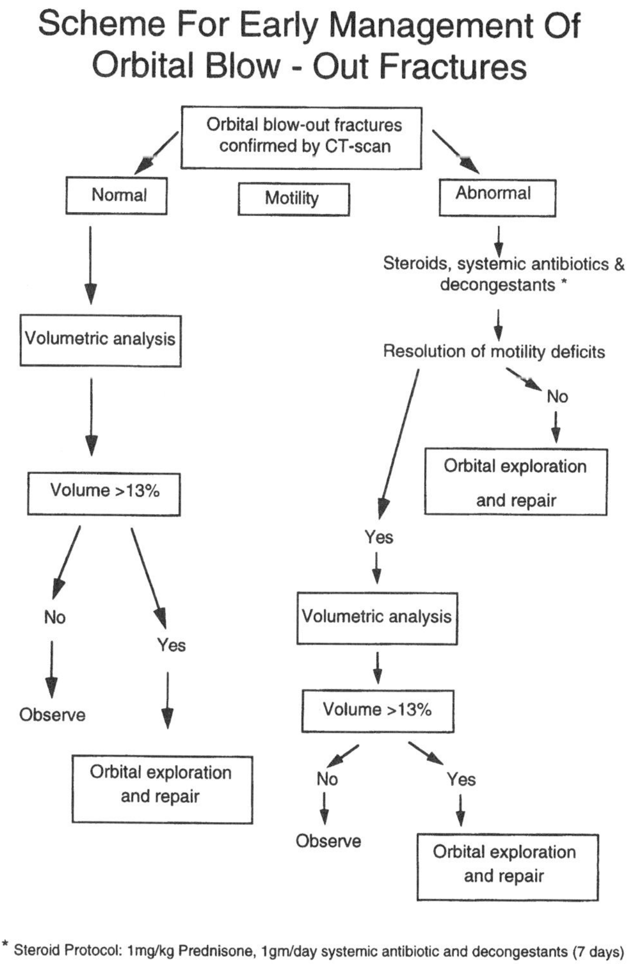

FIGURE 4.—Scheme for early medical and surgical management of acute orbital blowout fractures, based upon volumetric expansion. *Asterisk* indicates steroid protocol: 1 mg/kg prednisone, 1 g/day systemic antibiotics, and decongestants (7 days). (Courtesy of Raskin EM, Millman AL, Lubkin V, et al: Prediction of late enophthalmos by volumetric analysis of orbital fractures. *Ophthal Plast Reconstr Surg* 14:19-26, 1998. Copyright American Society of Ophthalmic Plastic & Reconstructive Surgery.)

volume changes are. The difficult decision involves the patients without diplopia and determining which patients will develop cosmetically significant diplopia. With volumetric analysis, an objective value is obtained for making this decision simpler. The number of patients in this study is small, and a larger study for confirming these findings is needed. Looking specifically at patients without need for repair because of entrapment and trying to predict which will develop enophthalmos may be able to be done in a prospective, randomized manner.

Another problem with this study is the subjective manner used to determine the orbital volume. The outlines of the orbital margins were drawn, which leaves significant room for variability depending on who was doing the drawing. This potential variability can certainly affect the volume changes used as a basis for the study.

The question of which patients will be disturbed by enophthalmos may not be as easy to answer. I find that patients often have trouble understanding the concept of enophthalmos until they see it themselves. An important factor in enophthalmos is downward displacement. Three millimeters of enophthalmos may not bother a patient if there is no downward displacement. However, with 1 to 2 mm of downward displacement, 2 mm of enophthalmos may be quite disfiguring. Medial wall fractures usually cause enophthalmos only, whereas large floor fractures also cause significant downward displacement. These factors must be considered in addition to the actual volume change.

Unlike late repair of orbital fractures with entrapment, surgery for enophthalmos can be very successfully performed months after the injury. For this reason, there is no real urgency to repair a fracture if potential enophthalmos is the only concern. The objective numbers this study offers are certainly a help in the management of orbital fractures. However, allowing a patient to visualize the cosmetic changes before deciding on surgical correction does not prevent successful correction.

R.B. Penne, M.D.

Long-term Efficacy of Local Doxorubicin Chemomyectomy in Patients With Blepharospasm and Hemifacial Spasm

Wirtschafter JD, McLoon LK (Univ of Minnesota, Minneapolis)
Ophthalmology 105:342-346, 1998 6–17

Background.—Studies of rabbits, monkeys, and humans have shown that direct doxorubicin injection into the eyelids results in a significant loss of muscle fiber number and cross-sectional area. The long-term outcomes of patients undergoing doxorubicin injections for blepharospasm and hemifacial spasm were investigated.

Methods.—Eighteen patients with blepharospasm and 9 with hemifacial spasm were treated in a nonrandomized, clinical trial. At intervals of 10 weeks or more, eyelids were injected repeatedly until the spasms were relieved or the patient wanted to stop treatments.

Findings.—Nine patients with blepharospasm completed treatment and are judged to be cured after 1 to 6 years. Six patients with hemifacial spasm completed treatment; 5 of them are considered cured after more than 4.5 to 6 years. Significant amelioration was noted in 1 patient with blepharospasm and 1 with hemifacial spasm. Although these patients have been untreated for more than 3 years, they sometimes request botulinum toxin supplementation. The minimum effective dose per treated eyelid ranged from 1 to 4.2 mg. Discontinuations of treatment were prompted by skin inflammation. Four of the 14 cured patients needed surgical revision of 1 eyelid.

Conclusion.—Doxorubicin chemomyectomy, an evolving technique, is effective in the treatment of essential blepharospasm and hemifacial spasms of the eyelid. Fifty-nine percent of the initial 27 patients in this study completed treatment and all are apparently cured. Although the treatment seems to be reasonably safe compared with surgical myectomy, further research is needed on co-treatments to minimize the associated acute skin changes and to maximize long-term efficacy.

► The introduction of botulinum toxin for the treatment of blepharospasm and hemifacial spasm was a dramatic advance in the treatment of these diseases. The problem with the treatment is that it must be repeated every 3 to 6 months indefinitely. This paper investigates the results of a long-term treatment for use in patients responsive to botulinum toxin but who desire a more prolonged response.

The ideal treatment would be a 1-time treatment with permanent resolution of the spasm and no adverse effects. Doxorubicin is certainly a step toward this goal; however, I do not think that the current approach will become widely used. Although botulinum toxin must be repeated multiple times a year, the risks are few and when side effects do occur, they are temporary. In the doxorubicin approach, despite cautious treatment by a single examiner, nearly 15% of patients required surgical treatment of injected lids as the result of side effects. This is not an acceptable rate of adverse effects when a good alternative treatment exists. This rate would be higher in general use with less experienced practitioners using it.

A population that may benefit from this form of treatment is patients who do not respond to botulinum toxin, although these patients would not be easy to study.

The concept of permanent treatment of facial spasms is very attractive. This study certainly takes a step toward that goal. Hopefully, with modification of the treatment protocol or with other agents, the effectiveness and side effects can be improved.

R.B. Penne, M.D.

7 Pediatric Ophthalmology

Adult Strabismus Surgery Is Really Reconstructive Surgery

by Leonard B. Nelson, M.D.

Managed care has significantly penetrated the health care arena in recent years. This has been accomplished in an attempt to control escalating health care costs and, at the same time, provide high-quality medical care. In evaluating the cost-benefit ratio of various procedures, insurers designate which type of services are covered and which are not. Purely cosmetic surgery is usually not covered by most managed care organizations (MCOs).

These companies often consider adult strabismus surgery as cosmetic surgery and therefore do not reimburse for it. They argue that strabismus surgery improves the alignment of an individual's eyes, and thus the person's appearance, making it a cosmetic procedure. *Cosmetic* means "beautifying; tending to preserve, restore or confer comeliness." *Reconstruct* means "to rebuild or make over." Surgical correction of strabismus does not restore or confer beauty but rebuilds or brings the patient's abnormal eye alignment to normal. Thus, it is, by definition, reconstructive.[1,2]

Cosmetic surgery improves the appearance of a person who does not have a specific disease or abnormality. Reconstructive surgery eliminates a disease, abnormality, or defect. Orthophoric is the only normal configuration for ocular alignment. It indicates that the ocular motor apparatus is in exquisite equilibrium so that the eyes remain coordinated and aligned in all positions of gaze at all distances.

Therefore, adult strabismus surgery, which, again, is designed to straighten the eyes from an abnormal alignment, should be considered reconstructive, regardless of the visual or sensory outcome. It is imperative that ophthalmologists agree on these terms and not refer to the correction of adult strabismus as cosmetic.[3] If ophthalmologists refer to strabismus surgery as cosmetic, so will MCOs.

Many MCOs will authorize adult strabismus surgery only if fusion can be achieved or to correct diplopia. They assume that unless perfect (bifoveal) fusion can be obtained, there is no benefit to be gained to warrant surgery. Kushner and Morton[4] tested for binocularity preoperatively and postoperatively in a series of 359 adults who underwent strabismus surgery. Regardless of the type of deviation present preoperatively, the duration of strabismus, or the depth of amblyopia in the deviating eye, fusion developed in the majority of patients.

Adults with long-standing or recurrent childhood strabismus usually do not report diplopia (seeing the same object in two places). Instead, a suppression scotoma develops that blocks the image from the non-fixating eye. However, these patients are frequently aware of visual confusion (the perception of two different images in the same visual direction).

These patients often report seeing two different objects that overlap in the same place. The goal of strabismus surgery would be to reduce the angle of strabismus where suppression would correct the visual confusion.

The binocular peripheral field is contracted in esotropia. Using Goldmann perimetry before and after strabismus surgery, Wortham and Greenwald[5] found in every case an expansion of the peripheral visual field. Subjective improvement in peripheral vision was appreciated by a number of patients. Contraction of the peripheral field in esotropia has obvious functional significance, particularly in relation to motor vehicle operation. In one study, subjects with binocular visual field loss had a traffic accident and conviction rates more than twice as high as that of age- and sex-matched controls with normal fields.[6]

The psychological implications of strabismus on an individual's life have been documented.[7,8] These patients with strabismus have difficulty with self-image, in securing employment, with interpersonal relationships, with school work and sports. These effects can be reversed by successful strabismus surgery.[8]

Adult strabismus surgery corrects a malalignment of the eyes and should be considered reconstructive surgery. It reduces diplopia and visual confusion, establishes binocularity, enhances peripheral visual field, and improves psychosocial functions.

References

1. Metz HS: Strabismus surgery is reconstructive surgery. *J Pediatr Ophthalmol Strabismus* 25:263, 1988.
2. Nelson LB: Strabismus surgery is reconstructive surgery. 1994 YEAR BOOK OF OPHTHALMOLOGY, pp 351-354.
3. Rosenbaum AL: The goal of adult strabismus surgery is not cosmetic. *Arch Ophthalmol* 117:250, 1999.
4. Kushner BJ, Morton GV: Postoperative binocularity in adults with long-standing strabismus. *Ophthalmology* 99:316-319, 1992.
5. Wortham E 5th, Greenwald MJ: Expanded binocular peripheral visual fields following surgery for esotropia. *J Pediatr Ophthalmol Strabismus* 26:109-112, 1989.
6. Johnson CA, Keltner JL: Incidence of visual field loss in 20,000 eyes and its relationship to driving performance. *Arch Ophthalmol* 101:371-375, 1983.
7. Satterfield D, Keltner JL, Morrison TL: Psychosocial aspects of strabismus study. *Arch Ophthalmol* 111:1100-1105, 1993.
8. Burke JP, Leach CM, Davis H: Psychosocial implications of strabismus surgery in adults. *J Pediatr Ophthalmol Strabismus* 34:159-164, 1997.

Clinical Characteristics and Long-term Postoperative Results of Infantile Esotropia and Myopia

Shauly Y, Miller B, Meyer E (Rambam Med Ctr, Haifa, Israel; Technion-Israel Inst of Technology, Haifa)

J Pediatr Ophthalmol Strabismus 34:357-364, 1997 7–1

Background.—Myopia occurs in only 5% to 11% of infants with esotropia, and little data exist about results of surgery in this group. These authors studied the short- and long-term effects of surgery in patients with infantile esotropia and moderate or high myopia.

Methods.—The control group consisted of 100 patients with no myopia. Patients with myopia were categorized as having moderate myopia (refractive error −2.0 to −5.0 D; n = 13) or high myopia (refractive error −8.0 D or greater; n = 14). All patients had been diagnosed with esotropia before 6 months of age and had undergone refraction with 1% cyclopentolate before 1 year of age. Initial surgery had been completed by 2 years of age, and at least 4 years of follow-up data were available. Both the short-term (6 months) and long-term (4 years) results of surgery on binocular vision, microtropia, and small-angle and large-angle deviation were assessed.

Findings.—At 6 months, all patients with high myopia had large-angle deviation (>20 prism D), compared with 28% of the control group and 27% of the patients with moderate myopia. Furthermore, in a subset of 23 patients with amblyopia who underwent monocular recession/resection, large-angle deviation was again significantly more prevalent in the high myopia group (7 of 7 patients, 100%) than in the control group (5 of 14 patients, 36%). At 4 years after the last surgery, the results of surgery were equally good in the control group (80% favorable results) and the patients with moderate myopia (77%). However, none of the patients with high myopia had good long-term results, with 10 patients (71%) having large-angle esotropia and 4 patients (29%) having small-angle esotropia. Differences in large-angle deviation were significant when the high myopia group (71%) was compared with the control group (20%) and the moderate myopia group (23%). For all patients, the greater the deviation before surgery, the more effect surgery had (on a per millimeter basis). However, responses to surgery in the high myopia group were smaller than in the other 2 groups, and showed much more variation. Persistent preoperative amblyopia that recurred after surgery was significantly more common in the high myopic group than in the other 2 groups, and postoperative mean visual acuity was significantly lower in the high myopia group also.

Conclusions.—Patients with infantile esotropia and high myopia had significant large-angle deviation, significantly poorer responses to surgery, more persistent amblyopia, and worse visual acuity. Recession or resection of muscles should be increased in these patients, because surgery has less effect in them than is generally appreciated. It seems that, long-term, the constant efforts to create accommodative convergence cause the esotropia to recur.

▶ The authors found an unacceptable postoperative result of large-angle esotropia to be more frequent among the high myopic patients than among patients in the control and more moderate myopia groups. The authors suggest increasing the conventional amount of surgery in cases of infantile esotropia and high myopia. In this study, the high myopic group was quite small, and further studies with more patients are needed before making a recommendation to change the surgical approach to these patients. It has not been my experience that patients with high myopia and large-angle esotropia do less well postoperatively than other patients with large-angle esotropia. I do agree with the authors that careful attention should be directed toward reversing amblyopia and correcting refractive errors in the preoperative period.

L.B. Nelson, M.D.

Theoretic Refractive Changes After Lens Implantation in Childhood

McClatchey SK, Parks MM (Naval Med Ctr, San Diego, Calif; Children's Natl Med Ctr, Washington, DC)

Ophthalmology 104:1744-1751, 1997 7–2

Background.—Children with aphakia were formerly treated with contact lenses or spectacles that changed as vision changed with growth. Now this disorder is also being treated with implanted intraocular lenses (IOLs), which correct the hyperopia. But how much refractive correction is needed to result in emmetropic adult vision? This article examines the refractive changes in children with aphakia and projects the long-term refractive effects of pseudophakia.

Methods.—Eyes were eligible for study if the cataract had been removed before age 10 years, if no more than 3 months had elapsed between cataract removal and postoperative refraction, and if at least 7 years of follow-up data between the first and last refractions were available. Ninety-three eyes met these criteria, and their data were mathematically modeled to calculate the IOL powers that would have been required to result in emmetropia when the cataracts were removed. These data were compared with the final pseudophakic refractions calculated from the aphakic refractions at last follow-up.

Findings.—Over a mean of 11 years of follow-up, the calculated pseudophakic refraction at last follow-up ranged from −36.3 to +2.9 D (median, −6.6 D). The myopic shift was significantly greater in children whose surgery was performed before 2 years of age (11.9 D) than in those whose surgery was performed later (4.7 D). The mathematic model was substantially more accurate in predicting myopic shift in the older children, giving a prediction within 3 D of the final refraction in 24% of eyes in children younger than 2 years old versus 77% of eyes in children older than 2 years old. Myopic shift was less when the IOL was implanted to give moderate hyperopia rather than emmetropia.

Conclusions.—All children experience a myopic shift as they grow. However, this shift is greater in children with pseudophakia. Also, the range of refractive changes is greater in these children, because the aphakic refractive changes vary widely depending on the high-power IOL used and the child's age. An IOL that leaves the child initially hyperopic is preferable to striving immediately for emmetropia. The ophthalmic surgeon must be aware of the long-term variance in myopic shift, and be prepared to treat excessive myopia with contact lenses, spectacles, or even further IOL or refractive cornea surgery.

► The use of IOLs to correct pediatric aphakia has become more popular in recent years. One concern with the use of IOLs in young children is the variance in long term myopia shift. When contact lenses or spectacles are used to correct pediatric aphakia, these optical corrections can be adjusted easily to match a new refraction. Intraocular lenses provide a permanent correction, and therefore, when a significant change in the hyperopic occurs, the resulting refractive error must be managed with contact lenses, spectacles, or perhaps refractive cornea surgery. The use of IOLs in young children must be approached with considerable caution.

L.B. Nelson, M.D.

Prevalence and Causes of Amblyopia in an Adult Population

Attebo K, Mitchell P, Cumming R, et al (Univ of Sydney, Australia; Australian Natl Univ, Canberra, Australia)

Ophthalmology 105:154-159, 1998 7–3

Background.—The most common cause of unilateral visual loss in adults is amblyopia, defined as a loss in visual acuity that has no identifiable organic cause and that responds to therapy. When vision in the good eye is present, amblyopia is not much of a problem. However, amblyopia in 1 eye may increase the risk of blindness (mainly from trauma) in the other eye. These authors examined the prevalence and causes of amblyopia in older adults.

Methods.—Data were collected from 3,647 individuals (57% women) at least 49 years old. The participant's medical history, particularly any family history of eye disease, was noted. Clinical measurements included tests for visual acuity, myopia, emmetropia, hypermetropia, astigmatism, and strabismus. Unilateral amblyopia was defined as best-corrected visual acuity in 1 eye of 20/30 or worse with no identifiable structural abnormality of the visual pathway or eye. Anisometric amblyopia was defined as a difference of at least 1 D between the 2 eyes when no strabismus was present. Strabismic amblyopia indicated that strabismus was present in the absence of anisometropia or high refractive error. Mixed amblyopia was defined as both anisometric and strabismic amblyopia. Stimulus deprivation amblyopia was assigned as the cause if the patient had congenital cataract, ptosis, corneal opacities, other media opacities, or uncorrected high refractive errors during childhood that had influenced vision.

Findings.—One hundred eighteen of the participants had amblyopia, a prevalence of 3.2%. No preferences for gender or for left versus right eye were found. Participants with amblyopia were not at significantly increased risk of bilateral blindness or visual impairment compared with participants without amblyopia. The amblyopia was typically diagnosed during childhood (mean age at diagnosis, 8.8 years), and 53% of these participants were wearing spectacles by age 12 years. Occlusion therapy had been used by 31 participants (26%). Anisometria was the most common cause of amblyopia (59 participants, or 50%), followed by strabismus (22, or 19%), mixed (32, or 27%), and stimulus deprivation (5, or 4%). The most common type of strabismic amblyopia was esotropia (59%), and the most common type of refractive error in amblyopic eyes was hypermetropia (50%). Visual acuity was poorest in patients with stimulus deprivation amblyopia (< 20/200), then strabismic amblyopia (20/125), then mixed (20/80), then anisometropia (20/60). Trauma was not the cause of decreased vision in the fellow eye; rather, the cause was age-related eye disease.

Conclusions.—Adult amblyopia occurred in 3.2% of this population, and affected men and women and left and right eyes equally. In this study, anisometropic amblyopia was the most common cause of amblyopia, a finding which is in conflict with those of other reports citing strabismic amblyopia as most common.

▶ Amblyopia is a more frequent cause of monocular visual loss in adults than diabetic retinopathy, glaucoma, macular degeneration, or cataract. It is an asymptomatic condition that often goes undetected unless an adequate visual screening program has been instituted in childhood. Adults with amblyopia may not be able to pursue certain occupations because of visual requirements. Unilateral low vision from amblyopia is considered only a mild handicap, but loss of vision in the good eye is the real tragedy. Therefore, it is vital that amblyopia be detected early and treated vigorously so that complications of unilateral visual loss are kept to a minimum.

L.B. Nelson, M.D.

Strabismus in Premature Infants in the First Year of Life

Bremer DL, for the Cryotherapy for Retinopathy of Prematurity Cooperative Group (Ohio State Univ, Columbus; et al)

Arch Ophthalmol 116:329-333, 1998 7–4

Background.—Premature infants are at risk for retinal detachment and blindness, but even if they avoid this serious complication, they remain at risk for strabismus. The Multicenter Trial of Cryotherapy for Retinopathy of Prematurity (ROP) prospectively collected visual motility data on premature infants with birth weights less than 1,251 kg. This study group was used to determine the overall prevalence of strabismus and to analyze factors that may be predictive of strabismus in premature infants at 3 and 12 months.

Study Design.—The study group consisted of 4,099 premature infants born during 1986 and 1987, from 23 centers. The infants had eye examinations after birth and then at 3 and 12 months. These follow-up examinations included evaluation of fixation behavior, ocular motility, anterior segment, refractive error, and fundus findings. The ROP severity was based on the worse eye.

Results.—Motility status could be observed at 3 months in 3,030 infants. Of these, 299 were strabismic. The incidence of strabismus increased as birth weight and gestational age decreased. Retinopathy of prematurity was a significant predictor of strabismus at 3 months, and more severe ROP increased this risk. Of the 2,449 infants who had ocular motility evaluations at both 3 and 12 months, 11.% had strabismus at 12 months. Acute-phase ROP was a significant predictor of strabismus at 12 months. Strabismus at 3 months was a significant predictor of strabismus at 12 months. Both abnormal fixation behavior and unfavorable retinal structure at 3 months were significant predictors of strabismus at 12 months. Abnormal retinal structure in 1 eye was a significant predictor of strabismus, while abnormal retinal structure in both eyes was not. The presence of anisometropia and delayed development at 3 months also significantly predicted strabismus at 12 months.

Conclusions.—Ocular alignment data were prospectively collected from a large group of premature infants. Premature infants had a higher rate of strabismus than full-term infants. The presence of acute-phase ROP was a strong predictor of strabismus within the first year. Incidence of strabismus increased with increasing severity of ROP. Anisometropia, unfavorable retinal structure, abnormal fixation, poor neurological development, and strabismus at 3 months were all predictive of strabismus at 12 months in this group of premature infants.

▶ As documented by other investigators, premature infants have a higher rate of strabismus than full-term infants. As the severity of ROP increases, the incidence of strabismus increases. The presence of strabismus at 3 months of age was found to be a highly significant prediction of strabismus at 12 months of age. It is important that infants with ROP be carefully screened for strabismus. Even when the ROP has resolved, these children are at a greater risk for developing strabismus and amblyopia.

L.B. Nelson, M.D.

Baltimore Vision Screening Project: Phase 2

Preslan MW, Novak A (Univ of Maryland, Baltimore; Maryland Society for Sight, Baltimore)

Ophthalmology 105:150-153, 1998 7–5

Background.—The primary goal of pediatric vision screening is to permit early treatment intervention. Usually, obtaining evaluation and treatment has been the responsibility of the parent or guardian. In urban inner cities, such care may be difficult to obtain. To define the extent of visual abnormalities in inner-city school children, a program was developed to sample preschoolers at an elementary school located in West Baltimore. The results of the initial survey revealed a relatively high prevalence of visual abnormalities. This article describes the results of 1-year follow-up, which re-examined the prevalence of visual abnormalities and rescreened those children from the previous study population who remained at the school.

Methods.—The study group consisted of 285 children enrolled in prekindergarten and kindergarten in Steuart Hill Elementary School in inner-city West Baltimore. Approximately half of the original study population was available to be rescreened at 1-year follow-up. Children were examined with a standard visual screening protocol and those with abnormal results were provided with initial treatment at the school.

Results.—Of the 285 children screened the previous year, 49 initially had abnormal ophthalmic evaluation results and were referred for evaluation. Ophthalmologic abnormalities were detected in 40 of these children at evaluation. When the children were examined at 1-year follow-up, 30% of those needing spectacles were wearing them and fewer than 20% passed follow-up visual screening.

Conclusions.—This follow-up study of inner-city children provided with appropriate ophthalmic care revealed that many were no longer wearing their spectacles after 1 year. This may be due to the lack of insurance in this population or to lack of parent education about the importance of ophthalmic treatment.

► Potentially treatable visual abnormalities can be identified through vision screening in pre-school and school age children. After these children have been identified by the screening process, they are typically referred to appropriate eye care providers. However, many of these children have not complied with the recommended treatment, even though they were provided with immediate access to ophthalmologic care. In this inner-city vision screening program, there were many socioeconomic factors which may have hindered the compliance with care for these children. Better methods of educating parents and primary care physicians regarding the implications of vision-screening failure, the importance of early treatment, and the need for careful follow-up should be a priority. Perhaps the school nurse should be made more available to monitor and/or oversee the referral of children to ophthalmologists in situations in which the family structure has broken down and the affected child is not cared for properly.

L.B. Nelson, M.D.

Development of Tearing in Preterm and Term Neonates

Isenberg SJ, Apt L, McCarty J, et al (Univ of California, Los Angeles)

Arch Ophthalmol 116:773-776, 1998 7–6

Introduction.—Studies have not been conducted to differentiate between basal and reflex tear secretion in preterm infants and term newborns. Early diagnosis of tear deficiency diseases such as familial dysautonomia or congenital absence of the lacrimal gland may benefit from the differentiation. Newborns with little reflex secretion may not be able to dilute topical medication by reflex tear production, allowing the medication to remain more concentrated. Corneal clarity may quickly decrease during ophthalmologic examination or during the treatment of intraocular structures. Nasolacrimal duct obstruction may also go unnoticed because of a lack of reflex secretion. To determine the developmental pattern of tear production, basal and reflex tear secretion was measured in preterm infants and in term newborns.

Methods.—There were 70 infants, of which 36 were preterm (30-37 weeks after conception) and 34 were term (38-42 weeks). The evaluation of tear secretion was conducted by applying Schirmer tear test strips to the inferior fornix for 5 minutes before applying a topical anesthetic agent to determine reflex plus basal secretion and after applying a topical anesthetic agent to determine basal secretion.

Results.—The mean basal tear secretion was in preterm infants 6.2 ± 4.5 mm and 9.2 ± 4.3 mm in term infants. With increasing weight, there was increasing basal tear secretion for all newborns. The mean reflex tear secretion was 7.4 ± 4.8 mm in preterm infants and 13.2 ± 6.5 mm in term infants. For all newborns, reflex tear secretion increased with increasing weight.

Conclusion.—Reduced reflex and basal tear secretion is seen in preterm infants. Diagnosis of a nasolacrimal duct obstruction may be masked by reduced reflex and basal tear secretion, which may also lead to concentration of topically applied medications and may cause corneas to quickly become dry during ophthalmologic examination and treatment. By the time infants reach term, their tear production is similar to that of adults.

▶ Basal and reflex tear secretion is reduced in preterm infants. The low level of tears in preterm infants may allow topical eye medications to remain more concentrated, resulting in an increased local or systemic effect. Therefore, topical medication doses need to be monitored carefully in these infants. Because these infants often require ophthalmologic evaluations to rule out retinopathy of prematurity, the lower tear levels may cause corneal dryness quicker. It is important to lubricate the cornea while performing retina examinations on these infants.

L.B. Nelson, M.D.

Needle Sterility During Strabismus Surgery

Olitsky SE, Vilardo M, Awner S, et al (State Univ of New York, Buffalo)

J AAPOS 2:151-152, 1998 7–7

Introduction.—Postoperative endophthalmitis after strabismus surgery is uncommon. Its cause is unknown, even when the host conjunctiva is a major source of infection, and is hard to determine because it occurs so rarely. Most pediatric ophthalmologists directly instill 5% povidone-iodine just before surgery. No method completely sterilizes the conjunctiva in all patients. If scleral perforation is involved in the mechanism of infection, then needle sterility becomes a key issue. The sterility of needles used during strabismus surgery was assessed.

Methods.—Sixty-one patients underwent strabismus surgery. One hundred six of the 110 needles used in the surgery were recovered and cultured.

Results.—Cultures were positive in 16 of 106 eyes (15.1%) and in 15 of 61 patients (24.6%). There were no postoperative infections. The organisms cultured closely resembled indigenous bacterial flora.

Conclusion.—Most trials addressing postoperative endophthalmitis after strabismus surgery have assumed that the patient's natural flora is the source of postoperative infection. Bacteria grown from the needles used in this trial closely resembled culture results of normal conjunctiva flora. It is understandable to speculate that the needles used during strabismus surgery could cause infection. Yet, the introduction of bacteria into the suprachoroidal or deeper spaces of the eye do not equate with the known rate of clinical infection. Immunity, blood flow, bacterial virulence, and amount of inoculation, are examples of other relative infectivity factors. Because there were no preoperative conjunctival cultures performed, the source of contaminated needles cannot be determined. Cultures were also not performed on needles not used for surgery. Given these limitations, it seems that needle contamination should be considered during surgery for strabismus.

► Endophthalmitis after strabismus surgery is rare and its cause remains unknown. It is assumed that the patient's own bacterial flora, either normal low virulent types or transient higher virulent types, is the source of postoperative infection. Somehow, a patient's own bacterial flora is introduced into the eye and results in an increased risk for the development of an intraocular infection. Fifteen percent of the needles used during strabismus surgery were cultured positive. The organism received from the needles closely resembled indigenous bacterial flora.

While needle contamination should be a concern for the strabismus surgeon, other infectivity factors must also be present for endophthalmitis to occur.

L.B. Nelson, M.D.

Traumatic Hyphema: Outcomes of Outpatient Management

Shiuey Y, Lucarelli MJ (Harvard Med School, Boston; Univ of Wisconsin, Madison)

Ophthalmology 105:851-855, 1998 7–8

Introduction.—In the first several days after blunt ocular trauma, rebleeding is of major concern. Secondary hemorrhages are usually more severe and may predispose the patient to vision-threatening complications. Many physicians recommend hospitalization and strict bed rest for patients with hyphema. The efficacy of hospitalization has not been determined in a controlled trial. Outcomes of outpatient and inpatient management of layered hyphema were retrospectively compared.

Methods.—Medical records of all patients treated between January 1991 and January 1995 in an emergency ward were compared with a historical control group of patients hospitalized and treated at the same institution between July 1986 and February 1989 (154 vs 119 patients). Rebleed rates, visual acuity, and causes of best-corrected visual acuity worse than 20/30 were analyzed. Fifty-three percent of the historical group received oral aminocaproic acid to prevent bleeding.

Results.—Rebleed rate for the study group was 4.5%; for controls, it was 5.0%. In study patients who did not receive aminocaproic acid, the rebleed rate was 3.3%, compared to 4.8% for a subset of historical control subjects who received aminocaproic acid. A final best-corrected visual acuity of 20/30 or better was achieved by 96% of the study group. The most frequently occurring complication of hyphema was elevated intraocular pressure (31%). Rebleeding was the second most common complication; 7 patients (4.5%) experienced rebleeding. Rebleeding was the most common cause of readmission in the study group (4%).

Conclusion.—There were no significant differences in the rebleed rate of patients treated initially as outpatients and controls who were admitted (3.4% vs 5.0%). Rebleed rates were similar for controls treated with aminocaproic acid and study patients who did not receive this drug. Ninety-two percent of the control group was white, but race of the study group was unknown. The black population historically has a higher rate of hyphema-related complications than other racial groups. Thus, these findings may not be applicable to predominately black populations. With close follow-up, most patients with hyphema may be safely and cost-effectively managed on an outpatient basis without increasing the rate of rebleeding.

▶ Patients with traumatic hyphemas have traditionally been treated as inpatients. The outpatient management of this condition offers several advantages. Outpatient care is generally preferred to admission by most patients and families. Additionally, outpatient management is cost-effective. These authors showed that close outpatient follow-up of traumatic hyphemas appears to be safe and effective. The incidence of rebleeding does not appear to increase with outpatient management.

The authors pointed out several limitations of their study. First, the race of the study group was not available. Therefore, the findings in this study may not be applicable to populations with markedly different racial compositions. Second, this study was performed in a retrospective manner. It would be better to compare inpatient to outpatient management in a prospective, randomized, controlled study instead. Finally, the average age of the historical and control groups was approximately 23. The treatment of hyphemas including strict bed rest may be more difficult for an outpatient in the pediatric age group.

L.B. Nelson, M.D.

▶ This study follows 154 patients in whom traumatic hyphema developed between January 1991 and November 1995. This was done retrospectively and was compared with a group of 119 patients seen earlier as a historical control group. The authors found that treating these patients without hospitalization was as efficacious as hospitalizing patients, as far as rebleeding is concerned. Rebleeding is one of the most important aspects of traumatic hyphema, and hospitalizing these patients did not alter this criteria. It was also interesting that the use of oral aminocaproic acid as a prophylaxis for rebleeding did not show a statistical difference between the overall rebleed rate of the study group who did not receive aminocaproic acid and that of the historical control patients who received aminocaproic acid. If a rebleed occurred, the patients in the study group were given aminocaproic acid, but they were not uniformly given this medication to prevent rebleeding.

Whether patients with hyphema should automatically be given aminocaproic acid to prevent rebleeding is still a controversial fact. Since hospitalization is required for the use of aminocaproic acid, and as this study does not show a statistically significant difference in rebleeds with patients who are hospitalized or not hospitalized, the use of this medication is left only for the more severe hyphemas with other confounding factors such as elevated intraocular pressure. These patients are automatically hospitalized after hyphema anyway.

P.R. Laibson, M.D.

The Accuracy of Experienced Strabismologists Using the Hirschberg and Krimsky Tests

Choi RY, Kushner BJ (Univ of Wisconsin, Madison)
Ophthalmology 105:1301-1306, 1998 7–9

Background.—Successful surgical treatment of strabismus relies on accurate evaluation of the angle of misalignment. The standard for evaluation is the alternate prism and cover test. For uncooperative patients or those with deep amblyopia, the Hirschberg or Krimsky test must be employed. This study compared the accuracy and interobserver reliability of a group of experienced strabismologists who applied the Hirschberg and Krimsky tests to photographs of patients whose angles of strabismus had been previously determined by the alternate prism and cover test.

Study Design.—Sixteen strabismologists, with an average of 22.8 years of experience since completion of formal training, estimated the angle of deviation from photographs of 4 patients, using the Hirschberg and Krimsky tests. These results were compared with those of an alternate prism and cover test.

Findings.—Using the Hirschberg test, participants underestimated at least 1 patient by at least 10Δ. The participants also tended to underestimate both large- and small-angle esotropic and exotropic patients, with error increasing with angle of strabismus. Using the Krimsky test, the majority of participants overestimated at least 1 patient by 10Δ and had difficulty in determining differences of 5Δ. The responses of participants were not consistent.

Conclusions.—The Hirschberg test for angle of misalignment in strabismus was not very accurate, even when employed by a group of experienced strabismologists. It was less accurate for larger deviations than for smaller ones and a large angle kappa decreased accuracy further. The Krimsky test was more accurate than the Hirschberg test, but it was also inaccurate and inconsistent. These findings suggest the need for additional tests for those patients with strabismus for whom the prism and cover test cannot be used for determining angle of misalignment.

► Different tests are used to assess ocular alignment. For patients who are uncooperative or have amblyopia, the angle of strabismus must be determined by using the Hirschberg or Krimsky test. Potential pitfalls, especially with the Hirschberg test, include eccentric fixation and an abnormal angle kappa. Therefore, I am not surprised that the authors found inconsistencies among the participants who measured angles of strabismus using the test based on the corneal light reflex. I agree with the authors that there is a need for a more accurate means of measuring the angle of strabismus, especially in young children with large deviations.

L.B. Nelson, M.D.

Success Rates of Nasolacrimal Duct Probing at Time Intervals After 1 Year of Age

Robb RM (Harvard Med School, Boston)

Ophthalmology 105:1307-1310, 1998 7–10

Background.—There is some controversy over the timing of probing procedures for congenital nasolacrimal duct obstruction. Some physicians prefer to perform this procedure during the first year, when it can be done

TABLE 1.—Results of 280 Nasolacrimal Duct Probings at Various Ages: No.(%)

	Group I (12-14 mos)	Group 2 (15-17 mos)	Group 3 (18-23 mos)	Group 4 (24-35 mos)	Group 5 (36+ mos)
Cured	96 (88.9)	61 (96.8)	49 (90.7)	27 (96.4)	25 (92.6)
Improved	10 (9.3)	0 (0)	3 (5.6)	1 (3.6)	0 (0)
Failed	2 (1.8)	2 (3.2)	2 (3.7)	0 (0)	2 (7.4)
Incomplete follow-up	10	3	6	2	2

(Published courtesy of *Ophthalmology*, from Robb RM: Success rates of nasolacrimal duct probing at time intervals after 1 year of age. *Ophthalmology* 105:1307-1310, 1998.)

with a local anesthetic, even though many cases will resolve spontaneously by the age of 1 year. Others prefer to wait until after the first year to allow spontaneous resolution to occur and then perform the procedure, if necessary, while the patient is under general anesthesia. There is some evidence that the success of the procedure declines with increasing age. To evaluate the success of nasolacrimal duct probing beyond the first year of life, records were reviewed at Children's Hospital in Boston.

Study Design.—The 1971 to 1997 records of 303 nasolacrimal duct probings in 252 children older than 1 year were reviewed. Adequate follow-up was available for 280 probings in this series. Individual ducts were evaluated independently. For analysis of procedure success, the children were divided into 5 categories according to age at probing—12 through 14 months, 15 through 17 months, 18 through 23 months, 24 through 35 months, and older than 36 months.

Results.—The overall cure rate of nasolacrimal duct probing in this older pediatric cohort was 92.1%. The cure rate ranged from 88.9% to 96.8% in the various age groups. These differences were not statistically significant (Table 1). Eight ducts were not improved by probing and were cured by secondary procedures.

Conclusions.—Probing for congenital nasolacrimal duct obstruction was very successful in this cohort of children over the age of 1 year. The cure rate did not decrease with advancing age.

► Congenital nasolacrimal duct obstruction is the most common abnormality of the entire lacrimal system in children and occurs in up to 6% of newborns. The decision to proceed with a probing is based primarily on the severity of symptoms, age, and parental concern. Standard of practice within the medical community also plays a part in the decision. It has been shown repeatedly that most nasolacrimal duct obstructions clear spontaneously after conservative management with topical antibiotics and massage. Many authors have reported a spontaneous resolution of more than 90% by 1 year of age. Probing in a hospital setting, with the patient under general anesthesia, offers a controlled environment for the procedure. Many ophthalmologists prefer to probe in this manner because the immobility of the infant allows one to use the fine tactile sensations required for a successful probing. The author has confirmed the findings of others that there is no increased incidence of failure if the probing is delayed beyond 1 year of age.

L.B. Nelson, M.D.

A Randomized Clinical Trial of the Nonsteroidal Eyedrop Diclofenac After Strabismus Surgery

Apt L, Voo I, Isenberg SJ (Harbor-Univ of California, Los Angeles)

Ophthalmology 105:1448-1454, 1998 7–11

Introduction.—To decrease inflammation, topical corticosteroids are frequently prescribed after strabismus surgery. However, because of their side effects, there is a search for less risky anti-inflammatory agents. One nonsteroidal anti-inflammatory drug is diclofenac sodium ophthalmic solution 0.1%, which has been shown to be even more effective than corticosteroids, and which can offer an additional benefit to patients who have strabismus surgery. Pain after eye surgery was found to be significantly reduced with diclofenac, without long-term reduction of sensitivity or impairment of corneal wound healing.

Methods.—There were 52 patients who had strabismus surgery for 80 eyes. The eye that was operated on received 1 drop of prednisolone or diclofenac 4 times a day for 1 week after surgery in this prospective, double-masked, randomized, 2-center clinical trial. On postoperative days 3 and 7, patients were examined for signs of inflammation, such as erythema, edema, discharge, patient comfort, and conjunctival incisional healing.

Results.—In eyes that received prednisolone on postoperative day 7, the conjunctival defects were more frequent and larger. In the inflammatory scores, there were no statistically significant differences between eyes that received prednisolone and those that received diclofenac. In the diclofenac-treated eyes or those treated with bilateral surgery, however, there was less postoperative erythema and edema.

Conclusion.—In controlling inflammation and discomfort, topical diclofenac proved at least as effective as prednisolone in the first week after strabismus surgery, with less delay in incisional wound healing. Topical diclofenac, a nonsteroidal anti-inflammatory agent, may be considered for use after strabismus surgery, in place of corticosteroids. Its anti-inflammatory effect and ability to reduce postsurgical pain are caused by its decreasing prostaglandin levels and prevention of a concurrent rise in leukotriene levels.

► Topical corticosteroids are commonly prescribed to reduce pain and the inflammatory process after strabismus surgery. However, this medication does have potential side effects, including steroid-induced glaucoma, facilitation of microbial infection, and delayed wound healing. Topical diclofenac has been shown to be at least as effective as corticosteroids in reducing inflammation and pain, with less delay in incisional wound healing. Therefore, topical diclofenac should be considered as an alternative to topical corticosteroids in the postoperative management of pain and inflammation following strabismus surgery.

L.B. Nelson, M.D.

Refractive Changes After Pediatric Intraocular Lens Implantation

Enyedi LB, Peterseim MW, Freedman SF, et al (Duke Univ, Durham, NC)

Am J Ophthalmol 126:772-781, 1998 7–12

Introduction.—Intraocular lens (IOL) implantation is being used with increasing frequency in children undergoing cataract surgery. It is not known how pseudophakia affects subsequent eye growth. Some trials suggest that increasing myopia occurs in pseudophakic eyes of children. Long-term evaluation is needed. Refractory changes after cataract surgery and IOL implantation were assessed in infants and children in an ongoing prospective investigation.

Methods.—The refractory errors of patients younger than 18 years undergoing IOL implantation were evaluated at 6 weeks, 3 months, 6 months, 1 year, and yearly thereafter.

Results.—Eighty-three eyes in 81 patients were examined. Cataracts were traumatic in 32 eyes and developmental in 42 eyes. Mean age at implantation was 6.3 years. Mean follow-up was 26.6 months. Patients who were 0 to 2 years of age at the time of surgery had significantly greater predicted myopic shift and a greater variance in the predicted refractive change than those who were older than 2 years at the time of surgery. In agreement with earlier findings, the myopic shift was greatest in younger children and continued until at least 8 years of age, with a marked variability in postoperative refraction. The rate of change varied with age; in young children, the refraction changed by more than 1 D per year (Table 1).

Conclusion.—In children undergoing IOL implantation, there is a trend toward increasing postoperative myopia, which is greatest in the youngest

TABLE 1.—Total Change and Rate of Change in Refraction (Spherical Equivalent) in the Operated-on Eye and the Fellow Eye

			Operated-on Eye		Fellow Eye	
Age at IOL (yrs)	No. of Eyes	Mean Follow-up After IOL (yrs)	Total Change, Mean ± SD (diopters)	Rate of Change, Mean ± SD (diopters/mo)	Total Change, Mean ± SD (diopters)	Rate of Change, Mean ± SD (diopters/mo)
0-2	12	2.5	−3.00 ± 2.7	−0.10 ± 0.07	−0.85 ± 1.1	−0.01 ± 0.01
2-4	23	2.2	−1.50 ± 2.7	−0.05 ± 0.07	0.25 ± 3.2	0.00 ± 0.03
4-6	16	1.9	−1.50 ± 2.3	−0.06 ± 0.14	−0.73 ± 1.5	−0.01 ± 0.03
6-8	9	3.0	−1.80 ± 2.9	−0.04 ± 0.10	−0.64 ± 1.0	0.00 ± 0.01
>8	23	1.8	−0.37 ± 1.6	−0.03 ± 0.12	−0.06 ± 0.5	0.00 ± 0.01

age group and persists until at least 8 years of age. Postoperative refractive changes vary greatly, making it difficult to predict when and where refraction may stabilize for an individual patient. The myopic shift in pseudophakic eyes may be due to excessive axial elongation caused by visual deprivation. It is possible that eyes with corneal opacities or unilateral cataracts may undergo excessive axial elongation or that amblyopic pseudophakic eyes have greater increases in axial length than pseudophakic eyes with normal vision. It is likely that the trend of myopia in these eyes is caused by normal eye growth with a fixed IOL power. Younger children have a greater myopic shift than older children because their eyes elongate more. The eye that has been operated on demonstrates a greater myopic shift than its untreated fellow eye. The IOL power is stable; the normal phakic lens power changes to compensate for axial elongation. Rate of change in refraction does not follow a predictable pattern, reflecting the diversity of actual refractions. These findings support undercorrection in young children at the time of surgery, in anticipation of a significant myopic shift over time. Patients who are 1 or 2 D myopic as adults may then enjoy good uncorrected near acuity, binocularity at near, and reasonably clear uncorrected distance vision.

▶ Many studies have demonstrated that IOL implantation to correct pediatric aphakia is a safe and effective means of providing a clear visual axis and optical correction. Although the anatomical results are encouraging, amblyopia remains the major obstacle to a good functional result, even in the case of an IOL. Although an IOL provides a considerable convenience not afforded by the use of a contact lens, there are no studies showing that an IOL will provide better visual outcome. Because of the changing refractive error of the developing eye, the choice of the IOL power to implant poses a dilemma, as pointed out by the authors. Some surgeons use an implant power to take into account the expected growth of the eye, the refractive error present in other family members, and, in the case of unilateral cataract, the refractive error of the fellow eye. Other surgeons believe that correction to emmetropia is preferable to allow for maximal treatment of amblyopia. The earlier in life a lens is implanted, the greater this dichotomy becomes. More studies will have to be presented to determine the appropriate IOL power to implant to correct aphakia during the amblyogenic age.

L.B. Nelson, M.D.

Refractive Changes Associated With Scleral Buckling and Division in Retinopathy of Prematurity

Chow DR, Ferrone PJ, Trese MT (William Beaumont Hosp, Royal Oak, Mich)

Arch Ophthalmol 116:1446-1448, 1998 7–13

Introduction.—The initial goal in the treatment of retinal detachments associated with retinopathy of prematurity (ROP) is anatomic reattachment of the retina. The ultimate goal is maintenance or improvement of visual function. Scleral buckling induces axial and lenticular myopia: thus, follow-up is important for treatment of these optical changes. The refractory changes associated with scleral buckling and subsequent division of the scleral buckle were evaluated retrospectively in infant eyes with ROP.

Methods.—Medical records were reviewed in infants in whom ROP was managed with an encircling scleral buckle that was subsequently divided in whom refraction was evaluated during and after division of the scleral buckle.

Results.—The average spherical equivalent was −11.1 D (range, −5 to −25 D) after placement of the scleral buckle. These refractions were recorded an average of 12 weeks after placement of the scleral buckle. The average induced anisometropia was −9.5 D in eyes with unilateral scleral buckles. The average spherical equivalent was −5.7 D (range, 1.25 to −14.5 D) after division of the scleral buckle. The induced refractive changes after division of the scleral buckle averaged a hyperopic shift of 5.5 D (range, 2-10.5 D). This was a significant change from the refractions recorded with the scleral buckle.

Conclusion.—Large myopic shifts after scleral buckling in infants with ROP are significantly diminished after revision of the scleral buckle. This underscores the importance of repeated refraction testing in infants after placement and division of the scleral buckle to avoid refractive amblyopia. These infants are in a critical period of visual development at the time of surgery. They are at risk of organic amblyopia and refractive and strabismic amblyopia. The 2 most likely causes of myopic refractive changes in infants are axial elongation induced by the encircling silicone band and a forward shift of the lens that induces lenticular myopia. Neonates with scleral buckling in 1 eye only are at risk of anisometropic amblyopia (average, 9.5 D). It is recommended that all infants be sent to a pediatric ophthalmologist for refractive evaluation and appropriate management within 4 to 6 weeks of surgery. Subsequent division of the scleral buckle helps reduce the risk of intrusion and promotes eye growth. It also reduces induced refractive error. It is further recommended that infants be evaluated by a pediatric ophthalmologist after division of the scleral buckle to make appropriate changes in optical correction. The retinal surgeon and the pediatric ophthalmologist need to collaborate to maximize visual outcome in infants with ROP retinal detachments who are subjected to scleral buckling.

▶ Although the number of patients in this study was small, the findings confirm the observations of others that scleral buckling in infants with ROP often results in large myopic shifts. Dividing the scleral buckle to reduce the risks of intrusion and to promote eye growth has been shown to reduce the myopic shift significantly. These changes in refractive errors can result in refractive amblyopia. There is also the risk of anisometropia or amblyopia when these infants are subjected to scleral buckling in only one eye. As the authors point out, it is important that there exist a close interaction between the pediatric ophthalmologist and the retina surgeon to maximize the visual results in infants with ROP retinal detachments who are subjected to scleral buckling.

L.B. Nelson, M.D.

The Natural History of Infantile Esotropia During the First Six Months of Life

Birch E, for the Pediatric Eye Disease Investigator Group (Retina Found of the Southwest, Dallas; et al)

J AAPOS 2:325-328, 1998 7–14

Introduction.—With the exception of a small number of infants who respond fully to hyperopic correction, infantile esotropia requires surgical intervention. Human and animal investigations have supported the strategy of early surgery in patients with esotropia. Even brief periods of 3 to 4 weeks of esotropia have resulted in permanent loss of binocular cortical cells. The natural history of ocular alignment in infantile esotropia at 2 to 4 months of age was examined in a prospective study of 80 infants enrolled at the Retinal Foundation of the Southwest (RFSW) and a retrospective study of 41 infants who were evaluated to provide pilot data for the Early Surgery for Congenital Esotropia Trial (ESCET).

Methods.—Seventy-nine of 80 children in the RFSW cohort were reassessed at age 4½ years or older to determine ocular alignment and stereopsis.

Results.—In infants with constant esotropia of 40 prism D (PD) or greater, none of 45 children in the RFSW cohort and none of 21 children in the ESCET cohort demonstrated resolution to orthophoria. Only 2 infants had a reduction in the angle of deviation below 40 PD (35 PD and 20 PD, respectively). Resolution to orthophoria was observed in a few infants who initially had small-angle or variable-angle esotropia. At follow-up at age 4½ years or older, 91% of the children in the RFSW cohort had alignment within 8 PD of orthoposition and 30% had stereoacuity of 3,000" to 60". Children who underwent surgical alignment at age 6 months had a greater incidence of coarse stereopsis than those who underwent alignment at 7 to 15 months.

Conclusion.—Infants in whom constant esotropia is observed at 2 to 4 months of age with constant esotropia of 40 PD or greater are candidates for surgical correction. Only a few infants, particularly those with small angle esotropia, experienced resolution to orthophoria. Patients who underwent surgical alignment at age 6 months had a higher rate of coarse stereopsis than those who underwent alignment at 7 to 15 months. This report supports earlier data suggesting that early surgical alignment may promote development of at least coarse stereopsis.

▶ The authors demonstrated that infantile esotropia that is equal to or greater than 40 PD without significant hyperopia noted at age 2 to 4 months rarely, if ever, resolves spontaneously. Although early surgical intervention for infantile esotropia improves binocular sensory outcome, further studies are necessary to determine whether surgical intervention by age 4 months will truly produce a higher grade of binocularity. This study will need to be performed in a prospective randomized manner with the results not available until these children can perform sensory tests adequately.

L.B. Nelson, M.D.

Suggested Reading

Holmes JM, Droste PJ, Beck RW: The natural history of acute traumatic sixth nerve palsy or paresis. *J AAPOS* 2:265-268, 1998.

▶ For acute traumatic sixth nerve palsy, the spontaneous recovery rate has been reported to be lower than for microvasular cases, ranging between 12% and 54%. Because of the low spontaneous recovery rate there has been much interest in early intervention of botulinum toxin. Injection of botulinum toxin into the ipsilateral medial rectus may reduce its contracture and increase lateral rectus recovery. In this prospective multicenter study, the overall recovery rate for traumatic sixth nerve palsies, particularly in unilateral cases, was much higher than previously reported. Further studies are needed to determine which patients with acute traumatic sixth nerve palsies will spontaneously recover and which would benefit from botulinum injections.

L.B. Nelson, M.D.

▶ This study demonstrates the power of proper study design and the critical importance of adequate sample size for investigating common clinical problems.

Holmes et al. found that the spontaneous recovery rate for unilateral sixth nerve palsies was 84% compared to rates in the literature ranging from 12% to 54%. The recovery rate here was related to the severity at the time of the initial examination. The previous data was based upon retrospective studies with a heterogeneous group of patients.

This work and other similar studies directed by the JAEB Center for Health Research, Tampa, Florida, should be regarded as the definitive methodology to investigate conditions with a controversial natural history.

R.C. Sergott, M.D.

8 Neuro-ophthalmology

Non-arteritic Ischemic Optic Neuropathy: Where Do We Stand, and Where Are We Going?

by Robert C. Sergott, M.D.

Ischemic disease of the optic nerve remains one of the major causes of blindness and visual disability in America. In contrast to cardiology and myocardial infarction and, more recently, neurology and stroke, neuro-ophthalmology has not moved beyond the clinical descriptive phase for the most common ischemic disease of the optic nerve, non-arteritic ischemic optic neuropathy (NAION).

In an effort to provide clinicians with a working template about NAION, I will review NAION and postulate the direction in which neuro-ophthalmologic research needs to move.

In my opinion, the clinical working knowledge about NAION is best illustrated by 2 studies. First, the work of Boghen and Glaser[1] described the natural history of NAION that most neuro-ophthalmologists still adhere to. Although published 28 years ago, this study gave us the following foundation:

- NAION is a disease of the vasculopathic age group.
- NAION is more common in patients with hypertension.
- Visual function in NAION is "monotonously static," with only 1 of 38 patients improving spontaneously.

Boghen and Glaser's observations were confirmed by other independent studies.[2-5]

Since 1971, the most useful new observation about NAION was made by Professor William Hoyt. Dr. Hoyt realized that most, if not all, patients with NAION displayed congenitally anomalous optic discs with a very small or absent central cup. This simple, but elegant, observation has been confirmed by other investigators.[6-8]

Although initially promising and supported by other independent studies,[9-11] the use of optic nerve sheath decompression (ONSD) for the select patients with progressive visual loss due to NAION became the subject of a vociferous debate, one frequently charged with inflammatory accusations. Fortunately, or unfortunately, depending upon your bias, ONSD was dismissed by the Ischemic Optic Neuropathy Decompression Trial (IONDT).[12-13]

From my perspective, the IONDT had several strengths and weaknesses:

Strengths

- Prospective design
- Randomized
- Expert epidemiologic support and analysis

Weaknesses

- Did not require that the contralateral optic disc demonstrate a congenitally anomalous appearance.
- MRI scans were not done. Therefore, inflammatory optic neuritis/papillitis could be misdiagnosed as NAION.
- Many surgeons were relatively inexperienced in ONSD.
- It was never considered that the postoperative loss of vision could be the result of poor surgical technique. The traction time upon the globe was not reported.
- A statistically significant greater number of patients with diabetes mellitus were in the non-operated group. The issue of possible diabetic papillopathy, a condition with a much greater rate of spontaneous improvement, was not considered.
- The 42% spontaneous improvement rate of NAION has not been the post-IONDT experience of most neuro-ophthalmologists.
- 80% of patients in the study had nonprogressive NAION. In the previous reports, surgery was recommended only for patients with progressive NAION.
- One center was eliminated from the final data analysis because of "protocol violations." (The center and the investigator were cleared of all charges by a university oversight committee.) That center allegedly had excellent surgical results.

Presently, surgery for NAION remains neuro-ophthalmologic napalm, and we do not advocate ONSD as a treatment option. However, we do recommend a critical reexamination of the data.

Where are we going now? I believe, based upon recent observations at Wills Eye Hospital, that neuro-ophthalmology needs to follow the lead of cardiology, especially in terms of lipid physiology. We have recently identified a subset of patients between the ages of 30 and 50 misdiagnosed with "papillitis" that have NAION.[14]

These patients have demonstrated statistically significant elevations in total serum cholesterol ($P < 0.001$), low-density lipoproteins ("bad" cholesterol, $P < 0.001$), and serum triglycerides ($P < 0.002$). No previous studies have considered that patients in this age group may develop ischemic disease of the optic nerve. Well-designed clinical studies have now shown that elevations of serum cholesterol and low-density lipoproteins are unequivocally associated with an increased risk of ischemic cardiovascular disease and stroke.[15]

These patients represent a distinct subset of NAION because:

- All patients had a congenitally anomalous "disc at risk" in the contralateral eye.
- All patients had gadolinium-enhanced, high-resolution MRI scans that showed no evidence of central nervous system or optic nerve demyelination.
- Patients followed the "monotonously static" natural history of Boghen and Glaser.

Some important implications evolve from this group with NAION and abnormal serum lipids.

- Hyperlipidemia may first present as NAION. The diagnosis of significant lipid pathology rests with the ophthalmologist and neuro-ophthalmologist
- Treatment of patients with hyperlipidemia prior to age of 50, rather than 5 or 10 years later, has great importance in possibly preventing myocardial infarction and stroke.
- Treatment of hyperlipidemia may decrease the risk of NAION in the contralateral eye.

Similar lipid abnormalities have not been seen in patients with acute NAION over the age of 50.

Based on these new data, I propose that further, well-designed investigations of lipid abnormalities and other optic neuropathies be undertaken. The optic neuropathies that merit further study include: (1) optic nerve drusen, (2) low-tension glaucoma, (3) primary open-angle glaucoma, and (4) branch or central retinal artery occlusions in young patients without cardiac or hematologic abnormalities.

References

1. Boghen DR, Glaser JS: Ischemic optic neuropathy: The clinical profile and natural history. *Brain* 98:689-708, 1975.
2. Repka MX, Savino PJ, Schatz NJ, et al: Clinical profile and long-term implications of anterior ischemic optic neuropathy. *Am J Ophthalmol* 96:478-483, 1983.
3. Kline LB: Progression of visual defects in ischemic optic neuropathy. *Am J Ophthalmol* 106:199-203, 1988.
4. Borchert M, Lessell S: Progressive and recurrent nonarteritic anterior ischemic optic neuropathy. *Am J Ophthalmol* 106:443-449, 1988.
5. Beri M, Klugman MR, Kohler JA, et al: Anterior ischemic optic neuropathy: VII. Incidence of bilaterality and various influencing factors. *Ophthalmology* 94:1020-1028, 1987.
6. Beck RW, Savino PJ, Repka MX, et al: Optic disc structure in anterior ischemic optic neuropathy. *Ophthalmology* 91:1334-1337, 1984.
7. Beck RW, Servais GE, Hayreh SS: Anterior ischemic optic neuropathy: IX. Cup-to-disc ratio and its role in pathogenesis. *Ophthalmology* 94:1503-1508, 1987.

8. Doro S, Lessell S: Cup-to-disc ratio and ischemic optic neuropathy. *Arch Ophthalmol* 104:1143-1144, 1985.
9. Sergott RC, Cohen MS, Bosley TM, et al: Optic nerve decompression may improve the progressive form of non-arteritic ischemic optic neuropathy. *Arch Ophthalmol* 107:1743-1754, 1989.
10. Kelman SE, Elman MJ: Optic nerve sheath decompression for nonarteritic ischemic optic neuropathy improves multiple visual function measurements. *Arch Ophthalmol* 109:667-671, 1991.
11. Spoor TC, Wilkinson MJ, Ramocki JM: Optic nerve sheath decompression for the treatment of progressive nonarteritic ischemic optic neuropathy. *Am J Ophthalmol* 15:724-728, 1991.
12. The Ischemic Optic Neuropathy Decompression Trial Research Group: Optic nerve decompression surgery for nonarteritic anterior ischemic optic neuropathy is not effective and may be harmful. *JAMA* 273:625-632, 1995.
13. Levin LA: Clarifying the treatment of nonarteritic anterior ischemic optic neuropathy (editorial). *JAMA* 273:666-667, 1995.
14. DeRamo V, Sergott RC, Savino PJ, et al: Non-arteritic ischemic optic neuropathy in young patients is associated with elevated lipid profiles, Submitted for publication.
15. Cleeman JI, Lenfant C: The National Cholesterol Education Program: Progress and prospects. *JAMA* 280:2099-2104, 1998.

The Fall and Rise of Carotid Endarterectomy in the United States and Canada

Tu JV, Hannan EL, Anderson GM, et al (Inst for Clinical Evaluative Sciences, Toronto; Univ of Toronto; State Univ of New York, Albany; et al)
N Engl J Med 339:1441-1447, 1998 8–1

Introduction.—Carotid endarterectomy is proven effective in the prevention of stroke when performed at regional centers of surgical excellence. However, it remains to be seen how clinical trials of carotid endarterectomy have affected clinical practice. Recent trends in the performance of carotid endarterectomy in the United States and Canada were analyzed.

Methods.—Discharge data from 1983 through 1995 were obtained for calculation of the annual rates of carotid endarterectomy in California, New York, and Ontario, Canada. The analysis focused on whether patients treated during the early 1990s were selectively referred to centers of surgical excellence—that is, hospitals with a high volume of cases and low hospital mortality rates.

Results.—From 1984 to 1989, carotid endarterectomy rates among adults aged 40 years and older fell from 126 to 66/100,000 in California; from 65 to 40/100,000 in New York; and from 40 to 15/100,000 in Ontario. This trend was related to studies showing unacceptably high complication rates. After subsequent studies demonstrating the benefits of carotid endarterectomy, the rates of this procedure rose again. By 1995, rates had risen to 99/100,000 in California, 96/100,000 in New York, and 38/100,000 in Ontario. This trend was not associated with any significant increase in referrals to high-volume, low-mortality centers.

Conclusion.—In response to clinical trials, the rates of carotid endarterectomy in North America have fallen and risen dramatically in recent years. The recent increase in carotid endarterectomy procedure has not been associated with selective referral to centers of surgical excellence. Thus, it is unclear whether the benefits of this procedure to the general population are the same as those achieved in the clinical trials.

► Since publication of the favorable results of carotid endarterectomy for stroke prevention, there has been a rapid increase in the number of procedures performed. These favorable results were obtained when the procedure was performed only at regional centers of surgical excellence. This study reports an unfortunate outcome of the successful carotid endarterectomy studies. Rather than being referred to surgical centers of excellence, the patients underwent endarterectomy at local hospitals. Therefore, the lack of selective referrals to centers with the lowest mortality rates indicates that the general population will undergo more surgery without necessarily experiencing the expected benefits of stroke prevention.

This insightful study demonstrates the dichotomy of theory and reality in American medicine. The financial pressures upon physicians, surgeons, institutions, and insurers in the current medical marketplace have coalesced to discourage referrals to centers of excellence. This scenario is a tragic outcome of the commercialization of medicine, with our patients' care often going to the "lowest bidder."

This collective behavior on the part of providers, hospitals, and managed care companies invites government oversight of practice patterns. Given the apparent lack of concern about the patients' welfare and the insurance industry's first loyalty to their profits and shareholders, it is only a matter of time until governmental oversight will occur. Physicians need to alert elected officials to this dilemma and demand that insurance companies pay for the best care, not necessarily the least expensive care. Numerous studies have demonstrated that the best care provided earliest in a patient's disease often is the least expensive in the long run.

R.C. Sergott, M.D.

Benefit of Carotid Endarterectomy in Patients With Symptomatic Moderate or Severe Stenosis

Barnett HJM, for the North American Symptomatic Carotid Endarterectomy Trial Collaborators (John P Robarts Research Inst, London, Ont; et al)

N Engl J Med 339:1415-1425, 1998 8–2

Objective.— Whether endarterectomy is beneficial for all patients with symptomatic carotid stenosis is controversial. Outcomes of carotid endarterectomy in patients with moderate stenosis enrolled from December 1987 through December 1996 in the North American Symptomatic Carotid Endarterectomy Trial were compared with those of patients with severe stenosis who enrolled through February 1991.

Methods.—Patients with symptomatic ischemia on the same side as the stenosis within 180 days before study entry were stratified by degree of stenosis (50% to 69% or less than 50%) and randomly allocated to the endarterectomy group (n = 1,108) or to medical care only (n = 1,118). Neurologic assessments were performed at baseline and at 1, 3, 6, 9, and 12 months and every 4 months thereafter. Brain imaging studies were obtained after suspected strokes. Duplex US was performed at baseline, 1 month later, annually thereafter, and after suspected strokes. Deaths and site, type, severity, and duration of strokes were outcome measures. Patients were followed for an average of 5 years.

Results.—At 5 years, ipsilateral stroke was detected in 22.2% of the high-moderate stenosis group receiving medical therapy and 15.7% of those undergoing surgery, and in 18.7% of the low-moderate stenosis group receiving medical therapy and 14.9% of those undergoing surgery. Disabling strokes occurred in 7.2% of high-moderate stenosis patients receiving medical therapy and in 2.8% of patients undergoing surgery, and in 4.7% of the low-moderate stenosis group receiving medical therapy and 4.6% of those undergoing surgery. According to the results of Cox regression analysis, surgery was most beneficial to men, recent stroke patients, those with recent hemispheric symptoms, and those taking 650 mg or more of aspirin daily.

Conclusion.—Endarterectomy did not confer a significantly decreased stroke risk on patients with moderate carotid stenosis. At 8 years, patients with severe stenosis (more than 70%) had a significant benefit from surgery.

▶ This trial examined a very important, and common, clinical problem: the benefit of carotid endartectomy in patients with symptomatic moderate stenosis (defined as stenosis of < 70%). In addition, the authors examined the 8-year follow-up and potential benefit of carotid endarterectomy in patients with 70% to 99% stenosis.

In a well-designed, clinically precise study, the authors have reported some very important results. First, with patients having severe stenosis (> 70%), there was a durable benefit of carotid endarterectomy at the 8-year follow-up point, with the primary measurement outcome being any fatal or nonfatal stroke ipsilateral to the stenosis. This benefit was greatest among men with a recent stroke and in patients with hemispheric symptoms. In patients with moderate stenosis (50%-69%), there was only a moderate reduction in stroke risk. Decisions about surgical intervention in these patients should be made considering risk factors and, according to the authors, "exceptional surgical skill is obligatory." Patients with stenosis of less than 50% did not benefit from endarterectomy.

Carotid endarterectomy, in my opinion, does have a place in the management of patients with severe stenosis, provided the procedure is performed by highly skilled surgeons with a low complication rate. Ophthalmologists confronted with patients with a transient ischemic attack in the distribution of either carotid artery must proceed promptly with US to evaluate the anatomy of the carotid system. If Doppler US demonstrates significant stenosis, then MR angiography should be done and evaluation arranged with a neurosurgeon with a low complication rate for carotid endarterectomy.

R.C. Sergott, M.D.

Importance of Hemodynamic Factors in the Prognosis of Symptomatic Carotid Occlusion

Grubb RL Jr, Derdeyn CP, Fritsch SM, et al (Washington Univ, St Louis; Jewish Hosp of St Louis)

JAMA 280:1055-1060, 1998 8–3

Background.—The role of hemodynamic factors in the pathogenesis of stroke has not been determined for patients with carotid artery occlusion. When cerebral perfusion pressure is normal, cerebral blood flow closely matches the tissue's metabolic rate and, thus, the oxygen extraction fraction (OEF) is fairly stable. As cerebral hemodynamic failure progresses, first blood volume increases to try to compensate for vasodilation, then (in stage II failure) OEF increases to maintain cerebral oxygen metabolism and brain function. These authors tested the hypothesis that increased OEF in the cerebral hemisphere distal to symptomatic carotic artery occlusion is a harbinger of stroke in these patients.

Methods.—The subjects were 81 patients with carotid artery occlusion who had transient ischemic neurologic deficits or had had a previous stroke in the territory of the occluded artery. All subjects underwent positron emission tomography to measure increases in regional OEF. Increased OEF in the cerebral hemisphere ipsilateral to the occluded carotid artery (i.e., stage II hemodynamic failure) was found in 39 patients (28 men and 11 women; mean age, 64 years), and 42 patients (30 men and 12 women; mean age, 66 years) were found to have normal OEF. Both groups of patients were followed with telephone calls every 6 months to elicit information on subsequent stroke, ipsilateral ischemic stroke, and death; follow-up averaged 31.5 months.

Findings.—Strokes were significantly more common in the patients with stage II hemodynamic failure: Twelve strokes occurred in these 39 patients (31%), 11 of which were ipsilateral. In comparison, 3 strokes occurred in the 42 patients with normal OEF (7%), 2 of which were ipsilateral. Multivariate analysis identified 2 independent predictors of stroke: increasing age and stage II hemodynamic failure. The patients with stage II hemodynamic failure had age-adjusted relative risk of ipsilateral ischemic stroke of 7.3 and of either ipsilateral or contralateral stroke of 6.0. Mortality rates in the 2 groups were similar, as 6 patients in each group died.

Conclusion.—Increased oxygen extraction is an independent risk factor for ischemic stroke in patients with symptomatic carotid artery occlusion.

Medical treatment in these high-risk patients had little effect, and, thus, surgical approaches should be considered. In particular, extracranial-intracranial arterial bypass surgery might be an appropriate approach to these patients, and it warrants further study.

► Dr. Powers and his team from Washington University in St. Louis, Mo. have been leaders in investigating cerebral ischemia and in providing a rational basis for therapeutic interventions. In my opinion, the present study is very well designed and identifies a subset of patients with carotid artery occlusions who are at increased risk for stroke. These patients may benefit from a much-maligned operation, the superficial temporal artery–middle cerebral anastomosis. The challenge not only for neuro-ophthalmology but also for all of medicine is precisely identifying patients who have the greatest chance to benefit from specific medical or surgical therapies.

The authors used positron emission tomography scanning to identify patients with increased cerebral OEF distal to an ipsilateral carotid occlusion. Strokes occurred in 12 of 39 patients with stage II hemodynamic failure and in 3 of 42 without failure ($P = 0.005$). Therefore, the authors discovered those individuals with carotid occlusion who are likely to have strokes despite maximal medical therapy.

Unfortunately positron emission tomography scanning is not universally available, but clinicians should consider referring patients with carotid occlusion for this procedure. A simpler reliable technique for measuring cerebral OEF (flow?, metabolism?) is now required.

R.C. Sergott, M.D.

High Risk of Cerebral-Vein Thrombosis in Carriers of a Prothrombin-Gene Mutation and in Users of Oral Contraceptives

Martinelli I, Sacchi E, Landi G, et al (Univ of Milan, Italy)

N Engl J Med 338:1793-1797, 1998 8–4

Introduction.—Patients with cerebral-vein thrombosis may also have headache, seizures, dysphasia, impaired consciousness, and focal deficits (motor or sensory). The severity of the symptoms and a high mortality rate make cerebral-vein thrombosis a frightening event. Risk factors of cerebral-vein thrombosis were assessed, including genetic risk factors (mutations in genes encoding factor V and prothrombin) and nongenetic risk factors (use of oral contraceptives).

Methods.—Risk factor prevalence was compared in 40 patients with cerebral-vein thrombosis, in 80 patients with deep-vein thrombosis, and in 120 healthy control subjects. Serum samples were obtained for DNA analysis of the G1691A mutation in the factor V gene and the G20210A prothrombin-gene mutation, which are known genetic risk factors for venous thrombosis.

Results.—Eight (20%), 14 (18%), and 3 (3%) patients, respectively, from the cerebral-vein thrombosis group, the deep-vein thrombosis group,

Reservation Card for the Year Book

Yes! I would like my own copy of ***Year Book of Ophthalmology***® at the price of **$84.00** (**$93.00** outside the U.S.) plus sales tax, postage, and handling. Please begin my subscription with the current edition according to the terms described below.* I understand that I will have 30 days to examine each annual edition.

Name ____________________

Address ____________________

City ____________________ State __________ ZIP __________

Method of Payment

Check (in U.S. dollars, drawn on a U.S. bank, payable to ***Year Book of Ophthalmology***®)

❑ VISA ❑ MasterCard ❑ Discover ❑ AmEx ❑ Bill me

Card number ____________________ Exp. date: __________

Signature ____________________

Prices are subject to change without notice. PMC-356

Subscribe to the related journal in your field!

Yes! Begin my one-year subscription to ***Journal of AAPOS (American Association for Pediatric Ophthalmology and Strabismus)*** (6 issues).

Name ____________________

Institution ____________________

Address ____________________

City ____________________ State __________

ZIP/PC __________ Country ____________________

Specialty ____________________
(Students/residents, please list Institution)

Subscription prices (through 9/30/99)

		USA	Canada*	Int'l
Individuals	❑	$110.00	$141.24	$132.00
Institutions	❑	140.00	173.34	162.00
Students, residents	❑	62.00	89.88	84.00

Method of payment

Enclose payment (check or credit card number) and we'll send an extra issue FREE!

❑ Check (in U.S. dollars, drawn on a U.S. bank, and payable to ***Journal of AAPOS***)

❑ VISA ❑ MasterCard ❑ Discover

❑ AmEx ❑ Bill me Exp. date __________

Card # ____________________

Signature ____________________

*Includes Canadian GST

Individual/student subscriptions must be in the name of, billed to, and paid for by the individual.

Airmail rates available upon request.
Prices subject to change without notice.

J075991YA

*Your Year Book service guarantee:

When you subscribe to the *Year Book*, you will receive advance notice of future annual volumes about two months before publication. To receive the new edition, you need do nothing—we'll send you the new volume as soon as it is available. If you want to discontinue, the advance notice allows you time to notify us of your decision. If you are not completely satisfied, you have 30 days to return any *Year Book*.

NO POSTAGE NECESSARY IF MAILED IN THE UNITED STATES

BUSINESS REPLY MAIL

FIRST-CLASS MAIL PERMIT NO 135 ST LOUIS MO

POSTAGE WILL BE PAID BY ADDRESSEE

SUBSCRIPTION SERVICES
MOSBY, INC.
11830 WESTLINE INDUSTRIAL DRIVE
ST. LOUIS MO 63146-9988

NO POSTAGE NECESSARY IF MAILED IN THE UNITED STATES

BUSINESS REPLY MAIL

FIRST-CLASS MAIL PERMIT NO 135 ST LOUIS MO

POSTAGE WILL BE PAID BY ADDRESSEE

SUBSCRIPTION SERVICES
MOSBY, INC.
11830 WESTLINE INDUSTRIAL DRIVE
ST. LOUIS MO 63146-9988

Want to speed up the process?

To order a *Year Book* or *Advances*, you also may call 1-800-426-4545

To subscribe to a journal today, call toll-free in the U.S.:
1-800-453-4351
or fax 314-432-1158
Outside the U.S., call: 314-453-4351

Visit us at: *www.mosby.com/periodicals*

Mosby, Inc.
Subscription Services
11830 Westline Industrial Drive
St. Louis, MO 63146 U.S.A.

Mosby

and control group were carriers of the prothrombin-gene mutation. Results were similar for the mutation in the factor V gene. Compared with control subjects, the proportion of oral-contraceptive users was higher among women with cerebral-vein thrombosis and deep-vein thrombosis (32%, 96%, and 61%, respectively). In women taking oral contraceptives and who had a prothrombin-gene mutation, the odds ratio for cerebral-vein thrombosis was nearly 150.

Conclusion.—There is a hypercoagulable state related to idiopathic cerebral-vein thrombosis in 35% of patients. The most commonly observed coagulation abnormality was the G20210A mutation in the prothrombin gene. Oral contraceptives were strongly correlated with cerebral-vein thrombosis. The combined effect of prothrombin-gene mutation and use of oral contraceptives notably increased the risk of cerebral-vein thrombosis. Their combination probably intensified their individual effects on coagulation. They both increased plasma levels of prothrombin, the zymogen responsible for thrombin formation. It is recommended that carriers of the prothrombin-gene mutation who have had an episode of thrombosis discontinue use of oral contraceptives. Women should probably be screened for prothrombin-gene mutation before oral contraceptives are prescribed. The efficacy and safety of oral anticoagulation therapy needs to be established in patients with cerebral-vein thrombosis.

► Cerebral-vein thrombosis is both a vision-threatening and life-threatening (mortality rate between 5% and 30%) disease that may first present to ophthalmologists because of papilledema. MRI scanning usually establishes the diagnosis. Prompt diagnosis and management by ophthalmologists, neurologists, and hematologists is essential.

This study establishes both a genetic and pharmacologic predisposition to this disorder. A mutation (G20210A) in the prothrombin gene increases the risk of the disorder by a factor of 10. Oral contraceptives also increase the risk by a factor of 20. Both the G20210A mutation and oral contraceptives increase plasma levels of prothrombin, the zymogen necessary for thrombin formation in the coagulation system.

In the future, screening for prothrombin gene mutations prior to the prescription of oral contraceptives may be worthwhile. The next extension of this work will be to search for the prothrombin gene mutations in venous thrombotic disease in other CNS and ophthalmic disorders.

R.C. Sergott, M.D.

Optic Neuropathy Associated With Sleep Apnea Syndrome

Mojon DS, Mathis J, Zulauf M, et al (Univ of Bern, Switzerland; Univ of Basel, Switzerland)

Ophthalmology 105:874-877, 1998 8–5

Introduction.—Sleep apnea syndrome (SAS) is typified by recurrent complete or partial upper airway obstruction during sleep. Ophthalmologic findings associated with SAS include floppy eyelid syndrome and keratoconus. Ophthalmologic examinations, including computerized perimetry, were performed to determine ocular abnormalities in 9 patients referred for suspected SAS.

Methods.—Patients underwent ophthalmologic examination, visual field data analysis, physical examination, neurologic examination, overnight polysomnography, chemical profile, and tests for fasting blood glucose levels. The respiratory disturbance index was calculated from the polysomnographic data.

Results.—Two patients were excluded: 1 because of optic nerve drusen with constricted visual fields and the other because of tilted discs with corresponding temporal visual field defects. Three patients with severe SAS and 1 with moderate SAS had relative nasal visual field defects. Two patients with severe mild-moderate SAS had visual fields within normal limits. There was a positive correlation between respiratory disturbance index and mean visual field defect and visual field loss variance. All 7 patients had normal clinical ophthalmologic examinations. Visual field defects remained stable over 18 months in 2 of 3 patients with severe SAS who were treated with continuous positive airway pressure (CPAP). One patient with optic nerve drusen and severe SAS had dramatic improvement in constricted visual fields after treatment with CPAP.

Conclusion.—Patients with SAS had visual field defects consistent with an optic neuropathy. Because these defects remained unchanged, they probably were permanent lesions. It may be that further field deterioration was prevented by CPAP therapy. Findings suggest an association between SAS and visual field defects.

► Sleep disorders have been a rapidly growing area of interest for neurologists and pulmonologists. As this article reports, ophthalmologists should consider sleep disorders in the pathogenesis of optic neuropathies in some patients.

Although this study is largely an anecdotal series of case reports, it provides the framework for future investigations. Of particular interest is the patient with optic nerve drusen whose visual fields improved with the use of CPAP. The authors correctly point out that, because of the observational character of their study, an association exists between SAS and optic neuropathy visual field defects. As of yet, a direct causal relationship cannot be established, and other factors may be involved.

R.C. Sergott, M.D.

Effect of Subtotal Thyroidectomy on Natural History of Ophthalmopathy in Graves' Disease

Abe Y, Sato H, Noguchi M, et al (Tokai Univ, Kanagawa, Japan; Ito Hosp, Tokyo)

World J Surg 22:714-717, 1998 8–6

Objective.—Studies relating the worsening of Graves' ophthalmopathy either to subtotal thyroidectomy or to treatment with radioactive iodine have given conflicting results. The effect of subtotal thyroidectomy on the outcome of Graves' ophthalmopathy compared with the effect of radioactive iodine treatment was examined in a long-term prospective study.

Methods.—Two hundred eighty-seven patients with Graves' disease were observed prospectively for 5 years; all patients were treated with antithyroid drugs. Nonresponders were treated with radioactive iodine (n = 67) or had subtotal thyroidectomy (n = 18). Thyroid function was assessed, and proptosis of the eyes were measured.

Results.—The average proptosis values increased over 5 years from 14.8 to 15.0 mm. Proptosis values increased in patients treated medically (+0.27) and in those treated with radioactive iodine (+0.89) but not in those receiving subtotal thyroidectomy (−0.07). The degree of proptosis was age-dependent (Fig 2). In patients treated with subtotal thyroidectomy, proptosis was unchanged in 77%, increased in 5.6%, and decreased in 16.7%. In patients treated with radioactive iodine, proptosis was unchanged in 86.6%, increased in 10.4%, and decreased in 3.0%.

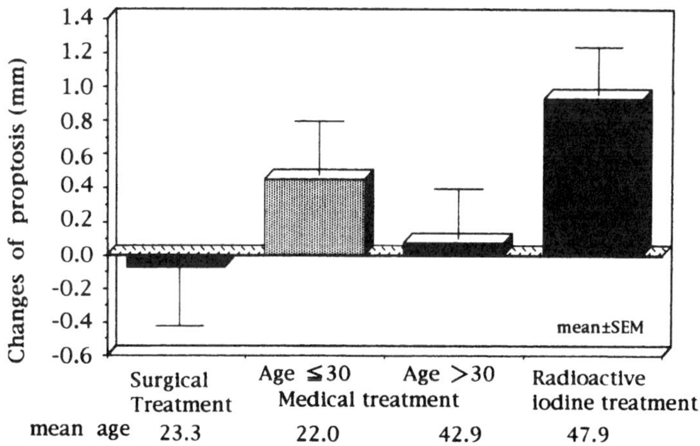

FIGURE 2.—Effect of treatment on the progression of proptosis in patients with Graves' disease. (Courtesy of Abe Y, Sato H, Noguchi M, et al: Effect of subtotal thyroidectomy on natural history of ophthalmology in Graves' disease. *World J Surg* 22:714-717. Copyright 1998, Springer-Verlag.)

Conclusion.—Surgery rather than treatment with radioactive iodine is a better choice for patients with ophthalmopathy as a result of Graves' disease.

▶ The literature continues to be deluged with "studies" reportedly elucidating the effect of thyroid treatment upon the clinical course of Graves' ophthalmopathy. This study does little to help us. Practicing ophthalmologists are strongly urged to read the letter to the editor published in *The New England Journal of Medicine* from Drs. Gorman and Offord,[1] which applies some much needed perspective to this debate. Drs. Gorman and Offord from the Mayo Clinic point out the shortcomings of another study[2] examining the same issue with special attention to radioactive iodine.

Both the surgical study and the radioactive iodine study are potentially dangerous. I have already been contacted by 2 plaintiffs' malpractice attorneys about potential claims of worsening eye problems after radioactive ablation of the thyroid gland.

As Drs. Gorman and Offord state that such studies are inconclusive because of serious methodologic flaws. Patients must be advised and counseled about the scientific shortcomings of these studies.

R.C. Sergott, M.D.

References

1. Gorman CA, Offord KP: Therapy for hyperthyroidism and Graves' ophthalmopathy [letter]. *N Engl J Med* 338:1546-1547, 1998.
2. Bartalena L, Marcocci C, Bogazzi F, et al: Relation between therapy for hyperthyroidism and the course of Graves' ophthalmopathy. *N Engl J Med* 338:73-78, 1998.

Pupil Involvement in Patients With Diabetes-associated Oculomotor Nerve Palsy

Jacobson DM (Marshfield Clinic, Wis)

Arch Ophthalmol 116:723-727, 1998 8–7

Objective.—Diabetes is a risk factor for ischemic oculomotor nerve injury. The size and reactivity of the pupil is an accurate indication of oculomotor function. The frequency of pupil involvement in patients with diabetes-associated oculomotor nerve palsy was estimated.

Methods.—Pupils in 26 diabetic patients were measured to estimate pupil diameters to the nearest 0.5 mm. Any anisocoria was recorded and used to define pupil involvement. Pupil diameters were assessed within 7 to 21 days after onset of diplopia in 22 of 26 patients.

Results.—Anisocoria, present in 14 patients at the beginning of the study, resolved completely in 7 during the study. Ten patients had internal ophthalmoplegia ranging from 0.5 to 2.5 mm with a degree of anisocoria 1 mm or less.

Conclusion.—Oculomotor nerve palsy occurs more frequently than previously suspected in patients with diabetes. This method detected anisocoria of ≥0.5 mm.

► Dr. Jacobson must be congratulated upon a meticulous clinical investigation demonstrating that mild anisocoria is more common than had been expected in diabetic oculomotor nerve palsies.

If you disregard editorials, this article is also unique because of its single authorship. The Transfer of Copyright form was probably thought to be incomplete when it arrived in the journal's office.

Most clinicians do not have the excellent equipment, skills, or knowledge necessary to record measurements as Dr. Jacobson has done. Therefore, clinicians may accept 1.0 mm of anisocoria, we must stress, under the proper historical circumstances.

In such a crucial differential diagnostic plot, pitting a benign ischemic process against a life-threatening aneurysm, clinicians must always use all possible information. I personally rely upon the patients' history of the circumstances about the onset of the palsy except when the pupil is clearly and unequivocally involved.

R.C. Sergott, M.D.

Benign Intracranial Hypertension and Recombinant Growth Hormone Therapy in Australia and New Zealand

Crock PA, McKenzie JD, Nicoll AM, et al (John Hunter Children's Hosp, Newcastle, England; Royal Children's Hosp, Parkville, Westmead, Austraila; Starship Hosp, Auckland, New Zealand; et al)

Acta Paediatr 87:381-386, 1998 8–8

Objective.—As of 1993, 23 cases of benign intracranial hypertension were identified in patients taking recombinant human growth hormone (rhGH). An additional 4 cases among children in Australia and New Zealand are described and possible pathophysiologic mechanisms and strategies to detect and avoid this complication are discussed.

Case 1.—Boy, 12.5 years, with short stature, was diagnosed with growth hormone deficiency (GHD). He was started on rhGH therapy at 14 IU/m^2/week. After 3 months, a right optic disc with hemorrhagic papilledema developed. rhGH therapy was stopped and the papilloedema resolved over the next month. The therapy was restarted 1 year later without further problems.

Case 2.—Girl, 10.5 years, with 45 XO Turner syndrome was treated with rhGH at a dosage of 28 IU/m^2/week. At 1 month, headache and swollen optic discs developed. She had a CSF pressure of 25 cm H_2O. rhGH therapy was stopped for 2 months until her CSF pressure normalized, and then the therapy continued uneventfully for 3 years.

Case 3.—Adolescent boy, 13 years, with GHD, received rhGH at 14 IU/m^2/week for 2 weeks when severe headache developed. Whereas there was no papilledema, a lumbar puncture revealed a pressure of 21.0 cm H_2O. rhGH therapy was stopped for 4 weeks and then resumed at half the original dose without recurrence.

Case 4.—Adolescent boy, 13.7 years, with diabetes, lethargy, and growth failure, was given rhGH 18.7 IU/m^2/week. After 2 weeks, headaches developed and lumbar pressure increased to 31.0 cm H_2O. The hormone therapy was stopped, and his condition resolved within 5 days. rhGH therapy was restarted 3 months later, but stopped again after several weeks when germinoma was diagnosed.

Results.—Four of 3,332 children treated with rhGH between January 1986 and 1996 displayed intracranial pressure for an overall incidence of 1.2/1,000. Children with biochemical GHD had an incidence of 6.5/1,000 or a relative risk of 18.4.

Conclusion.—Patients with GHD taking rhGH are at increased risk for the development of intracranial hypertension. Baseline and periodic ophthalmologic assessments are recommended for these patients particularly if headache, nausea, or edema are present. Patients can generally be safely restarted on rhGH therapy after the intracranial hypertension resolves.

▶ These authors provide an excellent clinical description and literature review of pseudotumor cerebri and rhGH therapy. My only problem with this work is the use of the term "benign intracranial hypertension." Certainly from a neuro-ophthalmologic perspective, there is absolutely nothing "benign" about this disease. The use of this word minimizes the potentially blinding complications of this disease to both patients and physicians.

It is most interesting, and most important, that cessation of the rhGH therapy produced resolution of the papilledema. Moreover, all the patients were able to be restarted on GH therapy at a lower dose and tolerated this regimen well without recurrent papilledema.

Although rare, this syndrome is of paramount importance to the individual patients, and an astute clinician can ease much stress and avoid excessive testing by being aware of this idiosyncratic complication.

R.C. Sergott, M.D.

Positive Temporal Artery Biopsy 6 Months After Prednisone Treatment

Guevara RA, Newman NJ, Grossniklaus HE (Emory Eye Ctr, Atlanta, Ga)

Arch Ophthalmol 116:1252-1253, 1998 8–9

Background.—Only rarely do histologic findings of giant cell arteritis (GCA) persist after long-term corticosteroid therapy. These authors reported on a temporal artery biopsy that produced positive findings for GCA after long-term treatment with high-dose prednisone.

> *Case Report.*—Woman, 71, was examined for severe headaches, joint pain, and tenderness of the temporal areas. She had experienced a sudden bilateral vision loss, but it had gradually improved. Her erythrocyte sedimentation rate (ESR) was greatly elevated (87 mm/hr). The patient was given a diagnosis of GCA and began taking prednisone, 60 mg/day. Her symptoms immediately improved; she had an ESR of 4 mm/hr after 2 months of therapy; at that time, the prednisone dosage was reduced to 30 mg/day. About 4 months after beginning treatment, the patient underwent successful cataract surgery in the left eye. One week after this surgery, she noticed tenderness in her scalp and temporal area. Her ESR was normal (5 mm/hr), but the prednisone dosage was increased to 40 mg/day until her symptoms abated; then she was tapered back to 30 mg/day. Because she had experienced a recurrence while taking 30 mg/day of prednisone, yet her ESR was normal, the initial diagnosis of GCA was revisited. A biopsy specimen from the left temporal artery revealed the presence of multinucleated giant cells centered around the inner elastic lamina and granulomatous inflammation.

Conclusion.—Both healed and active GCA are associated with substantial intimal thickening, disruption or loss of the internal elastic lamina, and thickening and scarring of the media and adventitia. In healed arteritis, there are only occasional foci of lymphocytes. However, active arteritis is characterized by an inflammatory infiltrate containing lymphocytes, macrophages, and multinucleated giant cells. This patient clearly had active arteritis, despite 6 months of treatment with large doses of prednisone and despite having a normal ESR and experiencing no symptoms. Thus, performing a biopsy in patients with "healed" GCA can provide important information and ensure that treatment is not merely symptomatic.

▶ The diagnosis and management of GCA persists as one of the major clinical challenges in neuro-ophthalmology. Prior to publication of this article, temporal artery biopsies performed 14 days after the initiation of corticosteroids were thought to be useless. This case report explodes that long-standing clinical dogma. Therefore, for patients in whom it is clinically difficult to assess disease activity, temporal artery biopsy later in the disease process may be helpful in management.

As an extension of this report, bilateral, simultaneous temporal artery biopsies should not be performed at the onset of the disease. In our experience at Wills Eye Hospital, bilateral, simultaneous biopsies have not enhanced our diagnostic accuracy (Danesh-Meyer et al., manuscript submitted for publication). We believe that the first temporal artery biopsy should be unilateral, with a 2- to 3-cm specimen, preserving the contralateral side for possible biopsy to assess disease activity.

R.C. Sergott, M.D.

A Relative Afferent Pupillary Defect Without Any Visual Sensory Deficit

Girkin CA, Perry JD, Miller NR (Johns Hopkins Hosp, Baltimore, Md)
Arch Ophthalmol 116:1544-1545, 1998 8–10

Background.—Sometimes afferent defects can be present even when no afferent visual deficit can be found. This case report described an afferent pupillary defect in a patient in whom no afferent visual deficit could be demonstrated.

Case Report.—Woman, 54, was the driver in a high-speed motor vehicle accident. She had not been wearing a seatbelt, and neuroimaging at hospital admission revealed a subarachnoid hemorrhage, a small subdural hematoma, and a basal skull fracture. She required intubation and remained in a coma for 8 days. As she recovered from her coma, marked left facial weakness and diplopia were evident. Six weeks after the accident, her visual acuity was 20/20 in each eye, and she had no color vision deficits. Afferent visual function was normal as measured by both kinetic and static perimetry. However, a moderate relative afferent pupillary defect was evident on the right side. The patient also had fourth, sixth, and seventh nerve pareses on the left side. She was found on MRI to have an infarction in the brachium of the left superior colliculus.

Conclusions.—Before reaching the lateral geniculate body, both afferent axons and visual axons provide information to the pretectal nuclei. The afferent fibers travel to the pretectal area via the brachium of the superior colliculus. Unilateral lesions of this brachium can cause a contralateral relative afferent pupillary defect, even though the affected eye has normal visual acuity, color vision, and visual fields. If the ipsilateral fourth nerve is also injured, fourth nerve palsy can occur in conjunction with these afferent defects.

► This case report is useful for 2 reasons: (1) it reviews the anatomy and physiology of the pupillary light reflex; and (2) it reviews and adds another case to the literature of a rare, nonafferent system mechanism for a Marcus Gunn "efferent" pupillary defect (efferent pupillary defect vs. afferent pupillary defect). The basis for the efferent pupillary defect is an infarction in the brachium of the left superior colliculus. Axons from the anterior visual pathway provide afferent information to the pretectal nuclei prior to the lateral geniculate body. These fibers travel through the brachium of the superior colliculus to the pretectal area. A lesion in this area will produce an efferent pupillary defect–afferent pupillary defect with or without a contralateral or ipsilateral fourth nerve palsy if the nucleus or fasciculus of this nerve is involved.

R.C. Sergott, M.D.

Migrainous Visual Accompaniments Are Not Rare in Late Life: The Framingham Study

Wijman CAC, Wolf PA, Kase CS, et al (Boston Univ; Natl Heart, Lung, and Blood Inst, Framingham, Mass)

Stroke 29:1539-1543, 1998 8–11

Background.—Epidemiologic questionnaires that ask about symptoms of transient ischemic attack often elicit transient visual phenomena called "migraine aura without headache." How common are these phenomena? These authors evaluated the sudden visual symptoms of more than 2,000 participants in the Framingham Study, and explored whether these visual symptoms are related to a greater risk of stroke.

Methods.—Over an 18-year period, 2,110 participants in the Framingham Study were questioned at least 6 times about any sudden visual symptoms they had experienced. First-ever episodes of sudden visual defect (SVD) were recorded and analyzed, and stroke incidence rates were compared between subjects with and without SVD.

Findings.—In total, 186 subjects (8.8%) reported a first-ever SVD during the study. The most common causes were stroke (n = 34), ocular disease (n = 32), and migrainous visual symptoms (n = 26). Subjects reporting migrainous visual symptoms (1.23% of all subjects) reported many different patterns of visual disturbances, including seeing heat rising, zigzag and geometric lines, halos, dancing spots, and "disco lights" (Table 2). Most of the subjects (17, or 65%) had stereotypic symptoms, and most (20, or 77%) had the first symptom after age 50 years. For 15 subjects (58%), the visual symptoms never occurred with headache, and, indeed, 11 subjects (42%) had no history of headache. Most of the subjects (18, or

TABLE 2.—Some of the Patterns of Migrainous Visual Disturbances Described by Subjects

- Heat rising off the ground and things jumping in front of both eyes followed by poor vision
- Loss of vision on the right associated with zigzag lines, moving visual phenomena, and a halo around the area
- Disco lights in front of both eyes and a bright silvery shape in the form of an eyebrow to the right of visual field
- Vision like looking through a kaleidoscope
- Bright lines in half of the visual field of both eyes interfering with ability to read
- Geometric figures consisting of squares with circles in them
- Bright wiggling lines in inferior left visual field advancing superiorly followed by left homonymous hemianopia
- Wavy vision as on television when the picture is not focused
- Vision is jumping like a film in an old film projector
- Dancing spots off to one side followed by blurring of vision and hemianopia on the same side
- Periphery of vision gets black and vision becomes as if looking through a pinhole followed by dancing black and white spots in front of both eyes
- Sudden white sheet descending in front of both eyes

(Courtesy of Wijman CAC, Wolf PA, Kase CS, et al: Migrainous visual accompaniments are not rare in late life: The Framingham Study. *Stroke* 29:1539-1543.

69%) had had 10 or more episodes, and the typical episode lasted either several minutes (7 patients, or 27%), or 15 to 60 minutes (13 patients, or 50%). Three subjects (11.5%) experienced a stroke 1, 3, and 27 years after the onset of the migrainous visual phenomena. Subjects in the same cohort with transient ischemic attack patients were much more likely to have stroke (33.3%) than subjects with migrainous visual phenomena.

Conclusion.—Transient visual phenomena that begin late in life are not uncommon, occurring in 1.33% of women and 1.08% of men. They often occur in the absence of headache or a history of headache; they can last up to an hour. These migrainous visual symptoms do not seem to be associated with an increased risk of stroke, and, thus, invasive diagnostic procedures or therapies to rule out stroke are usually not necessary.

▶ All ophthalmologists and neuro-ophthalmologists should feel some discomfort diagnosing migraine in elderly patients without a history of vascular headaches earlier in life. This study documents this occurrence but clinicians must be extremely cautious.

If the patients relate very stereotypical events over the course of 6 months or longer, then the clinical diagnosis of migraine in the elderly is secure. However, with the new onset of symptoms, clinicians must be aware of CNS ischemia, cerebral edema, or medications producing nonformed visual hallucinatory phenomena. We advocate a complete blood count, Holter monitoring, and MRI when a well-documented history of vascular headaches cannot be obtained.

R.C. Sergott, M.D.

Demonstration of Exclusive Cilioretinal Vascular System Supplying the Retina in Man: Vacant Discs

Parsa CF, Cheeseman EW JR, Maumenee IH (Johns Hopkins Hosp, Baltimore, Md)

Trans Am Ophthalmol Soc 96:95-109, 1998 8–12

Background.—On ophthalmoscopy, eyes with a combined cilioretinal arterial and venous supply have no vessels in the central portion of the retina; all vessels enter and leave the disc peripherally. An exclusive ciliary vascular supply of the retina is rare, and the diagnosis is based on suggestive signs rather than anatomical confirmation. These authors reported the first case of exclusive cilioretinal vessels that has been confirmed by fluorescein angiography and Doppler US.

Case Report.—Man, 69, was evaluated because he had noted progressively worse vision over the previous 57 years (since age 12). At age 20 years, visual acuity was 20/60 in the right eye and 20/80 in the left. His family history was remarkable for a maternal uncle whose retinitis pigmentosa sine pigmento had been confirmed only after extensive diagnostic tests at the National Institutes of

Health. Over the years, the patient had often experienced sudden visual loss that only partially resolved. Intraocular pressure readings were always normal, with no spikes; yet his best-corrected vision continued to deteriorate, even despite treatment. At the most recent evaluation, best-corrected visual acuity was 20/60 in the right eye and hand motion vision in the left eye. Ophthalmoscopy revealed that the diameter of the optical discs was normal, but the discs were centrally excavated and glial tufts were evident. Each disc was surrounded by a small zone of retinal pigment epithelium. In both eyes, the arteries and veins arose exclusively from the periphery, with substantial "hooking" of vessels over the extreme edge of the disc; this finding suggested a cilioretinal origin. Fluorescein angiography revealed that all arterial vessels filled simultaneous with the background choroidal flush. Color and power Doppler US failed to identify any central retinal vessels within the optic nerves; the central part of each disc was vacant. US also identified a renal anomaly: small kidneys with reduced renal parenchyma and chronic interstitial nephritis.

Conclusion.—The central retinal vessels were completely absent in both eyes; the retina was supplied exclusively by ciliary blood flow. Past authors have labeled the types of cavitary disc anomalies seen in this patient as "atypical" colobomas. However, in this case, the nomenclature is inaccurate in that the central vessels are displaced superiorly in colobomatous anomalies. In this case, the central vessels were completely absent (ie, dysplastic).

▶ This case report provides an interesting perspective about the "morning-glory" syndrome as well as recommending a more clinically accurate and useful nomenclature. Using IV fluorescein angiography and orbital color Doppler imaging, the authors prove that there is no measurable flow in the central retinal artery in this syndrome. The central retinal artery is probably absent. The blood supply to the retina must be entirely from the ciliary circulation.

I agree with the authors suggestion to use the word "dysplastic" or the phrase "vacant discs" to describe this optic nerve appearance. These patients may have renal and cerebellar abnormalities. The paper also includes an excellent review of the genetics of this condition.

R.C. Sergott, M.D.

Microvascular Decompression for Superior Oblique Myokymia: First Experience: Case Report

Samii M, Rosahl SK, Carvalho GA, et al (Nordstadt Hosp, Hannover, Germany; Med School, Hannover, Germany; Justus-Liebig-Univ, Giessen, Germany)

J Neurosurg 89:1020-1024, 1998 8–13

Introduction.—Superior oblique myokymia (SOM) is an uncommon disorder of eye movement with uniocular rotary microtremor caused by intermittent contractions of the superior oblique muscle. The term *myokymia* is derived from electromyographic recordings from the superior oblique muscle that exhibit spontaneous bursts of motor unit potentials that resemble myokymic discharges in chronic nerve compression syndromes. Nomenclature has been questioned, and it has been suggested that *superior oblique microtremor* may be a better term to describe the superior oblique movements. Reported is a patient with SOM who was referred as a candidate for microvascular decompression of the trochlear nerve root exit zone.

Case Report.—Man, 50, was referred because of intermittent nystagmus of the right eye of 17 years' duration. The intorsional oscillations of the eyeball happened several times every day, with a series of paroxysms that lasted 15 to 20 seconds and continued for up to 6 hours without intermission. During these episodes, he experienced oscillopsia, uniocular "shimmering," and frontal headaches. Mental stress and sometimes strong light exacerbated his condition. Medical history was unremarkable, except for poliomyelitis at age 4 years. The SOM was refractory to treatment with antiepileptic drugs and repeated injections botulinus toxin around the right eye. Symptoms became so severe that he patient could no longer work at a test driver for trucks. Improvement was achieved only when he closed or covered his right eye. He refused superior oblique tenectomy because of its uncertain outcome and destructive nature. The only pathologic findings on ophthalmic examination were intervals of intermittent unilateral, tonic intorsional nystagmus and phasic oscillations of the right eye, which lasted 10 to 20 seconds. Rotary movements could be evoked by moving the eye downward and medially. Enhanced and nonenhanced computerized tomography and magnetic resonance examination of the head and orbit showed small foci of demyelinization in the periventricular region. The basilar artery curved to the left, yet there were no pathologic abnormalities. Lumbar puncture, electroencephalography, brainstem auditory evoked potentials, visual evoked potentials, somatosensory evoked potentials, and transcranial Doppler sonography were normal. The patient underwent microvascular decompression of the fourth nerve at the root exit zone. He experienced temporary double vision that resolved 5 months after surgery. He had no recurrence of oscillopsia during a 22-month follow-up.

Conclusion.—This single observation shows that vascular compression of the trochlear nerve can be a significant pathophysiologic factor contributing to SOM. Some patients with SOM have had symptoms for up to 29 years. These patients usually have no abnormalities on neuroimaging. This syndrome may occur in association with a posterior fossa tumor or after removal of a cerebellar tumor. Cranial nerve vascular compression syndromes may share a variety of clinical features, with symptoms that are exacerbated by stress or fatigue and last only a few seconds. Microvascular decompression of the trochlear nerve at the brainstem exit zone may become the method of choice for selected patients with SOM who have disabling symptoms.

▶ An interesting case report concerning SOM, a rare but sometimes debilitating condition. In view of their success in treating hemifacial spasm and trigeminal neuralgia by eliminating compression by an artery on the fifth and seventh nerves, the authors report a similar operation on the trochlear nerve.

Obviously, since SOM can be a self-limited condition, a lateral suboccipital retrosigmoid craniectomy is not the first treatment option. A variety of medications, including Tegretol, Inderal, and Neurontin, have been used for SOM. Either medication or observation with the hope of spontaneous resolution should be the first management approach.

R.C. Sergott, M.D.

A Subgroup of Multiple Sclerosis Patients With Anticardiolipin Antibodies and Unusual Clinical Manifestations: Do They Represent a New Nosological Entity?

Karussis D, Leker RR, Ashkenazi A, et al (Hebrew Univ Hosp, Jerusalem)

Ann Neurol 44:629-634, 1998 8–14

Introduction.—Antiphospholipids are a heterogeneous family of autoantibodies that include the lupus anticoagulant and the anticardiolipin antibodies (ACL Abs). These antibodies may be a major risk factor for thromboembolic events. The immunoglobulin G isotype is linked to stroke. The relative risk of stroke increases in young patients with ACL Ab levels above 20. The presence of these antibodies has been reported in some patients who have multiple sclerosis (MS), particularly the neuromyelitic type. Bright T2-imaging foci (unidentified bright objects) are occasionally seen on brain MRI scans in patients with antiphospholipid syndrome. In a cohort of 100 patients who received a probable or definite diagnosis of MS, a subgroup of 20 patients who were consistently positive for ACL Abs were evaluated.

Methods.—Patients underwent brain MRI scanning and a complete autoimmune screening, with a follow-up of 1 to 3 years.

Results.—Nineteen patients had classic neuroimaging features of MS on MRI. The most common clinical findings were chronic, slowly progressing myopathy (15 patients) and optic neuropathy (6 patients). Eight patients had headache as a dominant symptom. Other less common symptoms included cognitive and psychiatric disorders and chronic fatigue. Mean levels of ACL Abs were 38.8 GPL (normal levels up to 7.5 GPL) in this cohort. Oligoclonal bands were detected in the cerebrospinal fluid of 3 patients. Treatment consisted of acetylsalycilic acid and occasionally short courses of steroids. Progression of chronic myelopathic/spinocerebellar syndrome was slower than assumed in MS (2 patients deteriorated and 4 improved during a mean follow-up of 20.8 months).

Conclusion.—Patients with probable or definite diagnosis of MS and consistently high levels of ACL Abs had a slower progression and some atypical features for MS (high incidence of headache and other pains and lack of oligoclonal antibodies in the cerebral spinal fluid). The dominant clinical characteristic in this subset of patients with MS was progressive myelopathy, spinocerebellar syndrome, or neuromyelitis optica. Other mechanisms may be involved in the pathogenesis of the neurological symptoms in these patients. Management may include antiplatelet or anticoagulant agents.

▶ The authors report a very stimulating study examining the possible relationship between MS and ACL Abs. These antiphospholipids are a heterogeneous group of antibodies considered to be a major risk factor for thromboembolic events. These strokes usually affect the moderately sized branches of the middle cerebral artery and are most common in young, female patients. The most common syndromes associated with ACL Abs and MS were chronic, slowly progressive myelopathy (15 of 20 patients) and optic neuropathy (6 of 20 patients). The progression of chronic myelopathy was slower in anticardiolipin antibody patients than in MS patients without these antibodies. These observations merit further investigation, especially in a large cohort of patients with optic neuritis. If patients demonstrate these antibodies, consideration should be given to treatment with antiplatelet and even anticoagulant agents.

R.C. Sergott, M.D.

Mydriatic Pupil as the Presenting Sign of Common Carotid Artery Dissection

Koennecke H-C, Seyfert S (Freie Universität Berlin)
Stroke 29:2653-2655, 1998 8–15

Introduction.—Transient and permanent paresis of ocular motor nerves with or without visual impairment is a novel finding in atherosclerotic carotid artery disease. Dissection of the internal carotid artery is sometimes associated with ipsilateral disturbance of oculomotor nerve function. Described is a unique patient in whom pupillary dysfunction from evolving paresis of the third nerve was the first clinical sign of acute dissection of the common carotid artery (CCA) and impending cerebral ischemia.

Case Report.—Woman, 44, underwent elective surgery for hypopharyngeal carcinoma. She was right-handed, nondiabetic, and had a history of alcoholism. A massive hemorrhage occurred from erosion of the right CCA during surgery and necessitated emergency tangential ligation of the vessel. The patient had no focal neurological deficit after surgery. On postsurgical day 1, the right pupil was fluctuating. The pupil was intermittently mydriatic and reacted poorly to bright light, then becoming 9 mm and fixing to light and near. An intermediate dilation to 10 mm was observed in the dark. The left pupil was 4 mm and had normal reactions to light, dark, and proximity. Twelve hours later, the patient developed complete right third-nerve palsy, visual hemiextinction to the left, and mild left brachiofacial hemiparesis. Head computed tomography was normal. Angiography showed occlusion of the right CCA to 2 cm below its bifurcation and left-to-right cross-flow to the right middle cerebral artery by the anterior communication artery. Right internal carotid artery filling was slow, in an antegrade fashion, through collaterals from the right vertebral artery connecting to the right external carotid artery. The proximal segment of the right posterior cerebral artery (PCA) was hypoplastic. Using controlled elevation of blood pressure, the right hemispheric syndrome resolved almost completely. The right third-nerve palsy persisted. The following day, reconstructive surgery of the CCA showed intimal dissection with occlusion at the level of the emergency ligation. The vessel was reconstructed with a saphenous graft before right-sided neck dissection. After surgery, the left hemiparesis resolved completely and the right pupil was fixed at 6 mm in light and dark, with no changes in ocular function. On postoperative day 2, the right pupil constricted to bright light and was slightly miotic. It did not dilate in the dark. In the next 4 weeks, the right ptosis partially resolved and all other extraocular muscles had normal function. At 5 weeks, the patient had normal neurologic status, with the exception of a right-sided Horner's syndrome, probably as a persisting deficit after neck dissection.

Conclusion.—A mydriatic pupil was the first unusual sign of a compromised carotid blood flow and impending cerebral ischemia in this patient. Carotid endarterectomy immediately and completely resolved all eye symptoms. Mitosis from oculosympathetic paralysis is the most frequent pupillary dysfunction in carotid dissection, even in patients with oculomotor disturbances. Blood supply to the oculomotor nerve is provided by small arteries that arise from the basilar artery, the PCA, and the posterior communicating artery. The combination of acute CCA occlusion and fetal origin of the PCA may explain this unusual susceptibility of the oculomotor nerve to ischemia.

▶ This case report is of great importance to general ophthalmologists, neurologists, and neuro-ophthalmologists. A miotic pupil with ptosis (oculosympathetic paresis, Horner's syndrome) is the usual pupillary abnormality with carotid dissection, even in cases with involvement of the oculomotor nerves. This is the first report of a dilated pupil as the presenting sign of common carotid artery dissection. The mydriatic pupil preceded by 12 hours the symptoms of an ipsilateral, complete third nerve palsy and cerebral ischemia. Cerebral angiography revealed occlusion of the CCA, with slow flow in the internal carotid and fetal origin of the posterior cerebral artery, implying a hemodynamic mechanism for an ischemic third nerve palsy. Carotid endarterectomy successfully reversed the third nerve palsy and cerebral ischemia. Therefore, carotid artery dissection must be added to the differential diagnosis of an isolated, unilaterally dilated pupil. If the pupil has been dilated for 12 hours without other signs of third nerve dysfunction and cerebral ishemia, the patient probably does not have a CCA dissection.

R.C. Sergott, M.D.

9 Imaging

Research and Peer Review

by Robert I. Grossman, M.D.

This has been the "Decade of the Brain," during which scientists and clinicians have witnessed exponential advances in our understanding of diseases of the brain. Imaging has been one of the areas of enormous growth. Surveying the literature for the YEAR BOOK provides a perspective on how specialties outside of radiology view and use imaging. It is clear that ophthalmology, as well as clinical neuroscience, has aggressively applied imaging, in particular, MR, to elucidate diseases and function of the brain. The engine that has fueled this research surge has been, in part, funding by the National Institutes of Health (NIH). The costs in performing research have escalated, and funding is essential to maintain the cutting edge.

Although it should not be necessary to justify imaging research, even in clinically busy academic departments, many question the essential nature of this commitment. I would point out that without research there is little need for specialization in medicine, be it radiology or ophthalmology. Stagnant knowledge and no excitement regarding new ideas or techniques condemns a specialty to slow, excruciating death or, to put it in economic terms, "loss of turf." Research is what attracts young and vibrant new investigators into the field. It also makes it difficult to fill high-level clinical positions by lower level technicians.

The NIH turns out to be critical in providing initiatives as well as funding investigator-initiated grants. For the past 4 years I have had the pleasure, and responsibility, of being a member of the Diagnostic Radiology Study Section, and I have acted as its chairman for the last 2 years. There is no question that it is a tremendous amount of work. The study section meets every 4 months. You are assigned usually between 6 to 10 grants that you review and critique according to the following criteria: significance, approach, innovation, investigator, and environment. At the meeting, where there are approximately 20 or more reviewers, you discuss in depth each of the proposals. Here, the reviewer serves as an advocate for his or her best grants. Everyone scores the proposal, and those with the best scores get funded (usually). I wish that every serious young investigator could sit in on the discussions at the study section. They would have a precise idea of what good science is all about and how grants should be written. I contend that the members of the study section should pay the NIH for the privilege of sitting, listening, and working in this environment. Before long you see and read some of the best science in your specialty. You are truly at the cutting edge.

What does it take to be funded? The answer is, hypothesis-driven research that will provide significant new information. The principal investigator must be meticulous in his or her approach. The proposal must be easy to read, even for someone who is not an expert in the field. The investigator must argue why the proposal should be funded and what will be accomplished within the funding period. Successful applications help to ensure the ability to achieve your research's specific aims, in spite of the vagaries of clinical revenues. Low-priority scores are depressing, and one feels that they have wasted an enormous amount of time and effort. This is particularly true for young investigators who need to be funded but also need to write papers. The young investigator also requires protected time to acquire data and write the proposal. It is very difficult to compete for funding when the employment environment is not supportive. Unfunded grants drive people out of research and into more lucrative areas of medicine. It is a unique feeling to have your research proposal pass the peer-review process and get funded. You have passed the most difficult test and have acquired the resources to accomplish your goals.

Peer review is an imperfect process. Yes, there are mistakes, but those are usually only in the proposals that don't get funded. The ball is in the investigators' court once they receive the resources to accomplish the specific aims. If investigators desire to have another opportunity for funding, they must be productive. Lack of productivity ensures the failure of subsequent proposals. The process is fair—you take the money, and you must do the work.

Research and the peer-review process are vital to your profession. While reading the articles selected to appear in this YEAR BOOK, you might just check the acknowledgments regarding support for the studies. The papers from investigators whose studies have been funded by the NIH should perhaps be viewed in a slightly different perspective, for they have not only passed the individual journal's peer-review process but have been subjected to an initial even more strenuous examination. You still may find fault with the paper and disagree with the results, nevertheless, these research groups are to be commended for advancing your specialty.

Combined Venous Lymphatic Malformations of the Orbit (So-called Lymphangiomas): Association With Noncontiguous Intracranial Vascular Anomalies

Katz SE, Rootman J, Vangveeravong S, et al (Univ of British Columbia, Vancouver)

Ophthalmology 105:176-184, 1998 9–1

Background.—Combined venous lymphatic vascular malformations (CVLVMs) of the orbit have been found in patients with vascular anomalies in the brain, such as intracranial hemorrhage. These authors retrospectively examined records of patients with orbital CVLVMs to examine the relationship of CVLVMs to intracranial vascular anomalies.

Methods.—Of 25 patients with CVLVMs for whom radiologic studies were available, 7 (28%) also had evidence of noncontiguous intracranial vascular anomalies. Computed tomographic scans and magnetic resonance images were used, when available, to describe the malformations in detail.

Findings.—Most of the noncontiguous intracranial vascular anomalies were located in the midbrain (Table 1). Developmental venous anomalies were found in 2 patients (Figs 1 and 2), and 1 patient had an intracranial hemorrhage. Orbital lesions had both superficial and deep components, with orbital bony expansion, in all 7 patients (Fig 3; Table 2). The superior orbital fissure was involved in all 7 patients, and the inferior orbital fissure was involved in 5 patients. The CVLVMs had been apparent at birth in 5 patients, and were noted because of intralesional hemorrhage in the 2 other patients, at ages 3 and 5 years. Six of 7 patients had eyelid swelling when first seen (Table 3), and 4 had unilateral ocular "prominence." At a mean of 13 years later, 6 of 7 patients still had eyelid thickening, and 6 of

TABLE 1.—Noncontiguous Intracranial Vascular Anomalies in Patients With Orbital Combined Venous Lymphatic Vascular Lesions (Lymphangiomas)

Case No.	Orbit	Location
1	R	Right peri-mesencephalic and trans-mesencephalic
2	L	Bilateral peri-mesencephalic
3	L	Left peri-mesencephalic and trans-mesencephalic
4	R	Bilateral peri-mesencephalic, trans-mesencephalic, right cerebellopontine angle, walls of 4th ventricle, extensive posterior fossa venous malformation with absence of the left transverse sinus, and presumed vascular lesion in the right lateral cerebellum representing either a cryptic arteriovenous malformation or venous angioma
5	R	Right basal ganglia and wall of right lateral ventricle
6	L	Right peri-mesencephalic, right cerebellopontine angle, walls of lateral ventricles bilaterally and left basal ganglia
7	R	Right basal ganglia

Abbreviations: R, right; *L*, left.

(Published courtesy of *Ophthalmology*, from Katz SE, Rootman J, Vangveeravong S, et al: Combined venous lymphatic malformations of the orbit [so-called lymphangiomas]: Association with noncontiguous intracranial vascular anomalies. *Ophthalmology* 105:176-184, 1998.)

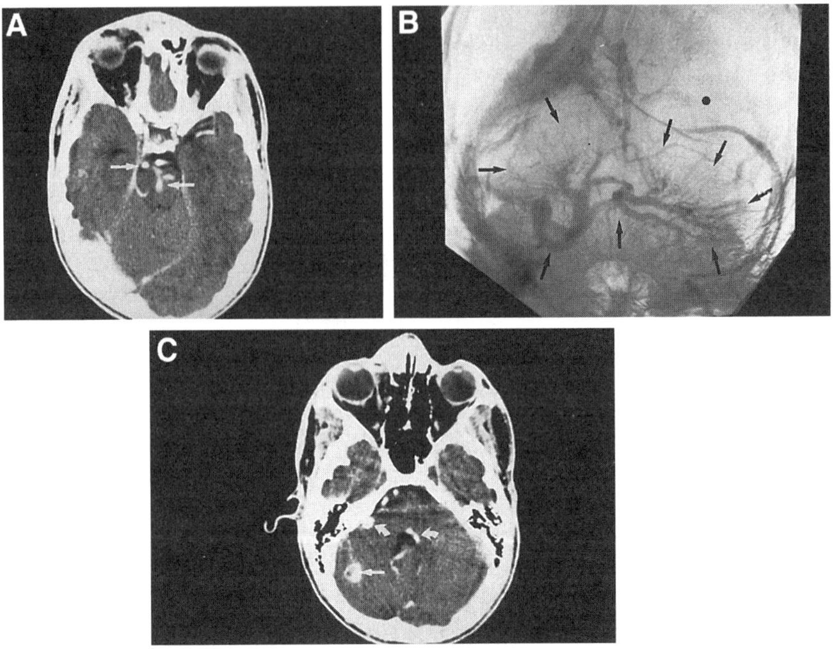

FIGURE 1.—Case 4. Noncontiguous anomalous right perimesencephalic and transmesencephalic vessels (*arrows*) are noted (**A**) in this 14-year-old boy with a right orbital lymphangioma. Extensive posterior fossa developmental venous anomalies (*DVA*) (*arrows*) with absence of the left transverse sinus (**B**, *dot*) and presumed vascular lesion in the right lateral cerebellum, representing either a cavernous hemangioma or cryptic arteriovenous malformation (**C**, *straight arrow*), were noted as well. Components of the DVA are seen as large vessels in the walls of the fourth ventricle and right cerebellopontine angle (*curved arrows*). (Published courtesy of *Ophthalmology*, from Katz SE, Rootman J, Vangveeravong S, et al: Combined venous lymphatic malformations of the orbit [so-called lymphangiomas]: Association with noncontiguous intracranial vascular anomalies. *Ophthalmology* 105:176-184, 1998.)

7 also had proptosis. While 3 eyes showed no visual loss, 4 eyes had visual acuity of 20/200 or less because of optic nerve compromise. The orbital CVLVMs in these 7 patients were likely to extend anteriorly into the soft tissues of the face and forehead, and other associated vascular lesions were common. Conversely, in patients without noncontiguous intracranial vascular anomalies, the orbital CVLVMs were less likely to extend into the soft tissues of the face, were associated with better visual outcome, were less diffuse, and were less likely to have associated vascular lesions.

Conclusions.—Noncontiguous intracranial vascular anomalies were found in 28% of patients with extensive orbital CVLVMs. Such anomalies included developmental venous anomalies and intracranial hemorrhage. Thus, radiographic studies in patients with diffuse orbital CVLVMs should encompass other areas of the brain to search for any abnormalities in other intracranial vasculature.

▶ The authors have observed an interesting possible association between vascular anomalies in the brain and what have been termed CVLVMs or lymphangiomas. CVLVMs of the orbit are derived from the venous anlage

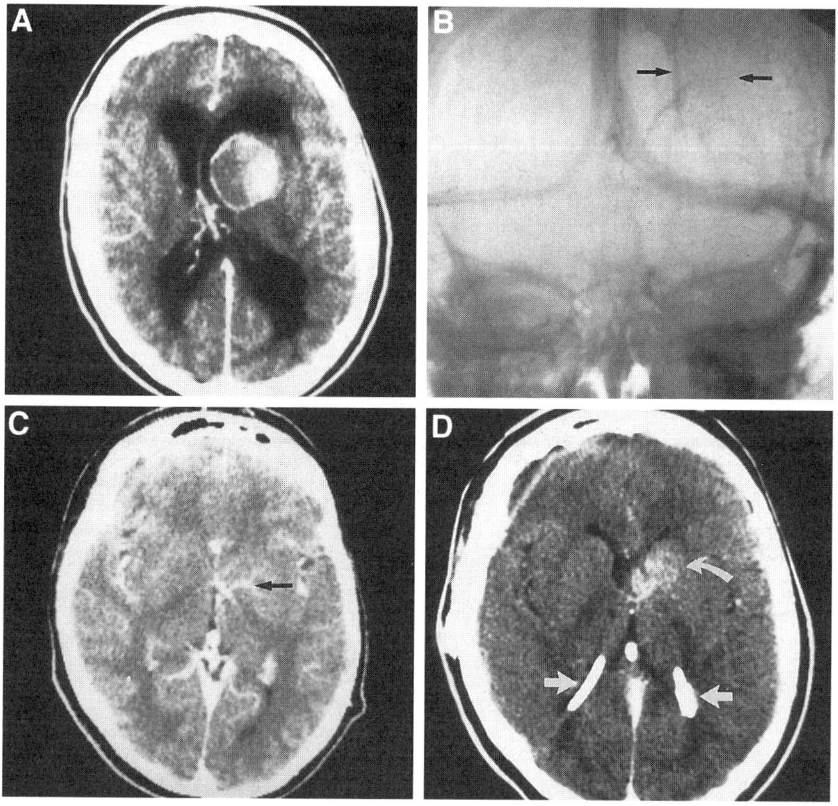

FIGURE 2.—Case 6. This 22-year-old woman had bare light perception on presentation with a diffuse left orbital lymphangioma. At age 27, obstructive hydrocephalus developed resulting from a left basal ganglia hemorrhage (**A**), requiring bilateral intraventricular shunts. Angiography showed a DVA in the left hemisphere (**B**, *arrows*). Retrospective review of prior enhanced computed tomographic scan showed a DVA in the left basal ganglia (**C**, *arrow*). A follow-up computed tomographic scan 3 years later showed bilateral interventricular shunts in place (*thick arrows*) and residual enhancement in the left basal ganglia (*curved arrow*) (**D**). (Published courtesy of *Ophthalmology*, from Katz SE, Rootman J, Vangveeravong S, et al: Combined venous lymphatic malformations of the orbit [so-called lymphangiomas]: Association with noncontiguous intracranial vascular anomalies. *Ophthalmology* 105:176-184, 1998.)

and have both venous and lymphatic components. Like other lymphangiomas within the body, they have a propensity to hemorrhage acutely, producing abrupt proptosis in the orbit or, in the case of cystic hygroma of the neck, sudden swelling. These lesions may enlarge slowly or may change quickly after expansion of the lymphoid elements in the lesion secondary to upper respiratory infection.

This article describes an association of CVLVMs with intracranial vascular malformation, beyond what would be expected by chance. Because of the retrospective nature of the observation and the lack of full vascular radiologic protocols in all of the CVLVMs cohort, the article does not sufficiently classify the intracranial vascular abnormalities. Nevertheless, most of the intracranial vascular lesions represent developmental venous anomalies,

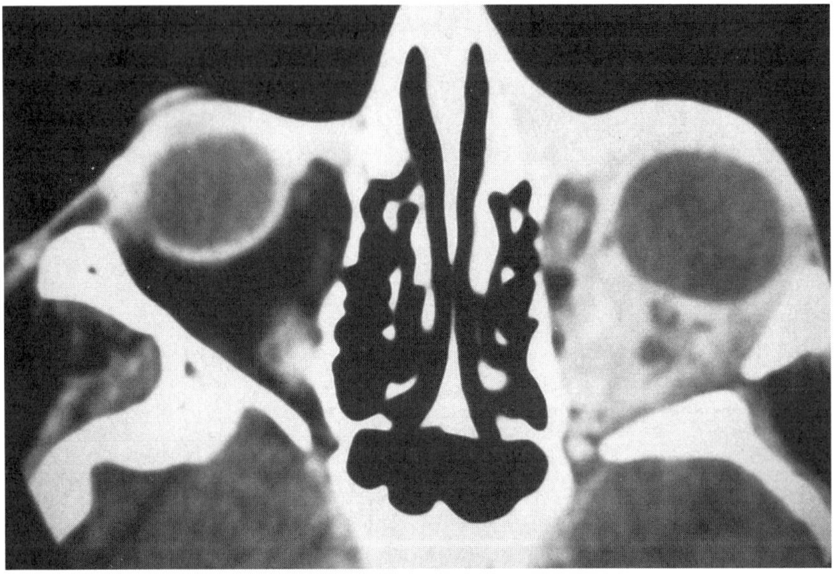

FIGURE 3.—Case 6. Contrast-enhanced axial CT shows a diffuse left orbital lymphangioma with both superficial and deep components extending into a slightly widened superior orbital fissure. Note the significant orbital expansion by this extensive lesion and the anterior extension into the soft tissues of the lateral nose. (Published courtesy of *Ophthalmology* from Katz SE, Rootman J, Vangveeravong S, et al: Combined venous lymphatic malformations of the orbit [so-called lymphangiomas]: Association with noncontiguous intracranial vascular anomalies. *Ophthalmology* 105:176-184, 1998.)

also termed venous angiomas, which the authors correctly describe as anatomic venous variants, representing normal venous drainage for that particular region of the brain. The authors cite an autopsy review of Jellinger, who found the incidence of developmental venous anomalies to be 0.26%.[1] The authors have also observed that the intracranial vascular anomalies were associated with CVLVMs that extended through the superior orbital fissure. The CVLVMs with intracranial vascular anomalies were more diffuse, often associated with bony expansion of the orbit, and more often associated with visual loss. One of the patients had an intracranial hemorrhage (Fig 2).

I have 1 minor disagreement with the article, regarding the possible association of intracranial hemorrhage in these cases. Developmental venous anomalies rarely bleed. I believe that the lesion in Figure 2 represents a cavernous malformation and an associated venous malformation. It is the cavernous malformation and not the venous malformation that has hemorrhaged. Thus, the increased incidence of venous angioma, while interesting, would have no significant effect upon any treatment and would not require any lifestyle alterations. The article indicates correctly that further studies are needed to delineate the precise nature of the intracranial vascular malformations associated with CVLVMs, and to understand why there is a relationship between CVLVMs and intracranial vascular malformations.

R.I. Grossman, M.D.

TABLE 2.—Radiologic Overview of Lymphangiomas Associated With Noncontiguous Intracranial Vascular Anomalies

	Location					Structural Involvement						Character				
Case No.	I/C	E/C	Sup	Mid	Deep	SOF	IOF	MCF	PPF	CS	ON	Locul	Homo	NHomo	Orbit Size (Enlrg)	Comments
1		Y	Y	Y	Y	Y	Y		Y			Y		Y	Y	
2		Medial Y	Y	Y	Y	Y		Y				Y		Y	Y	Vatrix component SR & MR
3		Medial Y	Y	Y	Y	Y		Y						Y	Y	Varix component SR & LR
4	Y	Medial Y	Y	Y	Y	Y	Y		Y					Y	Y	Varix component superomedial apex
5	Y	Y	Y	Y	Y	Y	Y		Y					Y	Y	
6	Y	Y	Y	Y	Y	Y	Y		Y			Y	Y		Y	
7	Y	Y	Y	Y	Y	Y	Y	Y	Y			Y		Y	Y	

Abbreviations: I/C, intraconal; *E/C*, extraconal; *Sup*, superficial; *Mid*, mid-orbit; *CS*, cavernous sinus; *IOF*, inferior orbital fissure; *MCE*, middle cranial fossa; *ON*, optic nerve; *PPF*, pterygopalatine fossa; *SOF*, superior orbital fissure; *Locul*, loculated; *Homo*, homogenous; *NHomo*, nonhomogenous; *Enlrg*, enlarged; *LR*, lateral rectus; *MR*, medial rectus; *SR*, superior rectus.

(Published courtesy of *Ophthalmology*, from Katz SE, Rootman J, Vangveeravong S, et al: Combined venous lymphatic malformations of the orbit [so-called lymphangiomas]: Association with noncontiguous intracranial vascular anomalies. *Ophthalmology* 105:176-184, 1998.)

TABLE 3.—Presentation, Management, and Outcome of Lymphangiomas Associated With Noncontiguous Intracranial Vascular Anomalies: University of British Columbia Orbit Clinic, 1976-1995

Case No.	Age (yrs)	Sex	Laterality	Presentation	Clinical Findings	Intervention	Follow-up (yrs)	Outcome
1	1.5	F	R	Thickening U & L lids at birth; gradual proptosis	Va fix and follow; no APD; globe displ. 5 mm ant, 4 mm lat, 3 mm down; inferomedial subconj. lymphangiectasis	Combined med and lat orbitotomy and debulking (age 5) after several bleeds; occlusion therapy; debulking lids & conj × 4	9.5	VA 20/60 (anisometropic amblyopia from 4 D induced hyperopia); residual proptosis 4 mm; mild ptosis
2	3	F	L	Sudden onset hemorrhage LUL with lid swollen shut; gradually resolved over 1 wk	Palpable 2.5 cm soft tissue mass medial LUL ext over glabella; VA 20/100 (+4.50 − 2.00 × 40°); no RAPD; L ptosis 4 mm; globe displ. 3 mm ant., 1 mm down; full ductions; large subcut vein L forehead	Superomed transconjunctival orbitotomy and partial excision with use of CO2 laser; patching CD	2.0	VA 20/50 (resid refractive amblyopia); no proptosis; slight ptosis remains
3	4	M	L	Intermittent progressive swelling LUL from birth	Soft tissue swelling lid, supraorbital and glabella; proptosis 1 mm; VA 20/40 OU; no APD; sup subconj lymphangiectasis; moderate decrease abd, up gazes	Med orbitotomy and debulking (age 12) after repeated episodes of orbital hemorrhage with pain, proptosis and strabismus; CO2 laser ablation superficial component	8.0	Mild ptosis; VA 20/20
4	14	M	R	Large soft tissue mass RUL, lateral nose and cheek at birth; previous debulking procedures × 5	Absence of eyebrow and portion of supraorbital rim; proptosis 2 mm; lymphangiectasis medial subconj and hard palate; VA 20/200; RAPD; moderate disc pallor	3 superficial cosmetic procedures	4.0	Improved cosmesis

5	18	M	R	Soft tissue mass lids and face at birth multiple orbital hemorrhages; status post 26 previous debulkings, cosmetic and strabismus procedures	Scarring UL; lymphangiectasis medial subconj; globe displ 6 mm ant, 9 mm lat, 6 mm down; upper scleral show 2 mm; lagophthalmos 4 mm; mild limitation abd, add, up; R esotropia 30D, VA 20/400 with RAPD; moderate disc pallor	Lateral orbitotomy and tumor debulking for cosmesis and corneal protection	0.35	Residual axial proptosis 2 mm with markedly decreased inferolateral displ; remains with poor lid closure and inferior SPK
6	22	F	L	Congenital lesion of medial conjunctiva and lids; episodic sudden proptosis from orbital bleeds; previous orbital XRT, vascular ligation (age 13), and debulking of lids (age 16)	L hemifacial atrophy; doughy thickening of lids; lymphangictasis inf fornix and hard palate; globe displ 6 mm ant, 10 mm lat, 7 mm down; significant ophthalmoplegia all fields of gaze; wide angle exotropia; VA bare LP with RAPD and severe disc pallor; dense cataract	Lateral orbitotomies × 2 within 1 year; unilateral recess-resect procedure; third orbital debulking (age 31)	13.0	Less displ of globe inferolat, slight enophthalmos; spontaneous L basal ganglia hemorrhage (age 27) requiring bilateral ventricular shunts
7	30	F	R	Sudden proptosis (age 5) treated with XRT, carotid ligation, orbital debulking of the lesion; multiple orbital hemorrhages	VA CF 1'; fullness UL; superior fornix subconj lymphangiectasis; ophthalmoloplegia all fields of gaze; large angle esotropia; hypoglobus 10 mm; UL entropion; RAPD with serevere disc pallor	Lateral orbitotomy and debulking of tumor with subsequent ptosis and entropian repair elsewhere	0.5	Resolution of 5 mm proptosis

(Published courtesy of *Ophthalmology*, from Katz SE, Rootman J, Vangveeravong S, et al: Combined venous lymphatic malformations of the orbit [so-called lymphangiomas]: Association with noncontiguous intracranial vascular anomalies. *Ophthalmology* 105:176-184, 1998.)

Reference

1. Jellinger K: Vascular malformations of the central nervous system: A morphological overview. *Neurosurg Rev* 9:177-216, 1986.

Absence of the Abducens Nerve in Duane Syndrome Verified by Magnetic Resonance Imaging

Parsa CF, Grant PE, Dillon WP Jr, et al (Univ of California, San Francisco; Salk Inst, San Francisco)

Am J Ophthalmol 125:399-401, 1998 9–2

Background.—Duane syndrome is a congenital unilateral horizontal abduction deficit in which attempted adduction shows retraction of the globe. Every autopsy of patients with Duane syndrome shows anomalous innervation of the lateral rectus muscle on the affected side by the ipsilateral oculomotor nerve, and also a lack of the abducens nerve on the side with the duction failure. These authors report this latter finding in vivo.

> *Case Report.*—High-resolution, 3-dimensional spoiled gradient recalled acquisition magnetic resonance imaging was used to examine a woman, 36, with typical left-sided type 1 Duane syndrome. High-matrix thin-slice sections were adjusted so that the relevant structures were best seen, and these data were reformatted into oblique axial sections to follow the course of the abducens nerve. Sequential axial sections showed portions of the abducens nerve on the right, but not on the left (Fig 1). Reformatting data to parallel the course of the right abducens nerve confirmed that it was present in its entirety, but the left abducens nerve was completely absent (Fig 2).

Conclusions.—The absence of the abducens nerve on the affected side can be shown by high-resolution, 3-dimensional spoiled gradient recalled acquisition magnetic resonance imaging and high-matrix thin-section volumetric images.

▶ This is a short article demonstrating that high resolution imaging can be critical to confirming clinical impressions. Duane syndrome represents a congenital unilateral horizontal abduction deficit accompanied by retraction of the globe on attempted adduction. Autopsy studies have demonstrated the unilateral absence of the abducens nerve, associated with anomalous innervation of the affected lateral rectus muscle by the ipsilateral oculomotor nerve at the level of the superior orbital fissure. With high resolution MR images, the authors have demonstrated this abnormality.

I chose the article to suggest how crucial correct imaging is to producing the correct answer. Focused MR protocols are essential in searching for small abnormalities around the orbit and at the base of the skull. This

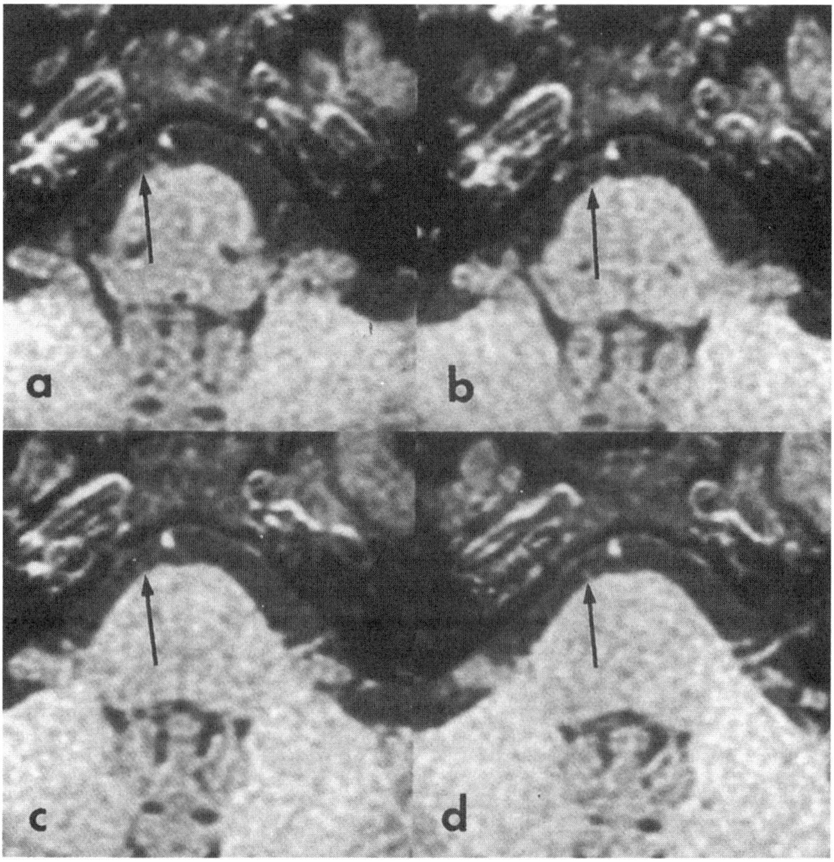

FIGURE 1.—Four consecutive axial images from a 3-dimensional spoiled gradient recalled acquisition in the steady state (repetition time, 35 msec; echo time, minimum; flip angle, 32 degrees; matrix, 256 × 192 pixels; number of excitations, 1; thickness, 0.7 mm) beginning at the inferior pons (**a**) and continuing superiorly (**b**, **c**, and **d**). The right abducens cranial nerve is identified as a linear soft tissue density structure leaving the inferior pons and coursing in a superior and oblique fashion toward the clivus (*arrows*). No equivalent structure is identified on the left side. (Reprinted by permission of the publisher from Parsa CF, Grant PE, Dillon WP Jr, et al: Absence of the abducens nerve in Duane syndrome verified by magnetic resonance imaging. *Am J Ophthalmol* 125:399-401. Copyright 1998 by Elsevier Science Inc.)

requires excellent MR techniques and high field magnets to produce optimal resolution. It also requires the referring physician to provide adequate information to tailor the radiologic investigation. Without appropriate history and examination results, it is difficult to detect the small but extremely significant lesions. In most cases, clinical input determines the quality of the radiologic output.

R.I. Grossman, M.D.

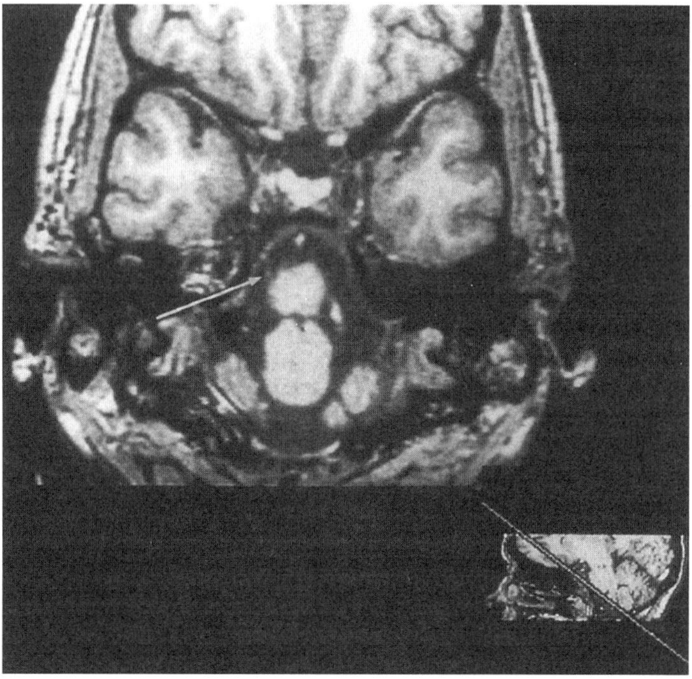

FIGURE 2.—An oblique reformation of the axially acquired 3-dimensional spoiled gradient recalled acquisition images along the course of the right abducens nerve in Fig 1. The entire subarachnoid course of the abducens nerve from the inferior pons to the posterior aspect of the clivus (region of Dorello canal) is identified on the right (*arrow*). No equivalent structure is identified on the left. (Reprinted by permission of the publisher from Parsa CF, Grant PE, Dillon WP Jr, et al: Absence of the abducens nerve in Duane syndrome verified by magnetic resonance imaging. *Am J Ophthalmol* 125:399-401. Copyright 1998 by Elsevier Science Inc.)

Terson Syndrome: Results of Vitrectomy and the Significance of Vitreous Hemorrhage in Patients With Subarachnoid Hemorrhage

Kuhn F, Morris R, Witherspoon CD, et al (Helen Keller Eye Research Found, Birmingham, Ala; Univ of Pécs, Hungary)

Ophthalmology 105:472-477, 1998 9–3

Background.—Intraocular hemorrhage reportedly occurs in 18% to 41% of adults with subarachnoid hemorrhage; the rate for children may be as high as 70%. If vitreous hemorrhage also occurs, the condition is termed Terson syndrome; reports state that 3% to 5% of patients with subarachnoid hemorrhage also have this condition. These authors performed 2 studies, 1 to evaluate surgical results of vitrectomy, and the second of patients with subarachnoid hemorrhage to describe the incidence of Terson syndrome.

Methods.—The first study was a chart review of 33 eyes (27 patients, aged 6 months to 69 years) in whom vitrectomy was used to treat vitreous hemorrhage caused by subarachnoid hemorrhage. Standard pars plana

TABLE 1.—Selected Clinical Data on 33 Eyes Vitrectomized for Terson Syndrome

Case No.	Eye	Age (yrs)	Time to PPV (mos)	Follow-up (mos)	Preoperative Visual Acuity	Final Visual Acuity	Comments
1	R	<1	1	96	N/A	20/60	SDH, HMC
	L		1	96	N/A	20/400	HMC
2	R	21	15	65	HM	20/25	SDH, HMC
3	R	<1	1	9	N/A	N/A	EMP
	L		2	10	N/A	N/A	SDH, HMC
4	R	49	3	4	HM	20/25	
5	R	66	19	6	CF	20/50	Pre-existing cataract
6	L	46	6	48	20/120	20/20	
7	R	69	6	21	HM	20/30	Cataract development
	L		7	20	HM	20/30	Cataract development
8	R	40	3	9	HM	20/25	EMP
9	R	43	4	6	20/200	20/20	
10	R	49	3	6	HM	20/20	EMP
	L		4	7	HM	20/20	EMP, exudative RD
11	L	43	2	5	HM	20/25	EMP
12	R	47	3	13	CF	20/25	HMC
	L		4	12	CF	20/20	
13	R	36	3	8	HM	20/20	HMC
14	L	48	4	5	CE	20/20	Subhyaloid hemorrhage later breaking into vitreous
15	R	67	4	6	CF	20/50	Pre-existing cataract
16	R	43	4	5	HM to 20/30	20/20	
17	L	5	23	27	20/400	20/200	SDH, HMC, amblyopia
18	R	60	30	67	20/60	20/25	
19	R	61	6	14	20/160	20/80	Pre-existing cataract
20	L	54	1	8	HM	20/20	HMC, cataract development
21	L	32	3	6	20/200 to 20/60	20/20	HMC
22	R	46	12	6	HM	20/50	Pigment disturbance in macula
23	L	34	4	1	HM	20/20	HMC
24	L	40	12	3	20/200	20/30	SDH, EMP, seizures
25	L	48	3	6	LP	6/200	HMC, giant retinal tear, RD, and cataract 1 month postoperatively; successful reoperation
26	R	<1	1	6	N/A	N/A	SDH, child abuse case
	L	<1	1	6	N/A	N/A	HMC
27	R	24	3	5	HM	20/20	SDH, HMC

Abbreviations; CF, count fingers; *EMP*, epimacular proliferation; *HM*, hand motion; *HMC*, hemorrhagic macular cyst; *L*, left eye; *LP*, light perception; *N/A*, not applicable; *PPV*, pars plana vitrectomy; *R*, right eye; *RD*, retinal detachment; *SAH*, subarachnoid hemorrhage; *SDH*, subdural hemorrhage.

(Published courtesy of *Ophthalmology*, from Kuhn F, Morris R, Witherspoon CD, et al: Terson syndrome: Results of vitrectomy and the significance of vitreous hemorrhage in patients with subarachnoid hemorrhage. *Ophthalmology* 105:472-477, 1998.)

vitrectomy was the surgical method, and most patients also had hemorrhagic macular cysts and epiretinal membranes removed. The outcome measures of interest were the extent and speed of visual recovery and whether any operative complications occurred. Mean follow-up was 21 months. The second prospective study involved 100 patients with subarachnoid hemorrhage caused by cerebral aneurysm who underwent neurosurgery. Patients who died preoperatively, perioperatively, or postoperatively were excluded from the study. Any intraocular hemorrhage was

TABLE 2.—Preoperative and Postoperative Lens Status of 33 Eyes Vitrectomized for Terson Syndrome

Lens Status				
Preoperatively	Postoperatively	Number (%) of Eyes	Average Length of Follow-up (mos)	Average Age (yrs)
Clear	Clear	25 (76)	20	31
Clear	Clear	4 (12)	22	60† 64‡
Cataract	No progression	2 (6)	6	67
Cataract	Progression	2* (6)	41	61
Total		33 (100)		

*Both patients developed cataract in the fellow eye, which has not undergone vitrectomy.
†Includes 1 eye with cataract formation in an eye that developed retinal detachment.
‡Excluding the patient with retinal detachment.
(Published courtesy of *Ophthalmology*, from Kuhn F, Morris R, Witherspoon CD, et al: Terson syndrome: Results of vitrectomy and the significance of vitreous hemorrhage in patients with subarachnoid hemorrhage. *Ophthalmology* 105:472-477, 1998.)

noted during a dilated pupil fundus examination, and no patient had previous pars plana vitrectomy.

Findings.—In the first study, vitrectomy significantly improved visual rehabilitation (Table 1). Visual acuity was 20/200 or less in 21 of 26 adult eyes (78%) before vitrectomy, and improved to 20/30 or greater in 21 of 26 adult eyes (81%) after surgery. However, visual acuity for all 7 infant eyes was 20/60 or less. There were no intraoperative complications, and the complications after surgery were giant retinal tear, retinal detachment, and cataract (Table 2). In the prospective study, 17 eyes (17%) had intraocular hemorrhage; vitreous hemorrhage was present in 8 (8%) of these. Coma was significantly more likely in all 8 of the patients with Terson syndrome, and in 8 of the 9 patients (89%) with other intraocular hemorrhage, than in patients with no intraocular hemorrhage.

Conclusions.—In adult patients with Terson syndrome, vitrectomy can significantly improve visual acuity, with few complications. The poor results in infants may be attributable to a higher incidence of amblyopia or to direct traumatic brain damage. Any type of intraocular hemorrhage was associated with a higher incidence of coma, which indicates a poorer prognosis for these patients. Also, Terson syndrome may be more common than previously reported (8% incidence here).

Small Retinal Hemorrhages as the Only Sign of an Intracranial Aneurysm

Kiriakopoulos ET, Gorn RA, Barton JJS (Univ of Toronto; Harvard Med School, Boston)

Am J Ophthalmol 125:401-403, 1998 9–4

Background.—The authors describe a patient with subarachnoid hemorrhage whose only presenting signs were 2 small retinal hemorrhages.

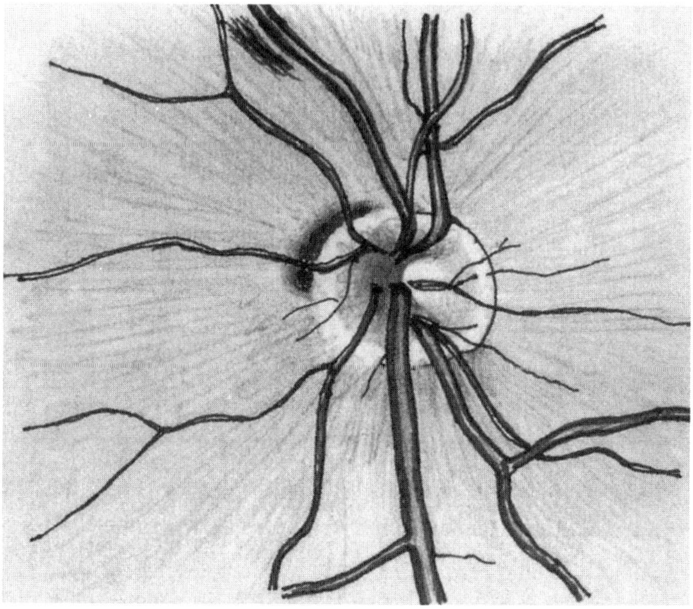

FIGURE 1.—Retinal hemorrhage. **Left**, illustration of the location of the nerve fiber layer hemorrhage and circumpapillary subretinal hemorrhage in the patient's left eye at initial examination. (Reprinted by permission of the publisher from Kiriakopoulos ET, Gorn RA, Barton JJS: Small retinal hemorrhages as the only sign of an intracranial aneurysm. *Am J Ophthalmol* 125:401-403. Copyright 1998 by Elsevier Science Inc.)

Case Report.—Woman, 42, underwent a routine eye examination, at which time she was found to have 2 retinal hemorrhages. She had experienced no vision problems, but she did report a recent, sudden headache, in the occipital region, that recurred in milder form for 2 weeks. Eye movements, visual acuity, and fields were normal in both eyes. In the left fundus, there was a circumpapillary subretinal hemorrhage and a hemorrhage in the superonasal nerve fiber layer near the disk (Fig 1). No papilledema was present, and no aberrations in neurologic tests, blood pressure, serum glucose level, platelet count, prothrombin time, and partial thromboplastin time were noted. An aneurysm in the right middle cerebral artery was noted on magnetic resonance imaging (Fig 2), and surgery was performed to clip the aneurysm. At 1 month after surgery, the nerve fiber layer hemorrhage had resolved, but traces of the circumpapillary hemorrhage remained.

Conclusions.—Up to 40% of patients with subarachnoid hemorrhage are first seen with fundal hemorrhages. The fundal hemorrhage is believed to be caused by a sudden rise in intracranial pressure transmitted into the distal optic nerve sheath. This pressure compresses the central retinal vein and causes the intraocular hemorrhage. Note that the only neurologic sign

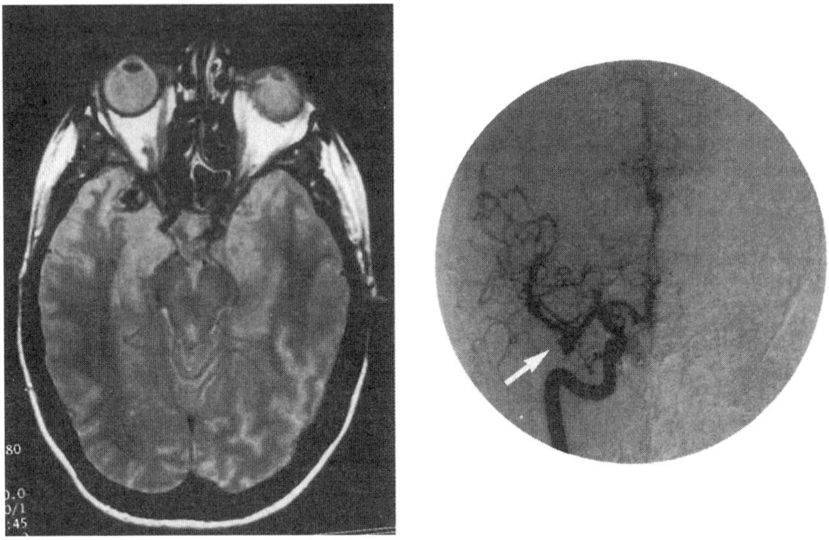

FIGURE 2.—Right middle cerebral artery aneurysm. **Left**, axial magnetic resonance image showing aneurysm as dark lobulated flow void at tip of right anterior temporal lobe, adjacent to orbital complex. **Right**, cerebral angiogram, anterior view, right carotid injection, showing same aneurysm (*arrow*). (Reprinted by permission of the publisher from Kiriakopoulos ET, Gorn RA, Barton JJS: Small retinal hemorrhages as the only sign of an intracranial aneurysm. *Am J Ophthalmol* 125:401-403. Copyright 1998 by Elsevier Science Inc.)

in this patient was a recent history of severe headache that recurred in a milder form over 2 weeks.

▶ These 2 articles (Abstracts 9–3 and 9–4) discuss the association of subarachnoid and subdural hemorrhage with intraocular hemorrhage. The intraocular hemorrhages may be preretinal, retinal, or subretinal, and may extend into the vitreous being termed Terson syndrome. The Kuhn et al., article describes the results of vitrectomy in Terson syndrome, but also reviews a prospective study of the incidences of intraocular hemorrhage and Terson syndrome in patients with subarachnoid hemorrhage. In this study, the incidence of intraocular hemorrhage was 17%, with Terson syndrome in 8%. The authors note that intraocular hemorrhage is associated with a history of transient or prolonged coma, and thus detection of intraocular hemorrhage indicates a generally poorer prognosis. Intraocular hemorrhage occurs in only 7% of patients with grade 1, but in 40% of those with worse grades. Unfortunately, in many cases such intraocular hemorrhages go undetected because fundoscopic examination was not performed. Additionally, the examination may be performed by clinicians not sufficiently skilled in detection of these lesions. Additionally, from this article it is clear that in adults vitrectomy is effective in clearing the vitreous hemorrhage and hastening visual rehabilitation.

Why do these patients get intraocular hemorrhage? Kiriakopoulos et al., state that it occurs as a result of the sudden rise of intracranial pressure, with this pressure being transmitted into the distal optic nerve sheath, compressing the central retinal vein, and producing venous congestion and intraocular hemorrhage. They state that fundal hemorrhages occur in 20% to 40% of patients with ruptured intracranial aneurysms. I do not believe that all of the patients with these intraocular hemorrhages had enough intracranial acute pressure rises to produce venous congestion. I wonder if, indeed, it results in some cases from subarachnoid blood traversing the subarachnoid space around the optic nerve and seeping into the fundus and other intraocular locations. Perhaps the vitreal hemorrhage is caused by abrupt venous congestion associated with raised intracranial pressure.

From the radiological perspective, I have observed the optic nerve sheath complex to be denser on CT in many cases of subarachnoid hemorrhage, and have attributed this to blood tracking along the optic nerve subarachnoid space. I believe it would be interesting to investigate this more thoroughly with CT or MR to see if we could detect intraocular hemorrhage more often. At present, it is clearly underappreciated radiologically.

R.I. Grossman, M.D.

In Vivo CT and MR Appearance of Prosthetic Intraocular Lens

Kuo MD, Hayman LA, Lee AG, et al (Baylor College of Medicine, Houston)
AJNR 19:749-753, 1998 9–5

Background.—Cataract surgery is an extremely common procedure, with the vast majority of operations including intraocular lens (IOL) implantation. Thus, scanning studies of the orbits or brain in elderly patients will commonly show the presence of these devices. This study reports the in vivo radiologic appearance of IOLs.

Methods.—The retrospective study included 22 eyes of 20 patients with IOLs and 4 eyes of 3 patients with aphakia. All CT and MRI scans were performed according to standard protocols. A total of 6 CT and 43 MRI studies were done in 16 patients with 18 posterior IOLs, and 1 CT and 8 MRI studies were performed in 4 patients with 4 anterior IOLs. Eight MR and 2 CT studies were performed in the patients with aphakia.

Results.—On CT imaging, scans using 1-mm thick sections provided the best information on the exact position of the optic portion of the IOL. On MRI scans, the optic portion of the IOL was best localized by fat-saturated fast T2-weighted MR orbital coil studies (Figs 3, 4, and 5). These studies could not differentiate between the haptics and the ciliary body. Studies with image thicknesses greater than the diameter of the pupil—2.5 to 4.0 mm—had difficulty demonstrating the presence of aphakia (Table 3).

Conclusions.—Computed tomographic and MRI scans can identify the optic portion of an IOL in vivo. The devices are best demonstrated by fast T2-weighted images with or without fat saturation. The haptic portion of the lens cannot be visualized by these studies, however. If the axial sections include portions of the iris, with partial volume artifact obscuring the

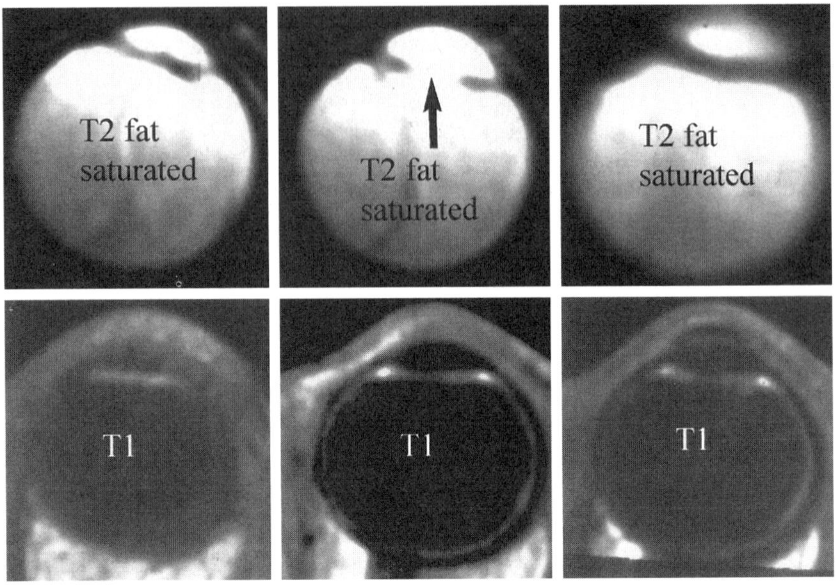

FIGURE 3.—Serial axial images in aphakia (no IOL) show the pupillary opening (*arrow*) in the fast T2-weighted fat-saturated images (**top row**). Companion serial T1-weighted images (500/15) (**bottom row**) show a partial volume artifact, which obscures the pupillary opening. On the T2-weighted fat-saturated images, the bright signal in the anterior globe, as compared with the posterior globe, occurs as a result of loss of signal as the tissue becomes farther removed from the surface of the coil. (Courtesy of Kuo MD, Hayman LA, Lee AG, et al: In vivo CT and MR appearance of prosthetic intraocular lens. *AJNR* 19[4]:749-753, 1998. Copyright by American Society of Neuroradiology.)

pupillary opening, the appearance of aphakic eyes can be similar to that of IOLs.

▶ The study described here included 20 patients with IOLs and 3 patients with aphakia (absence of a lens). The authors demonstrate the appearance of an IOL on CT and MR and note that aphakia sometimes is difficult to identify, especially if the imaging slice thickness is greater than the diameter of the pupil (2.5-4.0 mm). The haptic portion of the lens was not seen using either CT or MR.

Most of the time, identification of cataract surgery or lens implants is not a big deal or a particular challenge for radiologists. Occasionally, however, identification of the lens becomes important. This is particularly true in ocular trauma, because of concern about the position of the lens or about whether the patient has one. Normally, the lens can be seen as an ovoid mass with a convex posterior surface. The lens has the greatest concentration of protein in the body and is readily seen on CT as a high-density ovoid area in the anterior globe. If the position of the lens is in question, I generally prefer CT. The authors make an interesting observation that in cases of aphakia, one should be able to demonstrate the pupillary opening.

R.I. Grossman, M.D.

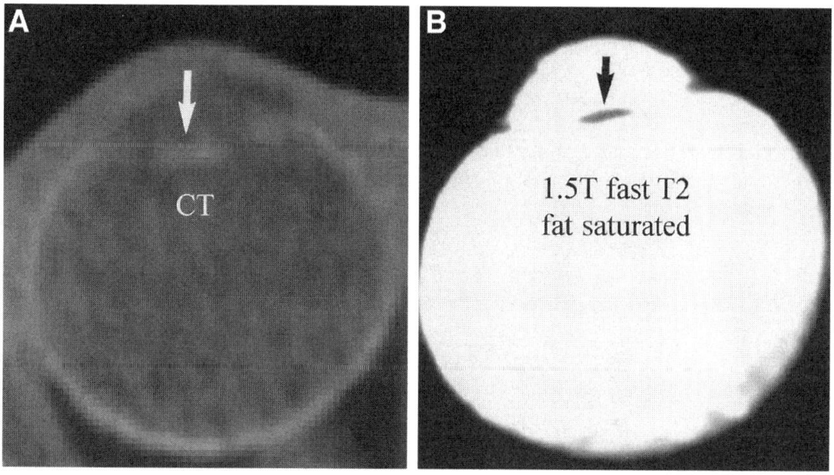

FIGURE 4.—Axial images through iris show a posterior IOL (*arrow*) on companion CT scan (**A**) and fast T2-weighted fat-saturated MR image (40000/102) (**B**). *Dotted lines* on the MR image indicate the position of the unseen haptics, and *dashed lines* show the invisible lens capsule. Note that the latter has been opened anteriorly to remove the native lens and allow the insertion of the IOL. (Courtesy of Kuo MD, Hayman LA, Lee AG, et al: In vivo CT and MR appearance of prosthetic intraocular lens. *AJNR* 19[4]:749-753, 1998. Copyright by American Society of Neuroradiology.)

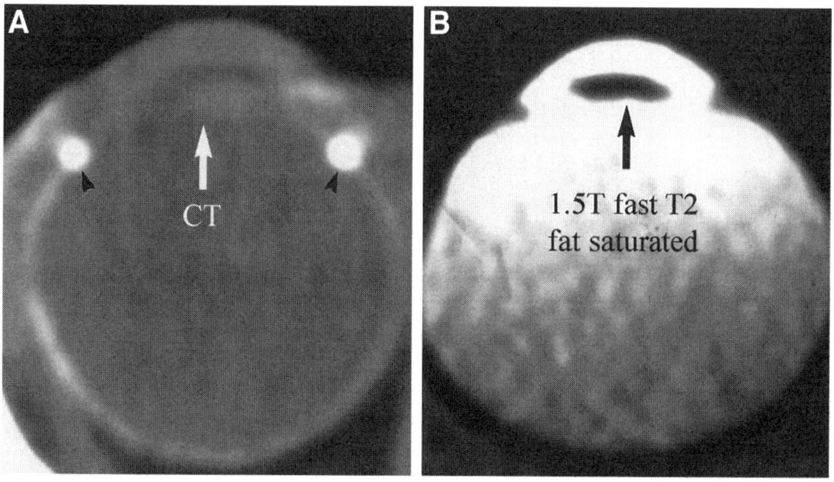

FIGURE 5.—Axial images through iris show an anterior IOL (*arrow*) on companion CT scan (**A**) and fast T2-weighted fat-saturated image (4000/102) (**B**). *Dotted lines* on the MR image indicate the position of the unseen haptics, which extend into the angle formed by the iris (posteriorly) and the cornea (anteriorly). The lens capsule has been surgically removed. The silicone band (*arrowheads*) seen on the CT scan is not visible on the MR image because of a lack of contrast between its signal void and the hypointense area at its outer margins. On the fast T2-weighted fat-saturated images, the brighter signal in the anterior globe occurs as a result of loss of signal as the tissue becomes farther removed from the surface of the coil. (Courtesy of Kuo MD, Hayman LA, Lee AG, et al: In vivo CT and MR appearance of prosthetic intraocular lens. *AJNR* 19[4]:749-753, 1998. Copyright by American Society of Neuroradiology.)

TABLE 3.—Comparison Between Slit-lamp Findings and Imaging Findings
(Number of Eyes With the Described Imaging Pattern/Number of Eyes in the Group)

Slit-Lamp Examination	CT	MR at 1.5 T (T1- and T2-Weighted Studies)	MR at 0.5 T (T2- and T1-Weighted Studies)
Aphakia	Continuous thin line (1/2) (partial volume of iris) Only absence of lens (1/2)	Centrally fenestrated thin line (5/8) (normal pupil anatomy) Continuous thin line (1/8) (partial volume of iris) Interpretation complicated by silicon oil tamponade (2/8)	…
Posterior IOL	Optic posterior to plane of iris (1/6) Only presence of optic detected (5/6)	Only presence of optic detected (3/5 Continuous thin line (1/5) (probably partial volume artifact of iris) Only absence of lens, no optic detected, (1/5)	Optic posterior to plane of iris (0/38) Only presence of optic detected (18/38) Only absence of lens detected (17/38) Continuous thin line (3/38) (probably partial volume of iris
Anterior IOL	Optic anterior to plane of iris (1/1)	Optic anterior to plane of iris (5/5)	Only absence of lens, no optic detected (3/3)

(Courtesy of Kuo MD, Hayman LA, Lee AG, et al: In vivo CT and MR appearance of prosthetic intraocular lens. *AJNR* 19[4]:749-753, 1998. Copyright by American Society of Neuroradiology.)

The Ophthalmology of Intracranial Vascular Abnormalities

Biousse V, Mendicino ME, Simon DJ, et al (Emory Univ, Atlanta, Ga; Lariboisière Hosp, Paris)

Am J Ophthalmol 125:527-544, 1998 9–6

Introduction.—Ocular signs and symptoms are sometimes the first clinical manifestations of intracranial vascular malformations. This article reviews the ophthalmologic manifestations of intracranial vascular lesions.

Aneurysms.—Visual loss may result from ruptured intracranial aneurysms, with subarachnoid hemorrhage leading to vitreous hemorrhage from Terson syndrome. For patients with unruptured aneurysms, the risk of rupture is approximately 6% per year. Third nerve palsy can result from unruptured aneurysms at the junction of the internal carotid artery and posterior communicating artery, as well as at other locations (Fig 1). Typical presenting signs include headache; ptosis; limited elevation, depression, and adduction; and a dilated or poorly reactive pupil (Fig 2). The

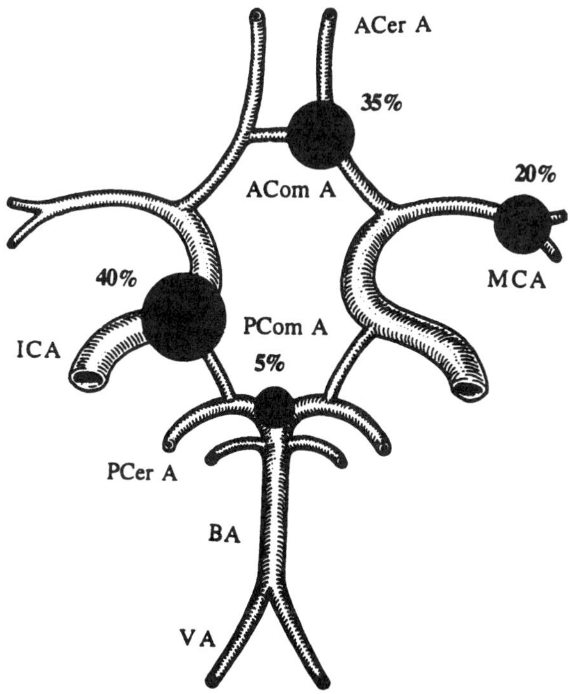

FIGURE 1.—Common sites and frequency of intracranial aneurysms on the circle of Willis at the base of the brain. The majority of aneurysms are located in the anterior circulation: 40% at the junction of the internal carotid artery (*ICA*) and the posterior communicating artery (*PCom A*), 35% at the junction of the anterior cerebral artery (*ACer A*), and 20% at the bifurcation of the middle cerebral artery (*MCA*). Approximately 5% are located at the bifurcation of the basilar artery (*BA*) into posterior cerebral arteries (*PCer A*), or the junction of the vertebral artery (*VA*) and the ipsilateral posterior inferior cerebellar artery. (Reprinted by permission of the publisher from Biousse V, Mendicino ME, Simon DJ, et al: The ophthalmology of intracranial vascular abnormalities. *Am J Ophthalmol* 125:527-544. Copyright 1998 by Elsevier Science Inc.)

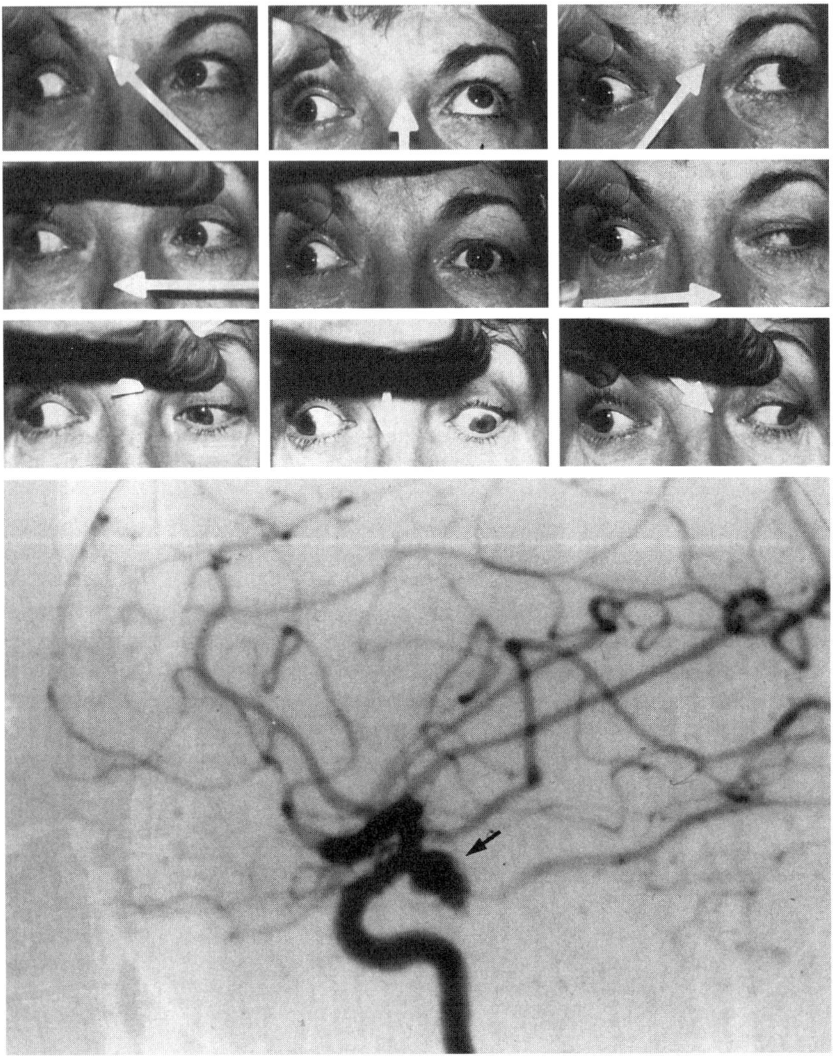

FIGURE 2.—Right third nerve palsy from right posterior communicating artery aneurysm. **Upper**, ocular motility in the 9 cardinal positions of gaze, showing limitation of elevation, depression, and adduction of the right eye, with pupillary dilatation. There was right upper eyelid ptosis. **Lower**, cerebral arteriography demonstrating a right posterior communicating aneurysm (*arrow*). (Reprinted by permission of the publisher from Biousse V, Mendicino ME, Simon DJ, et al: The ophthalmology of intracranial vascular abnormalities. *Am J Ophthalmol* 125:527-544. Copyright 1998 by Elsevier Science Inc.)

pupillary fibers are almost always involved because of their location along the subarachnoid portion of the third nerve. In a patient with complete paresis, the absence of pupillary involvement almost always means no aneurysm is present.

Isolated sixth nerve paresis rarely results from aneurysmal involvement in the subarachnoid space. Cavernous aneurysms producing sixth nerve

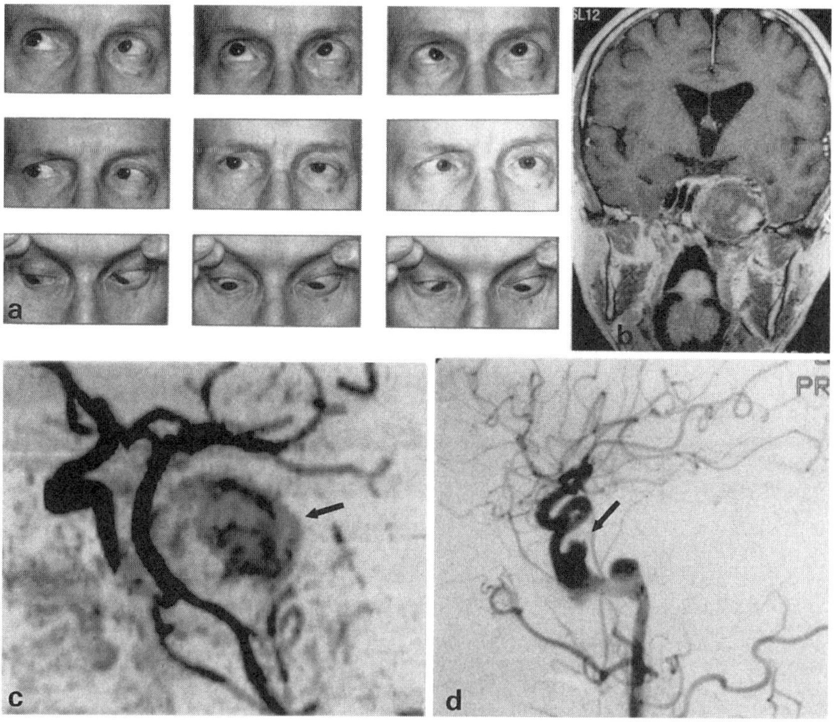

FIGURE 3.—Left sixth nerve palsy and Horner syndrome caused by left intracavernous giant aneurysm. **Top left, a,** ocular motility in the 9 cardinal positions of gaze, showing an abduction deficit in the left eye, with a smaller palpebral fissure and mild anisocoria (left pupil smaller than right), consistent with a left sixth nerve palsy and Horner syndrome. **Top right, b,** coronal contrast-enhanced T1-weighted magnetic resonance image of the brain disclosing a large lesion in the left cavernous sinus, with mass effect on the adjacent structures, consistent with a giant cavernous sinus aneurysm. **Bottom left, c,** magnetic resonance angiography demonstrating the carotid cavernous sinus aneurysm (*arrow*). **Bottom right, d,** conventional angiography showing the partially thrombosed aneurysm (*arrow*). (Reprinted by permission of the publisher from Biousse V, Mendicino ME, Simon DJ, et al: The ophthalmology of intracranial vascular abnormalities. *Am J Ophthalmol* 125:527-544. Copyright 1998 by Elsevier Science Inc.)

palsy often cause ipsilateral Horner syndrome (Fig 3). Abnormalities of trochlear nerve function typically go unnoticed because of combined palsies of the third and sixth nerves. Damage to the sympathetic fibers may cause the pupil not to dilate or to be small. Patients with a giant aneurysm at or near the ophthalmic artery origin commonly have an ipsilateral nasal field defect, sometimes with a contralateral upper temporal defect ("junctional scotoma"). The finding of Terson syndrome usually means subarachnoid hemorrhage resulting from aneurysmal rupture. The hemorrhage may be retinal or preretinal, commonly contained by the internal limiting membrane, but sometimes the hemorrhage breaks into the preretinal space or vitreous (Fig 4). Patients with unilateral or bilateral sixth nerve palsy may show papilledema.

Fistulas.—Dural fistulas are congenital arteriovenous connections that may open spontaneously or in the course of hypertension, diabetes, ath-

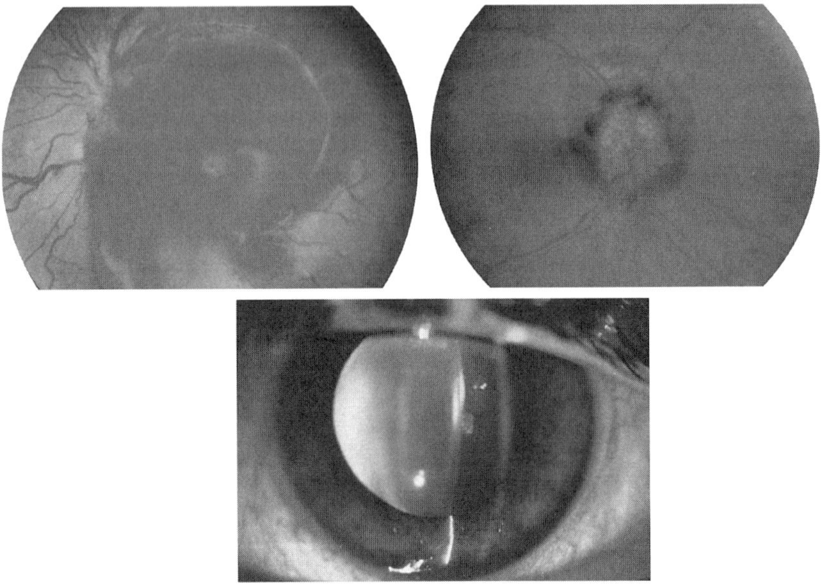

FIGURE 4.—Terson syndrome. **Top left**, preretinal hemorrhage breaking into the vitreous inferiorly. **Top right**, peripapillary hemorrhage and papilledema. **Bottom**, slit-lamp appearance of organizing vitreous hemorrhage. (All photographs courtesy of Steven A. Newman, M.D., printed by permission of the publisher from Biousse V, Mendicino ME, Simon DJ, et al: The ophthalmology of intracranial vascular abnormalities. *Am J Ophthalmol* 125:527-544. Copyright 1998 by Elsevier Science Inc.)

erosclerosis, collagen vascular disease, or childbirth. Carotid-cavernous fistula is associated with arterialization of the conjunctival vessels, the result of arterial blood flow into the orbital and conjunctival veins. Delayed visual loss may be caused by factors such as increased intraocular pressure, retinal venous stasis, choroidal detachment, or ischemic optic neuropathy. Patients with indirect or dural fistula may have mild proptosis, minimal eyelid swelling, and conjunctival chemosis. The retinal veins may be moderately dilated, and sixth nerve palsy may cause diplopia. These patients have chronic red eye, which may be mistaken for conjunctivitis. Visual loss is less common than in patients with direct carotid-cavernous fistulas, but delayed diagnosis can lead to severe, permanent visual loss.

Arteriovenous Malformations.—Most arteriovenous malformations involve the pial vessels only, though some malformations are purely dural in origin and others involve both pial and dural vessels. Headache is the most common presenting symptom, and may be mistaken for migraine. Symptoms may result from compression, ischemia, vascular steal, or other mechanisms. "Optic nerve apoplexy" refers to sudden loss of vision from lesions involving the intracranial optic nerve or chiasm. Neuroradiologic studies are indicated for patients with headaches occurring consistently on the same side, preceded by a visual aura lasting a few seconds, and with visual symptoms in the visual field contralateral to the headache.

Summary.—This article discusses the ophthalmologic manifestations associated with various types of intracranial vascular lesions. For some patients, the ophthalmologist is the first to notice the clinical signs of these abnormalities, which may cause permanent neurologic complications. Recognition and prompt diagnosis help to ensure appropriate treatment.

► This article acquaints the general ophthalmologist with intracranial vascular abnormalities seen with ophthalmic manifestations. The subject is clearly important, because the ophthalmologist may be the initial physician whom the patient contacts for these particular complaints. The article covers intracranial aneurysms, carotid-cavernous fistula/malformations, arteriovenous malformations, and cavernous malformations. Other vascular malformations, such as capillary telangiectasia and venous anomalies, are not discussed.

Salient features of these abnormalities, with discussion of both ophthalmologic presentations and pathophysiology, are presented. The ophthalmologist must be cognizant of the ophthalmic manifestations of intracranial vascular abnormalities. Clearly, intracranial cerebral aneurysm provides the highest risk for both the patient and the physician. The authors correctly state that early diagnosis is paramount to preventing a devastating subarachnoid hemorrhage. The combination of frontal headache with a complete third nerve palsy necessitates emergency neuradiological studies, including MRI and conventional angiography. The absence of pupil involvement in the setting of a complete paresis almost always excludes the diagnosis of aneurysm. However, when the extraocular muscles are incompletely involved, this rule does not apply. Although the absence of pain is unusual, it clearly does not totally exclude the diagnosis of aneurysm.

Carotid-cavernous fistula/malformation represents a group of vascular abnormalities around the cavernous sinus that may be related to trauma or may occur spontaneously. The authors present one classification scheme for this group of vascular lesions. Dural malformations are associated with older women and with hypertension, diabetes, atherosclerotic disease, childbirth, or collagen-vascular disease. The lesion produces elevated venous pressure, which is the source for arterialization of conjunctival vessels, chemosis, proptosis, angle-closure glaucoma, and diplopia. Dural malformations are, at times, associated with a chronic red eye, which is frequently misdiagnosed as chronic conjunctivitis, thyroid ophthalmopathy, scleritis, or orbital pseudo tumor. Both carotid-cavernous fistula and dural malformations, when significant, result in intracranial venous drainage. This can be a source of an acute subdural, subarachnoid, or intraparenchymal hemorrhage.

Intracranial arteriovenous malformations are seen with headache, which is often misdiagnosed as migraine. The ophthalmologist should be concerned when such migrainous headaches occur consistently on the same side, when the headache precedes the visual aura, when the visual aura lasts only a few seconds, and when the visual symptoms are always seen in the hemifield contralateral to the headache.

MRI has been extremely successful in diagnosing cavernous malformations of the brain. These are dilated vascular spaces filled with blood. They have an associated matrix and are quite stereotyped in their MR appearance. Although they occur sporadically, there is a familial form, characterized by multiple lesions and an autosomal mode of inheritance more frequently seen in the Hispanic population. A familial neuro-oculocutaneous syndrome has been described, in which cerebral cavernous malformations are associated with angiomas of the retina or optic disk or both. These lesions occasionally hemorrhage and produce symptoms based upon their location.

This report reviews some of the most important aspects of common vascular abnormalities of the brain and is worthwhile reading for all practicing ophthalmologists.

R.I. Grossman, M.D.

Posterior Leukoencephalopathy Without Severe Hypertension: Utility of Diffusion-weighted MRI

Ay H, Buonanno FS, Schaefer PW, et al (Harvard Med School, Boston)

Neurology 51:1369-1376, 1998 9–7

Introduction.—Characterized by headache, nausea and vomiting, visual disturbances, altered mental status, decreased alertness, seizures, and, occasionally, focal neurologic signs, posterior leukoencephalopathy syndrome is a rapidly evolving neurologic condition. It is usually associated with an abrupt and severe increase in blood pressure, such as eclampsia or renal disease, but it is also seen in patients taking immunosuppressive drugs. It is essential to recognize posterior leukoencephalopathy syndrome early. A new technique is echo-planar diffusion-weighted imaging, which contains diffusion and T2 components and appears as a signal that is markedly hyperintense to the normal brain tissue. Ischemic tissue is hypointense to normal tissue on apparent diffusion coefficient maps, which display the diffusion component only. Three patients with posterior leukoencephalopathy syndrome with only mild elevations in blood pressure were described.

Methods.—The 3 women's studies, included CT, standard MRI, diffusion-weighted imaging, apparent diffusion coefficient maps, and, in 1 case, perfusion-weighted imaging. All of the patients had a mild elevation in blood pressure and none had previously described risk factors for posterior leukoencephalopathy.

Results.—Large, abnormal, T2 hyperintense regions in the posterior cerebrum were seen on MRI, with corresponding hyperintensity on apparent diffusion coefficient maps, which are signal characteristics that are usually consistent with vasogenic edema (Fig 1). One patient had smaller, patchy posterior cortical regions with decreased apparent diffusion coefficient and bright diffusion-weighted imaging consistent with infarction (Fig 2). Another patient had a dramatic conversion of a large region to an ischemic pattern (Fig 3).

Conclusion.—Diffusion-weighted imaging and apparent diffusion coefficient maps can play a pivotal role in treatment decisions, as they can

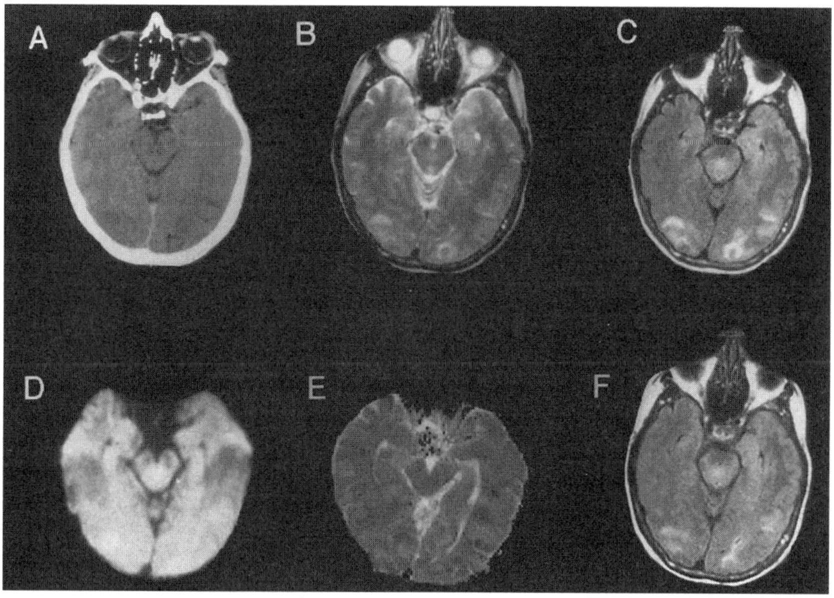

FIGURE 1.—Patient 1. **A,** non–contrast-enhanced axial CT demonstrates hypodensity in the posterior temporal and parietal lobes bilaterally. **B,** axial T2-weighted and **C,** axial fast fluid-attenuated inversion recovery (fFLAIR) weighted MR images, obtained 2 days later, demonstrate hyperintensity in the posterior parietal and occipital lobe white matter with some involvement of the overlying cortex. **D,** diffusion-weighted MR image demonstrates these regions to have signal slightly hyperintense to normal gray and white matter. **E,** apparent diffusion coefficient MR image demonstrates these regions to have signal subtly hyperintense to normal gray and white matter, consistent with increased diffusion and vasogenic edema. No definite areas of decreased diffusion to suggest infarction are identified. **F,** fFLAIR MR image obtained 2 days later demonstrates nearly complete interval resolution of the previously seen hyperintense abnormalities, consistent with reversible vasogenic edema. (Courtesy of Ay H, Buonanno FS, Schaefer PW, et al: Posterior leukoencephalopathy without severe hypertension: Utility of diffusion-weighted MRI. *Neurology* 51:1369-1376. Copyright 1998, American Academy of Neurology. Used with permission of Lippincott-Raven Publishers.)

successfully differentiate posterior leukoencephalopathy from early cerebral ischemia (Table). Posterior leukoencephalopathy is not always reversible and is associated with a wider variety of conditions than previously reported. A tissue stage of permanent brain injury is marked in patients with the syndrome who have hyperintense diffusion-weighted image signal.

► Posterior leukoencephalopathy syndrome is a rapidly evolving neurologic condition whose manifestations include headache, nausea and vomiting, altered mental status, seizures, and visual disturbances. The syndrome is acute and most often associated with hypertension. It has been controversial because some of the patients may not have severe hypertension; however, their elevations in blood pressure may be high relative to the blood pressure they normally run. On MRI, one may see high-intensity in the occipital region radiating into the parietal region. This is also seen on fast fluid-attenuated inversion recovery images. The authors of this paper have

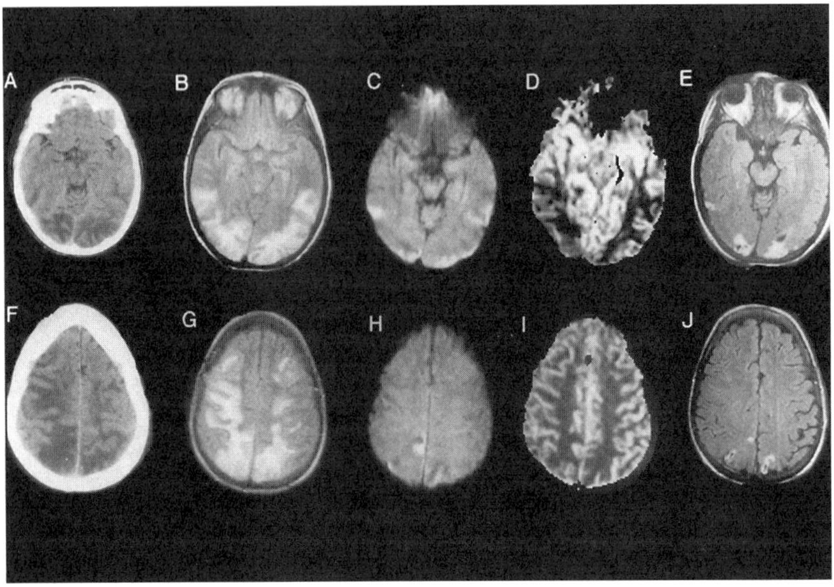

FIGURE 2.—Patient 2. **A** and **F**, Non–contrast-enhanced axial CT images demonstrate hypodensity in the posterior temporal and occipital lobes bilaterally as well as in the frontal and pareital lobes. The hypodensity predominantly involves white matter, but there is some involvement of the overlying cortex. **B** and **G**, fast fluid-attenuated inversion recovery (fFLAIR) weighted MR images obtained 4 days later demonstrate hyperintensity in similar regions. **C** and **H**, diffusion-weighted images at similar levels demonstrate hypodensity and isointensity, consistent with vasogenic edema, in the affected white matter. There is hyperintensity, consistent with cytotoxic edema, in some affected cortex. **D** and **I**, relative cerebral blood flow maps demonstrate decreased signal intensity, consistent with decreased flow, in the cortex, which is hyperintense on diffusion-weighted images **E** and **J**, fFLAIR weighted images obtained 9 days later demonstrate persistent hyperintensity in the cortex, which was hyperintense on diffusion-weighted images; this is consistent with infarcted tissue. The T2 hyperintensities characterized by increased diffusion (relatively decreased signal) on the earlier images have completely resolved. (Courtesy of Ay H, Buonanno FS, Schaefer PW, et al: Posterior leukoencephalopathy without severe hypertension: Utility of diffusion-weighted MRI. *Neurology* 51:1369-1376. Copyright 1998, American Academy of Neurology. Used with permission of Lippincott-Raven Publishers.)

applied diffusion-weighted imaging and also have made apparent diffusion coefficient maps.

I have chosen this paper to demonstrate an interesting application of diffusion-weighted imaging. This technique is sensitive to microscopic random motion (diffusion) of water molecules. With the development of cytotoxic edema, there is decreased diffusion of water molecules. This appears quite early and may be imaged by diffusion-weighted imaging and apparent diffusion coefficient maps. On diffusion-weighted imaging, one may see high signal intensity that may be the result of cytotoxic swelling or edema. The diffusion-weighted imaging contains both a diffusion component and a T2 component. Apparent diffusion coefficient maps which display the diffusion component only demonstrate hypointensity in ischemic tissue. In acute ischemia depletion of high-energy phosphates leads to cessation of the sodium/potassium pump, and water becomes trapped intracellularly with restricted motion. Decreased water diffusion is characterized by marked

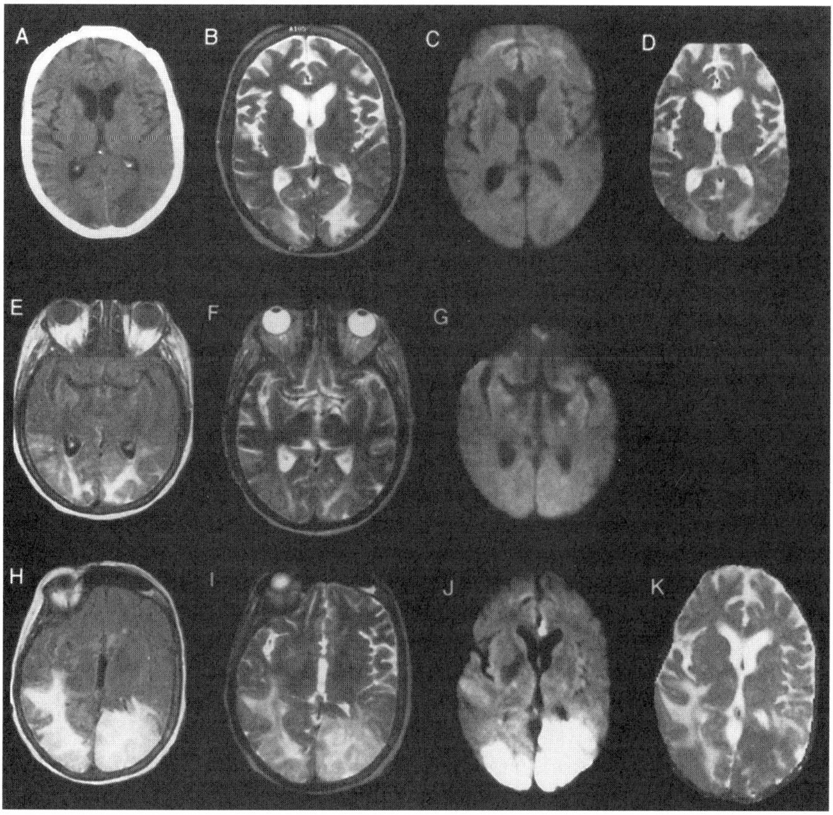

FIGURE 3.—Patient 3. **A,** non–contrast-enhanced axial CT demonstrates hypodensity in the occipital lobes bilaterally. **B,** axial T2-weighted MR image, obtained 1 day later, demonstrates hyperintensity in the occipital lobe white matter bilaterally with some involvement of the overlying cortex. **C,** axial diffusion-weighted image demonstrates hypointensity and **D,** axial apparent diffusion coefficient map demonstrates hyperintensity in these regions: these findings are consistent with vasogenic edema. **E,** axial fast fluid-attenuated inversion recover (fFLAIR) weighted, **F,** axial T2-weighted, and **G,** axial diffusion-weighted images obtained 9 days later demonstrate partial resolution of the previously seen abnormalities. **H,** axial fFLAIR and **I,** axial T2-weighted images obtained 2 weeks later demonstrate an increase in the hyperintensities with extension to involve the posterior temporal lobes and most of the adjacent cortex. **J,** axial diffusion-weighted images demonstrate homogeneous hyperintensity and **K,** axial apparent diffusion coefficient map demonstrates homogeneous hypointensity; these findings are consistent with decreased diffusion and cytotoxic edema. (Courtesy of Ay H, Buonanno FS, Schaefer PW, et al: Posterior leukoencephalopathy without severe hypertension: Utility of diffusion-weighted MRI. *Neurology* 51:1369-1376. Copyright 1998, American Academy of Neurology. Used with permission of Lippincott-Raven Publishers.)

hyperintensity on diffusion-weighted images and hypointensity on apparent diffusion coefficient maps. This is contrasted with vasogenic edema where there is markedly increased apparent diffusion coefficient with hypointense or isointense signal on diffusion-weighted imaging. The application of this technique offers the opportunity to separate vasogenic changes from cytotoxic changes.

Why is this important? In the differential diagnosis, there are many conditions in posterior leukoencephalopathy syndrome that are associated with

TABLE.—MRI Signal Intensities in Various Tissue States

	Vasogenic edema	Cytotoxic edema	Reversible PLES	Acute cerebral infarction
T2	↑	↑	↑	N, then ↑
FLAIR	↑	↑	↑	N, then ↑
DWI	↓, N or slight ↑	↑	↓	↑, then ↑ ↑
ADC	↑	↓	↑	↓

Note: Comparison of various MR signal intensities in vasogenic and cytotoxic edema, posterior leukoencephalopathy syndrome, and in early phases of acute cerebral infarction. In posterior leukoencephalopathy syndrome, as the irreversible injury (infarction) develops, signal intensity is increased on diffusion-weighted imaging (*DWI*) and decreased on apparent diffusion coefficient (*ADC*) maps. Note the ability of diffusion-weighted imaging/apparent diffusion coefficient techniques to depict the similarities between early infarction and cytotoxic edema.

Abbreviations: FLAIR, fluid-attenuated inversion recovery; *N*, normal; ↑, increased or hyperintense signal; ↓, decreased or hypointense signal.

(Courtesy of Ay H, Buonanno FS, Schaefer PW, et al: Posterior leukoencephalopathy without severe hypertension: Utility of diffusion-weighted MRI. *Neurology* 51:1369-1376. Copyright 1998, American Academy of Neurology. Used with permission of Lippincott-Raven, Publishers.)

infarction. These include emboli producing stroke, particularly an embolus at top of the basilar artery, venous thrombosis, and vasculitis. Diffusion imaging can separate conditions causing infarction from those that produce edema. Other disorders associated with these high intensity abnormalities include eclampsia, renal disease with hypertension, and reactions to immunosuppressive drugs such as cyclosporine, Tacrolimus, and α-interferon.

The most likely etiology of posterior leukoencephalopathy syndrome is related to hyperperfusion of the perforating arteries in the posterior circulation. There is a paucity of sympathetic innervation, particularly in the basilar artery and its branches. This makes the posterior circulation, particularly the occipital region, prone to these lesions. For the ophthalmologist, the visual component of the disease is extremely common. Furthermore, it is important to understand that these cases, although initially involving vasogenic edema, may progress to ischemic disease.

This paper demonstrates application of newer MRI techniques to aid in subcategorization of brain disease. The technology is being implemented in many centers throughout the United States and the world and will serve as another parameter to differentiate reversible from irreversible change. It is important for ophthalmologists to appreciate the power of this technique, not only for stroke but for other acute neurologic problems.

R.I. Grossman, M.D.

Unruptured Intracranial Aneurysms: Risk of Rupture and Risks of Surgical Intervention

Wiebers DO, for the International Study of Unruptured Intracranial Aneuryms Investigators (Mayo Clinic, Rochester, Minn)

N Engl J Med 339:1725-1733, 1998 9–8

Introduction.—In the general population, the overall frequency of intracranial aneurysm is as high as 9.9%, or as many as 15 million people in

TABLE 1.—Baseline Characteristics of the Retrospective Cohort

Characteristic	Group 1 (*N* = 727)	Group 2 (*N* = 722)	*P* Value
Age—yr			
Mean	56.0	49.4	<0.001
Range	9-87	13-80	
Female sex—no. of patients (%)	517 (71.1)	535 (74.1)	0.27
White race—no. of patients (%)	669 (92.0)	681 (94.3)	0.08
Single aneurysm—no. of patients (%)	545 (75.0)	540 (74.8)	NS
Multiple aneurysms—no. of patients (%)	182 (25.0)	182 (25.2)	
Total no. of aneurysms	977	960	
Diameter of largest aneurysm—mm			
Mean	10.9	5.7	<0.001
Range	2-60	2-35	
Size of largest aneurysm—no. of patients (%)			
2-5 mm	238 (32.7)	442 (61.2)	0.001
6-9 mm	186 (25.6)	199 (27.6)	
10-14 mm	113 (15.5)	65 (9.0)	
15-24 mm	120 (16.5)	13 (1.8)	
≥25 mm	70 (9.6)	3 (0.4)	
Location of aneurysm—no. of aneurysms (%)			
Cavernous carotid artery	165 (16.9)	91 (9.5)	<0.001
Internal carotid artery	242 (24.8)	171 (17.8)	<0.001
Anterior communicating or anterior cerebral artery	98 (10.0)	79 (8.2)	0.22
Mild cerebral artery	222 (22.7)	363 (37.8)	<0.001
Posterior communicating artery	136 (13.9)	163 (17.0)	0.06
Vertebrobasilar or posterior cerebral artery	64 (6.6)	56 (5.8)	0.51
Tip of basilar artery	50 (5.1)	37 (3.9)	0.18

Note: Patients in group 1 had no history of subarachnoid hemorrhage, and those in group 2 had a history of subarachnoid hemorrhage.

Abbreviation: *NS*, not significant.

(Reprinted by permission of *The New England Journal of Medicine*, from Wiebers DO, for the International Study of Unruptured Intracranial Aneurysms Investigators: Unruptured intracranial aneurysms: Risk of rupture and risks of surgical intervention. *N Engl J Med* 339:1725-1733.)

the United States. Most intracranial aneurysms, however, do not rupture. Because of a lack of understanding of the natural history of unruptured intracranial aneurysms and the risks of repairing them, their management remains controversial. The risk of rupture was determined, as well as the risks associated with the repair of unruptured intracranial aneurysms.

Methods.—There were 2,721 patients with an unruptured intracranial aneurysm who were retrospectively and prospectively reviewed. The natural history of unruptured intracranial aneurysms in 1,449 patients with 1,937 aneurysms was retrospectively reviewed; 727 of the patients had no history of subarachnoid hemorrhage from a different aneurysm (group 1), and 722 patients had a history of subarachnoid hemorrhage from a different aneurysm that had been repaired successfully (group 2) (Table 1). The treatment-related morbidity and mortality in 1,172 patients with newly diagnosed unruptured intracranial aneurysms were prospectively examined.

Results.—There was a less than 0.05% per year cumulative rate of rupture of aneurysms that were less than 10 mm in diameter at diagnosis in group 1. The rate was approximately 11 times as high or 0.5% per year

TABLE 3.—Baseline Characteristics of the Prospective Cohort

Characteristic	Group 1 (*N* = 798)	Group 2 (*N* = 197)	*P* Value
Age—yr			
Mean	53.0	47.2	<0.001
Range	19-91	24-78	
Female sex—no. of patients (%)	598 (74.9)	163 (82.7)	
White race—no. of patients (%)	735 (92.1)	175 (88.8)	
Total no. of aneurysms	1039	262	
Diameter of largest aneurysm—mm			
Mean	11.6	8.3	
Range	2-50	2-60	
Size of largest aneurysm—no. of patients (%)			
2-5 mm	128 (16.0)	65 (33.0)	<0.001
6-9 mm	262 (32.8)	79 (40.1)	
10-14 mm	203 (25.4)	39 (19.8)	
15-24 mm	148 (18.5)	11 (5.6)	
≥25 mm	57 (7.1)	3 (1.5)	
Location of aneurysm—no. of aneurysms (%)			
Cavernous carotid artery	24 (2.3)	3 (1.1)	0.24
Internal carotid artery	393 (37.8)	82 (31.3)	0.05
Anterior communicating or anterior cerebral artery	167 (16.1)	23 (8.8)	0.003
Middle cerebral artery	305 (29.4)	116 (44.3)	<0.001
Posterior communicating artery	43 (4.1)	15 (5.7)	0.27
Vertebrobasilar or posterior cerebral artery	50 (4.8)	15 (5.7)	0.54
Tip of basilar artery	57 (5.5)	8 (3.1)	0.11

(Reprinted by permission of *The New England Journal of Medicine*, from Wiebers DO, for the International Study of Unruptured Intracranial Aneurysms Investigators: Unruptured intracranial aneurysms: Risk of rupture and risks of surgical intervention. *N Engl J Med* 339:1725-1733.)

in group 2. In both groups, the rupture rate of aneurysms that were 10 mm or more in diameter was less than 1 % per year. But in group 1, the rate of rupture for giant aneurysms, those 25 mm or greater in diameter, was 6% in the first year. Independent predictors of rupture were the size and location of the aneurysm (Table 3) and (Fig 2). In group 1, the overall rate of surgery-related morbidity and mortality was 17.5% at 30 days. In group 2, the overall rate of surgery-related morbidity and mortality was 13.6% at 30 days (Table 4). At 1 year, the overall rate of surgery-related morbidity and mortality was 15.7% for group 1 and 13.1% for group 2. Surgical outcome was independently predicted by age.

Conclusion.—Among patients in group 1, the likelihood of rupture of unruptured intracranial aneurysms that were less than 10 mm in diameter was exceedingly low, but among those in group 2, the likelihood was substantially higher. Among patients in group 1 with unruptured intracranial aneurysms smaller than 10 mm in diameter, the risk of morbidity and mortality related to surgery greatly exceeded the 7.5-year risk of rupture (Fig 1).

▶ This is a most important study for ophthalmologists, as well as physicians in general, regarding the natural history of aneurysms. There is also an accompanying editorial.

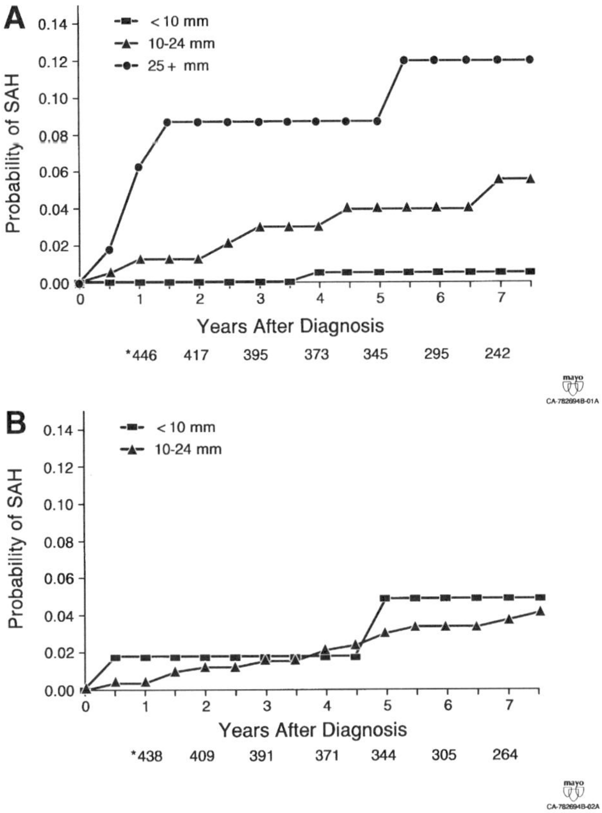

FIGURE 2.—Probability of subarachnoid hemorrhage over time in group 1 (**Panel A**) and group 2 (**Panel B**), according to the size of the aneurysm. In Panel B, no rates are shown for aneurysms in the largest category (25 mm or greater) because there were only 3 patients with aneurysms in this category. The *numbers* at the bottom of each panel are the numbers of patients not operated on who were at risk for a first hemorrhage. Data are from the retrospective cohort. (Reprinted by permission of *The New England Journal of Medicine*, from Wiebers DO, for the International Study of Unruptured Intracranial Aneurysms Investigators: Unruptured intracranial aneurysms: Risk of rupture and risks of surgical intervention. *N Engl J Med* 339:1725-1733. Copyright 1998, Massachusetts Medical Society. All rights reserved.)

This study is extremely well performed and demonstrates conclusively that the likelihood of hemorrhage from unruptured intracranial aneurysms that are less than 10 mm in diameter is exceedingly low in patients who have never had a ruptured aneurysm. It is even low (0.5% per year) in patients who have had a subarachnoid hemorrhage from a different aneurysm. The conclusion of the paper is that for aneurysms less than 10 mm in diameter, the risk of hemorrhage may be less than the risk of surgical treatment.

There are a great deal of data in this report. How does the physician decide whether to recommend surgery? Here, size and location of the aneurysm and a history or absence of history of previously ruptured aneurysms are extremely significant. The patient's medical condition also is important. However, it appears that from this study age is also very important. Surgery is a more obvious choice the younger the patient. This paper clearly provides

TABLE 4.—Surgical Outcome in Groups 1 and 2

Outcome	Group 1 (*N* = 798) No. of Patients	Group 1 (*N* = 798) % (95% CI)	Group 2 (*N* = 197) No. of Patients	Group 2 (*N* = 197) % (95% CI)
At 1 mo				
Surgery-related death	18	2.3 (1.3-3.3)	0	0 (0-1.4)
Disability	122	15.3	27	13.7
Rankin score of 3-5 only	29	3.6	6	3.0
Impaired cognitive status only	44	5.5	19	9.6
Both	49	6.1	2	1.0
Overall morbidity and mortality				
All patients	140	17.5 (15.5-20.5)	27	13.6 (8.0-17.2)
Patients with normal neurologic status at base line*	130	17.0	24	12.8
At 1 yr				
Surgery-related death	30	3.8 (2.4-5.4)	2	1.0 (0-2.6)
Disability	95	12.0	24	12.1
Rankin score of 3-5 only	26	3.3	3	1.5
Impaired congnitive status only	43	5.4	18	9.1
Both	26	3.3	3	1.5
Overall morbidity and mortality				
All patients	125	15.7 (13.2-18.2)	26	13.1 (8.0-17.2)
Patients with normal neurologic status at base line*	119	15.6	21	11.2

*Normal neurologic status was defined as a Rankin score of 1 and no cognitive impairment as measured by the Mini-Mental State Examination. There were 764 patients in group 1 and 188 in group 2 who had normal neurologic status at baseline.

Abbreviation: CI, confidence interval.

(Reprinted by permission of *The New England Journal of Medicine*, from Wiebers DO, for the International Study of Unruptured Intracranial Aneurysms Investigators: Unruptured intracranial aneurysms: Risk of rupture and risks of surgical intervention. *N Engl J Med* 339:1725-1733.)

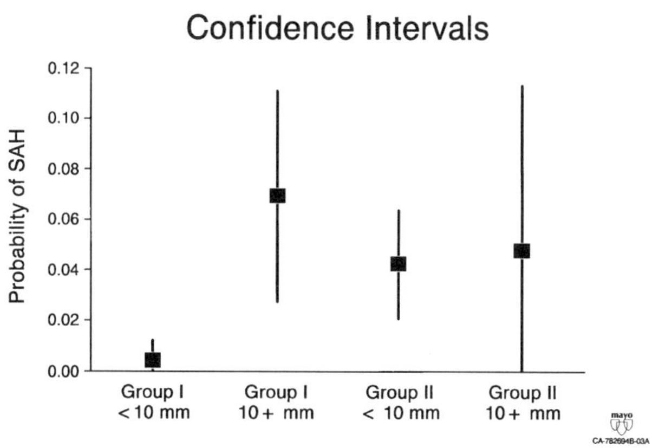

FIGURE 1.—Probability of subarachnoid hemorrhage 7.5 years after the diagnosis of unruptured intracranial aneurysm, according to the diameter of the aneurysm. Patients in group 1 had no history of subarachnoid hemorrhage from a different aneurysm, and those in group 2 did have such a history. Data are from the retrospective cohort. The *bars* represent 95% confidence intervals (Reprinted by permission of *The New England Journal of Medicine*, from Wiebers DO, for the International Study of Unruptured Intracranial Aneurysms Investigators: Unruptured intracranial aneurysms: Risk of rupture and risks of surgical intervention. *N Engl J Med* 339:1725-1733.)

important objective data for deciding whether a patient should undergo surgical treatment.

What was not discussed, and I believe important, was the use of nonsurgical interventional techniques for the treatment of aneurysms. This relatively new but important modality may impact significantly on treatment decisions. It offers high-risk patients an alternative to difficult surgery. The costs are markedly lower than for patients undergoing surgical treatment. There are clearly exceptions to neurovascular intervention and the data are clearly not available on the natural history of such treatment. Nevertheless, the advantages appear obvious.

Natural history studies, such as these comparing morbidity and mortality of surgical treatment vs. neurovascular interventional therapy, are critical. Such an alternative might significantly change the equation regarding aneurysmal treatment in all patients, but particularly in the elderly. I strongly recommend this article for ophthalmologists interested in understanding the implications of surgery versus conservative therapy in patients who have incidental aneurysms detected.

R.I. Grossman, M.D.

Ophthalmic Manifestations of Fibrous Dysplasia: A Disease of Children and Adults

Katz BJ, Nerad JA (Univ of Iowa Hosps and Clinics, Iowa City)

Ophthalmology 105:2207-2215, 1998 9–9

Background.—In fibrous dysplasia, normal bone is replaced by immature bone and osteoid in a cellular fibrous matrix. Pain, swelling, and disfigurement throughout the skeleton can result from the fibroblastic expansion of affected bones. The cause of fibrous dysplasia has not been defined. Malignant transformation is rare and often associated with previous irradiation. In about 20% of cases, craniofacial bones are involved. Most orbital lesions are monoostotic but frequently involve multiple skull bones and cross suture lines. Patients with fibrous dysplasia of orbital bones may seek treatment from an ophthalmologist because of facial deformities, loss of vision, or globe displacement, which may be the first clinical signs of the disease. Fibrous dysplasia is usually considered a disease of children and adolescents, but it can also occur in adults. The percentage of adults with ophthalmic complications of fibrous dysplasia was determined.

Methods.—In a retrospective study, 20 patients with fibrous dysplasia were investigated. Data were collected on patient demographics, major signs and symptoms, loss of vision, pattern of bone involvement, and radiographic appearance of fibrous dysplasia.

Results.—In contrast to previous reports, adults made up a significant percentage of patients with ophthalmic complications of fibrous dysplasia. Of the 20 patients, 9 were younger than 18 years and 11 were 18 years old

TABLE 1.—Patients With Biopsy-proven Fibrous Dysplasia

Patient No.	Case Report No.	Age at Presentation (yrs)	Age at Diagnosis (yrs)	Sex	Acuity or Field Loss	Facial Asymmetry	Major Symptom or Sign	Primary Location of Lesion
1	3	1	1	M	+	+	Multiple midfacial anomalies	Diffuse
2	1	1	1	M	–	+	NLD obstruction	Anterior orbit
3	–	6	6	F	–	+	Proptosis	Diffuse
4	–	7	7	M	–	+	Globe ptosis	Anterior orbit
5	–	9	3	F	–	+	Globe ptosis	Diffuse
6	–	12	11	M	–	–	Recurrent sinusitis	Orbital roof and sinuses
7	–	14	13	M	–	+	Facial asymmetry	Diffuse
8	7	16	16	F	+	+	NLP OD	Diffuse
9	–	16	16	M	–	+	Globe ptosis	Anterior orbit
10	–	18	23	F	–	+	Cheek mass	Maxilla
11	6	19	19	F	+	+	CF OD; CN V, VI palsies	Posterior orbit
12	–	21	20	M	–	+	Cheek mass	Maxilla
13	2	23	23	F	–	+	Proptosis	Posterior orbit
14	8	25	6	M	+	–	Homonymous field defect	Mandible
15	5	25	11	F	+	+	Central scotoma CD	Diffuse
16	–	28	17	M	–	+	Cheek mass	Zygoma
17	–	30	28	F	–	–	Blurred vision	Parietal
18	4	32	32	M	+	–	NLP OD	Posterior orbit
19	–	38	13	F	–	+	Cheek mass	Maxilla and sphenoid
20	–	72	72	F	–	+	Cheek mass	Orbital rim

Abbreviations: CF, counts fingers; *CN*, cranial nerve; *NLD*, nasolacrimal duct; *NLP*, no light perception.
(Published courtesy of *Ophthalmology*, from Katz BJ, Nerad JA: Ophthalmic manifestations of fibrous dysplasia: A disease of children and adults. *Ophthalmology* 105:2207-2215, 1998.)

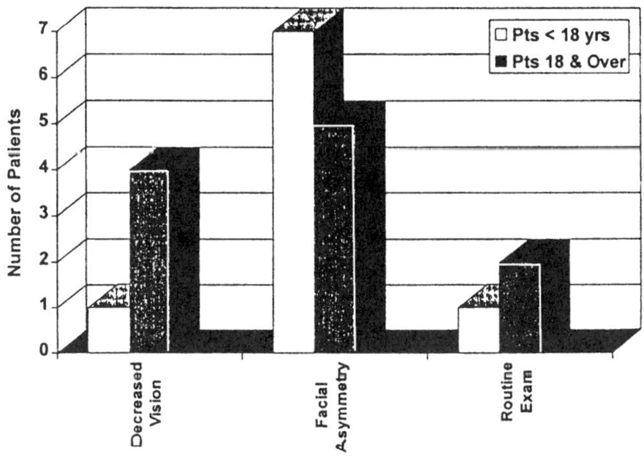

FIGURE 1.—Complaints of patients with biopsy-proven fibrous dysplasia. Only 1 complaint is noted per patient. (Published courtesy of *Ophthalmology*, from Katz BJ, Nerad JA: Ophthalmic manifestations of fibrous dysplasia: A disease of children and adults. *Ophthalmology* 105:2207-2215,1998.)

or older (Table 1). The most common signs and symptoms were changes in facial contour and symmetry (Figs 1 and 2). Five patients had acute visual loss; 4 of these patients were adults. The most commonly affected facial bone was the maxilla (Fig 3). In most patients, monoostotic lesions that crossed suture lines and involved multiple craniofacial bones were seen.

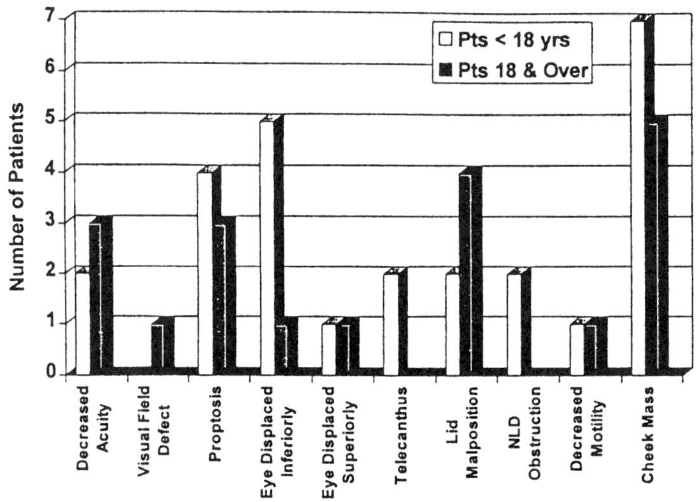

FIGURE 2.—Signs of patients with biopsy-proven fibrous dysplasia. More than 1 examination finding may be noted per patient. *Abbreviation*: *NLD*, nasolacrimal duct. (Published courtesy of *Ophthalmology* from Katz BJ, Nerad JA: Ophthalmic manifestations of fibrous dysplasia: A disease of children and adults. *Ophthalmology* 105:2207-2215,1998.)

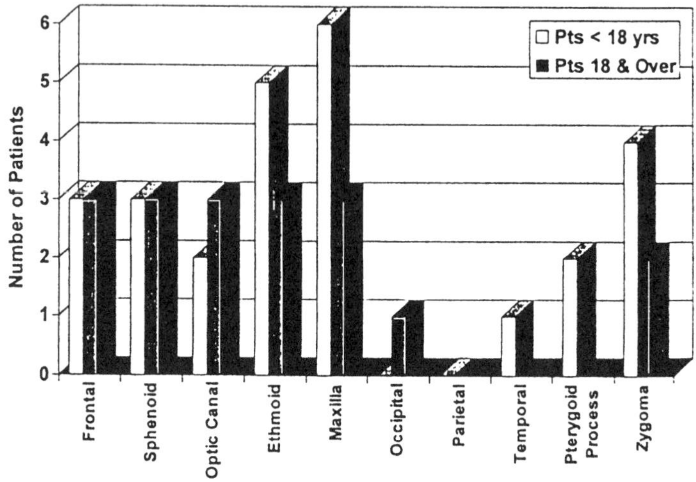

FIGURE 3.—Cranial bones involved. Of the 20 patients with biopsy-proven fibrous dysplasia, 13 had scans available for review. Seven scans were of patients younger than 18 years of age, and 6 were of patients 18 years of age and older. Each scan was evaluated for involvement of 8 of the cranial bones, the optic canals, and pterygoid processes. (Published courtesy of *Ophthalmology*, from Katz BJ, Nerad JA: Ophthalmic manifestations of fibrous dysplasia: A disease of children and adults. *Ophthalmology* 105:2207-2215,1998.)

CT results showed a characteristic pagetoid appearance with alternating areas of radiolucency and radiodensity in most of the lesions.

Discussion.—A diagnosis of fibrous dysplasia should not be ruled out on the basis of the age of the patient alone. Fibrous dysplasia of the orbital bones can cause significant dysfunction and disfigurement but is a treatable cause of blindness in both children and adults. In 1994, Bibby and McFadzean reported that 5 of 12 patients had progression of fibrous dysplasia beyond the teenage years. Also in 1994, Henderson reported that most patients with dysplasia of at least 2 cranial bones would probably have slow progressive disease indefinitely. The typical appearance of fibrous dysplasia on plain radiographs was originally described as a "ground glass" appearance. It can be difficult to differentiate fibrous dysplasia from meningioma because of their clinical and radiologic similarities. Both diseases involve slow, progressive globe displacement. Meningioma can induce a hyperostotic reaction in adjoining bone, making it resemble fibrous dysplasia on CT scans. The authors report that a pagetoid, heterogeneous appearance was seen in 12 of 13 CT scans of fibrous dysplasia, and in all cases, affected bones appeared "expanded" and had smooth, cortical boundaries. The hyperostosis of meningioma often shows a homogeneous thickening of bone with bone involvement often bowing into the temporalis fossa and with some feathering of bone surfaces. There is also soft tissue involvement in meningioma, seen more easily on MRI, that is rarely seen in fibrous dysplasia.

▶ Fibrous dysplasia is a disease where normal bone is replaced by immature bone and osteoid in a cellular fibrous matrix. The bony expansion can produce pain, swelling, and disfiguration. The orbital lesions are monoostotic but can often involve multiple skull bones and can cross suture lines. This article presents a series of biopsy-proven cases of fibrous dysplasia presenting with ophthalmic manifestations. The authors provide a nice table of the signs and symptoms as well as the location. The paper makes the point that one can see adults presenting with this problem, although it had been traditionally thought to be quiescent after puberty.

Radiographically, the disease produces a ground glass appearance or alternating areas of lucency and increased density (pagetoid lesion) on plain radiographs and CT with bone windows. The differential diagnosis involves meningioma, which produces homogeneous thickening of bone. Meningiomas also have a "feathered" appearance and may have a soft tissue component. Meningiomas enhance avidly and may have a tail of enhancement (dural tail).

This paper nicely presents a large series of ophthalmic manifestations of fibrous dysplasia and confirms that it is a disease of adults as well as children.

R.I. Grossman, M.D.

Ophthalmologic Manifestations of Internal Carotid Artery Dissection

Biousse V, Touboul P-J, D'Anglejan-Chatillon J, et al (Lariboisière Hosp, Paris; Versailles Hosp, Le Chesnay, France; Saint-Antoine Hosp, Paris)

Am J Ophthalmol 126:565-577, 1998 9–10

Background.—Dissection of cervical arteries is a common cause of ischemic stroke in young adults. Ophthalmologic signs and symptoms associated with extracranial internal carotid artery dissection were examined.

Methods.—The medical records of 146 consecutive patients with extracranial internal carotid artery dissection were reviewed. There were 79 men and 67 women, and the mean patient age was 45.5 years. The records of 29 patients from 1972 to 1984 were studied retrospectively, and the records of 117 patients from 1985 to 1997 were studied prospectively.

Results.—Of the 146 patients, 91 had ophthalmologic signs and symptoms, and in 76 patients, these were the signs and symptoms that were first seen. Painful Horner syndrome was seen in 65 patients and remained isolated in 32. Transient monocular visual loss was seen in 41 patients; this visual loss was painful in 31 patients, associated with Horner syndrome in 13 patients, and described as scintillations or flashing lights, often related to postural changes or exposure to bright lights, in 23 patients. These descriptions suggest acute choroidal hypoperfusion. Ischemic optic neuropathy was seen in 4 patients, one with diplopia (Table). Among the 76 patients with ophthalmologic signs and symptoms as the signs or symptoms first seen, 27 had a nonreversible ocular or hemispheric stroke within

TABLE.—Neuro-ophthalmologic Symptoms and Signs of 146 Patients with Extracranial Internal Carotid Artery Dissection

	Patients With Neuro-ophthalmologic Symptoms/Signs	
	Overall Frequency: *n* (%)	Frequency as Presenting Symptom/Sign: *n* (%)
Neuro-ophthalmologic symptoms/signs	91/146 (62.5)	76/146 (52)
Painful Horner syndrome	65/146 (44.5)	52/65 (80)
Isolated	32/65 (49)	32/32 (100)
With ischemic symptoms/signs	33/65 (51)	20/33 (60.5)
Transient monocular visual loss	41/146 (28)	25/41 (61)
Associated with pain	31/41 (75.5)	19/31 (61)
Associated with Horner syndrome	13/41 (31.5)	11/13 (85)
Described as "scintillations"	23/41 (56)	14/23 (61)
Permanent visual loss	4/146 (2.5)	0/4 (0)
Ischemic optic neuropathy	4/146 (2.5)	0/4 (0)
Ophthalmic artery occlusion	0/146 (0)	—
Central retinal artery occlusion	0/146 (0)	—
Ischemic ocular syndrome	0/146 (0)	—
Ocular motor nerve palsies	1/146 (0.007)	0/1 (0)

a mean of 6.2 days. Eighteen patients had a stroke within a week of onset of neuro-ophthalmologic symptoms, and 24 patients had a stroke within 2 weeks of the onset of such symptoms.

Discussion.—Ophthalmologic signs and symptoms often are associated with internal carotid artery dissection and are frequently the presenting features. Painful Horner syndrome or transient monocular visual loss indicates carotid artery dissection. Early treatment may help prevent ocular or hemispheric stroke.

▶ This paper presents a large series of patients with ophthalmic manifestations of internal carotid artery dissection. Ophthalmologists should be sensitive to the presenting symptoms or signs of this problem. They are enumerated in the Table provided. It is impressive that two thirds of the patients in this series with extracranial carotid dissections had ophthalmologic symptoms or signs.

What should the physician do who is concerned about this diagnosis? The first imaging study is the MR and MR angiography. This is a sensitive and specific test that can reveal hemorrhage in the wall of the vessel and narrowing of the vascular lumen. The radiologist needs to have the appropriate historic information to tailor the study.

The treatment of vascular dissection is somewhat controversial. The first issue is anticoagulation therapy to prevent emboli that occur as a result of the irregular intima and slower vascular flow. The authors mention hemodynamic stroke. In my experience, most of the strokes are embolic in nature. Early recognition is critical. Standard treatment includes anticoagulation therapy. However, if there is concern regarding hemodynamic occlusion or pseudoaneurysm formation, newer interventional procedures may be warranted, including stent placement.

Vascular dissection is an overlooked cause of stroke. Ophthalmologists can be in the front line in seeing these patients and referring them for emergent imaging and treatment. Their diagnostic acumen can save lives and prevent stroke.

R.I. Grossman, M.D.

10 Ocular Oncology

Developments in Ocular Oncology 1998

by James J. Augsburger, M.D.

During 1998, numerous papers on various topics related to ocular oncology appeared in the medical literature. Not surprisingly, most of these publications were case reports and descriptions of small series of cases. Although such papers help to expand our knowledge of the spectrum clinical findings in a particular lesion or disorder, inform us about a new diagnostic test or treatment method for a condition, or alert us to potentially important clinical associations with a particular lesion or disorder, they do not clarify the frequency of the described abnormalities or associations or provide scientifically valid information about the relative effectiveness of a proposed new diagnostic method or treatment compared to standard approaches. This does not mean that they are valueless. Some important insights occasionally come from such reports. In contrast, articles that present information based on case-control studies or a comparison of matched, statistically adjusted, or randomly assigned cases evaluated or managed by traditional versus new techniques generally provide much more valuable clinical insights about the disease or abnormalities of interest. This is because they address the standard biostatistical query, "Compared with what?"

One major randomized clinical trial was reported in 1998. The large tumor trial of the Collaborative Ocular Melanoma Study (COMS) found that there was no appreciable difference in the posttreatment survival rates of patients with a choroidal or ciliary body melanoma treated by enucleation alone versus by enucleation and presurgical external beam radiation therapy (radiation dose 20 Gy in five fractions of 4 Gy each) to the affected eye and orbit. This result was not surprising to me. I had predicted it many years ago in presentations to the American Academy of Ophthalmology and the Macula Society, in a scientific poster presented at the annual AAO meeting, and in the Ocular Oncology chapter in a prior volume of the YEAR BOOK OF OPHTHALMOLOGY. In fact, I objected to the expenditure of so much money by National Eye Institute on this study and to the recruitment of so many patients whose participation was unlikely to yield a clinically important differential result. My prior objections were based upon my own survival analyses of prospectively enrolled but non-randomly assigned patients treated by enucleation versus preenucleation radiation followed by enucleation. Another COMS trial, the medium size tumor trial comparing enucleation with I-125 plaque radiotherapy, completed its prespecified patient enrollment by the end of the year and is now closed to additional recruitment. One of the articles I reviewed for this year's YEAR BOOK (see abstracts and reviews that follow this introduction) was of my own group's study of long-term survival data on prospectively evaluated but retrospectively matched subgroups of patients treated by plaque radiotherapy versus enucleation for choroidal or ciliary body melanoma. We also found no clinically apparent or statistically significant survival differential between these subgroups. We expect that the COMS medium tumor trial results, when they are finally published (probably around 2004 or 2005), will also confirm these results and my prior predictions.

Several publications and presentations during 1998 concerned the role of intraocular fine-needle aspiration biopsy (FNAB) for the evaluation of suspected primary choroidal or ciliary body melanomas. My belief is that FNAB is a useful technique for confirming the cytologic character of many melanocytic choroidal lesions and that such a technique should be considered for borderline cases with both benign and malignant features. The biopsy of some form or another is routine prior to institution of treatment in virtually all types of suspected human cancers except skin lesions that are easily excised and intraocular tumors. My experience with more than 100 such biopsies revealed a high level of diagnostic accuracy and an acceptable level of local complications.

Several publications over the past 5 years have described the evaluation of chromosomal factors in uveal melanoma cells as possible prognostic indicators of future metastatic disease in patients with a primary choroidal or ciliary body melanoma. Various researchers have noted that uveal melanomas with deletion of a large portion of chromosome 3, duplication of chromosome 8, or both in a large proportion of tumor cells are associated with substantially greater posttreatment risk of metastasis and tumor-specific mortality than are uveal melanomas without such abnormalities. Such abnormalities can now be identified with relative ease by using a technique known as fluorescence in situ hybridization. During 1998, several groups reported the application of this technology or a similar methodology to microscopic tumor fragments obtained by means of intraocular FNAB. Evidence is accumulating that FNAB may provide a better distinction between true high-risk patients (those with substantially greater than a 50% chance of developing metastatic melanoma and dying from that condition within 3 to 5 years) and those with substantially lower risk than any combination of other currently evaluable clinical prognostic factors. If this is true, then ocular oncologists may be able to identify a high-risk group of uveal melanoma patients for whom clinical trials of adjuvant chemotherapy may be appropriate.

In the field of retinoblastoma, our understanding of the germinal factors associated with development of this disease continue to undergo refinement. A few years ago, it was generally believed that a loss or inactivation of both alleles at the q14 locus on chromosome 13 was all that was needed to make a cell at risk for developing retinoblastoma. New evidence reported in 1998 suggests that additional deletions or inactivations of other tumor suppressor genes may be a prerequisite for the development of retinoblastoma, at least in some affected families.

Treatment of choroidal and retinal hemangiomas continues to undergo refinement. Several years ago, circumscribed choroidal hemangiomas associated with macular subretinal fluid were treated almost exclusively by either intense generalized photocoagulation or multiple closely spaced argon laser burns to the surface of the lesion. The former treatment usually produced profound visual loss, unless the lesion was relatively small and located far from the central macula and optic disc. The latter treatment induced absorption of the exudative subretinal fluid in most cases but was frequently associated with subsequent reaccumulation of such fluid and ultimate visual loss. Most eyes with a diffuse choroidal hemangioma and visual loss due to progressive macular retinal degeneration, secondary exudative retinal detachment, or both had no effective form of treatment until recent years. Now, most central macular circumscribed choroidal hemangiomas are treated with plaque radiotherapy, and most extramacular or diffuse choroidal hemangiomas associated with serous retinal detachment and visual loss are treated with low-dose external beam radiation therapy. These treatments appear to preserve much more vision and prevent reaccumulation of subretinal fluid much more consistently than do the former treatments. Similarly, eyes with a large retinal capillary hemangioma (von Hippel tumor) were formerly treated in most cases by intense repeated transscleral cryotherapy or transscleral diathermy. Intractable tractional retinal detachment with irrevocable visual loss was a frequent complication. Eyes with such a tumor on the optic disc frequently developed a progressive retinal detachment, and no treatment was generally effective. In recent years, many tumors of the former type have been found to respond favorably to episcleral plaque radiotherapy, and many others in the latter category have been observed to regress satisfactorily following proton beam irradiation.

The past year has seen some revision of our understanding the spectrum of intraocular lymphoma. At least four specific types of intraocular lymphoma are now recognized. The first type is *metastatic lymphoma* from a solid visceral primary tumor that is usually in the abdomen or thorax. The intraocular lesions of this form of lymphoma resemble metastatic intraocular tumors from other primary cancer types. Most affected patients have a prior history or concurrent evidence of visceral lymphoma. In most cases, the affected patient has a single intraocular, uveal lesion in one eye. Intravitreal cells are uncommon. Such tumors frequently regress rapidly and completely in response to either systemic chemotherapy or ocular irradiation. The second type is *primary intraocular lymphoma* (formerly referred to as "ocular reticulum cell sarcoma"). The characteristic intraocular lesions in this form include diffuse intravitreal cells, yellow-white geographic subretinal pigment epithelial infiltrates, multifocal flat depigmentation or granularity of the extramacular retinal pigment epithelium, patches of retinal infiltration with hemorrhage simulating foci of cytomegalovirus retinitis, and retinal vascular occlusive disease. Almost all of these patients either have or subsequently develop independent foci of CNS lymphoma and die as a result of complications of that aspect of the disease. Almost all patients are affected bilaterally, although the intraocular involvement can be highly asymmetric and asynchronous in onset. Some patients show remarkable waxing and waning of intraocular lesions without treatment. Few of these patients have a history of visceral lymphoma in the thorax or abdomen or develop such tumors subsequent to detection of the intraocular disorders. The third type is a *primary uveal lymphocytic neoplasia or hyperplasia*. The clinical lesions in this form consist of localized nodules and diffuse thickening of the entire uveal tract. Diffuse intraocular lesions of this type are frequently associated with a solid epibulbar or retrobulbar orbital lymphoid infiltrate that frequently simulates extraocular extension of a diffuse, hypomelanotic uveal melanoma. Such lesions are almost always unilateral and unassociated with either visceral or CNS lymphoma. Pathologic study of the uveal infiltrates reveals lymphoid cells that can range from benign (lymphoid hyperplasia) to frankly malignant (lymphoma). The fourth type is *intraocular lymphocytic leukemia*. The typical intraocular features of this form include finely dispersed intravitreal white cells and occasional retinal infiltrates. Most patients with this form have elevated lymphocyte counts in the peripheral blood and other manifestations of lymphocytic leukemia. Most have a well-documented history of either chronic lymphocytosis or lymphocytic leukemia prior to the onset of the ocular abnormalities. Most patients I have encountered with this form of the disease ultimately developed bilateral ocular involvement.

The preceding paragraphs have outlined some of the advances that have occurred in clinical ocular oncology during the past year. What follows are abstracts of several pertinent papers on ocular oncology that were published in 1998 and my comments regarding those publications.

The Collaborative Ocular Melanoma Study (COMS) Randomized Trial of Pre-enucleation Radiation of Large Choroidal Melanoma. II: Initial Mortality Findings. COMS Report No. 10

The Collaborative Ocular Melanoma Study Group (COMS Coordinating Ctr, Baltimore, Md)

Am J Ophthalmol 125:779-796, 1998 10–1

Background.—Enucleation continues to be standard treatment for large primary choroidal melanoma. Although several studies of pre-enucleation radiotherapy (PERT) for choroidal melanoma have been reported, the small numbers of patients included and the absence of concurrent controls make it difficult to interpret the findings. Initial mortality findings from the Collaborative Ocular Melanoma Study (COMS), a randomized, multicenter, clinical trial of pre-enucleation radiation in patients with large choroidal melanoma, were reported.

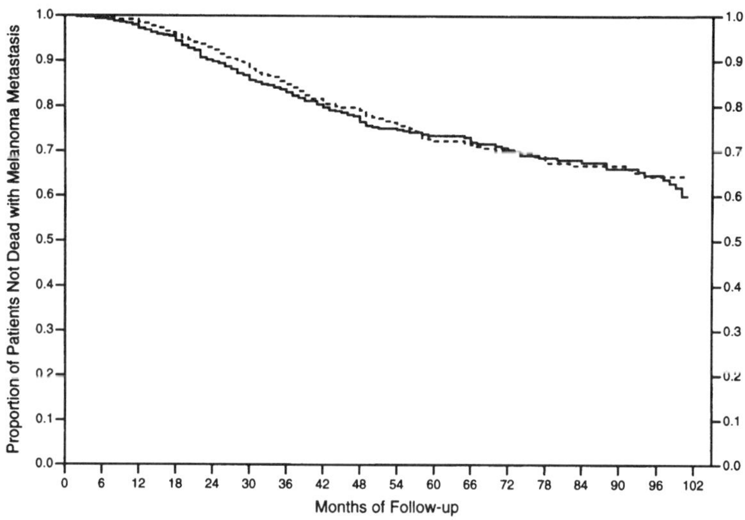

No. at Risk									
Std Enuc.	506	494	436	361	271	204	157	110	69
PERT	497	476	425	367	287	216	164	114	76

No. Censored									
Std Enuc.	-	8	28	41	67	45	41	40	38
PERT	-	11	14	28	56	56	45	44	33

FIGURE 2.—The proportion of patients who did not die with metastatic melanoma. *Sold line*, patients assigned to pre-enucleation radiation treatment (PERT); *dashed line*, patients assigned to enucleation alone. The numbers of patients at risk of death and numbers censored based on the date of enrollment are given at annual anniversaries of enrollment by random treatment assignment. Event is death with histologically confirmed metastatic melanoma. Patients who died of other causes were censored at time of death. (Reprinted by permission of the publisher from Hawkins BS, for the Collaborative Ocular Melanoma Study Group: The collaborative ocular melanoma study [COMS] randomized trial of pre-enucleation radiation of large choroidal melanoma. II: Initial mortality findings COMS report No. 10. *Am J Ophthalmol* 125:779-796. Copyright 1998 by Elsevier Science Inc.)

Methods.—Forty-three U.S. and Canadian centers enrolled 1,003 patients with confirmed diagnoses of choroidal melanoma. Five hundred six were assigned to enucleation only, and 497 were assigned to PERT.

Findings.—Five-year outcomes were known for 801 patients (80%). The estimated 5-year survival rates were 57% for patients undergoing enucleation only and 62% for those undergoing PERT. Age and longest basal diameter of the melanoma were the only baseline covariates analyzed that significantly affected prognosis. Compared with patients treated with enucleation alone, patients treated with PERT had a relative risk of death of 1.03 after adjustment for the baseline characteristics of patients, eyes, and tumors. Two hundred sixty-nine of 435 nonsurvivors classified by the Mortality Coding Committee had histologically confirmed melanoma metastases at the time of death. The estimated 5-year survival rates for this secondary outcome were 72% and 74% in the groups treated by enucleation only and by PERT, respectively (Fig 2).

Conclusions.—PERT appears to confer no survival benefit in patients with large choroidal melanomas. Although the statistical power of the current study may not have been great enough to detect smaller survival differences between the 2 treatment groups, a clinically meaningful difference in mortality from all causes or from metastatic melanoma is not likely.

▶ This study confirms previously reported evidence that adjuvant PERT (20 Gy in 5 fractions of 400 cGy) does not appreciably improve survival in patients with choroidal melanoma treated by enucleation. Because of the randomized nature of patient assignment, the reported result is likely to be a good estimate of the unbiased impact of PERT on survival in such patients. This article includes one sentence about orbital tumor recurrence after enucleation with versus without PERT, but it does not otherwise address this issue. Long-term follow-up of our nonrandomized comparison groups suggest that PERT substantially reduces the incidence of orbital recurrence after enucleation in patients with gross extrascleral extension of choroidal melanoma noted clinically before enucleation. We anticipate that longer-term follow-up of the patients in this study will confirm our findings about orbital tumor recurrence, just as this article confirms our previously reported finding of no significant benefit of PERT on overall patient survival.

J.J. Augsburger, M.D.

Histopathologic Characteristics of Uveal Melanomas in Eyes Enucleated From the Collaborative Ocular Melanoma Study COMS Report No. 6

Vine AK, for the Collaborative Ocular Melanoma Study Group (Kellogg Eye Ctr, Ann Arbor, Mich; et al)

J Am Optom Assoc 125:745-766, 1998 10–2

Background.—The histopathologic characteristics of uveal melanomas have been reported in large, retrospective studies. The current prospective study analyzed the main histologic findings in a series of enucleated globes from patients with choroidal melanoma enrolled in the Collaborative Ocular Melanoma Study (COMS).

Methods.—Three ophthalmic pathologists independently examined all 1,527 eyes with choroidal melanoma from patients in the COMS. Findings were recorded on a data form, and a composite of findings was developed.

Findings.—Five tumors in this series had been misdiagnosed (4 with metastatic adenocarcinoma and 1 with hemangioma). Of the confirmed choroidal and ciliochorodal melanomas, 86% were mixed cell; 9%, spindle cell; and 5%, epithelioid cell melanomas. Medium-sized tumors were found to be more posterior than large tumors. Local invasion was considerable, including rupture of Bruch's membrane in 87.7%, retinal invasion in 49.1%, tumor cells in the vitreous in 25.2%, vortex vein invasion in 8.9%, tumor cells in tumor vessels in 13.8%, and invasion into emissary canals in 55%. Overall, local invasion occurred in 81.1%, excluding rupture of Bruch's membrane. Scleral invasion was noted in 55.7% and extrascleral extension in 8.2%. Mitotic activity was significantly decreased in eyes that had been treated with pre-enucleation radiotherapy. The number of macrophages in the tumor increased with greater pigmentation and necrosis.

Conclusions.—These enucleated eyes with choroidal melanoma showed extensive local invasion. Pre-enucleation radiotherapy significantly decreased the number of mitotic figures. The presence of macrophages, level of pigmentation, and degree of necrosis were associated.

▶ This is the second published article dealing with diagnostic accuracy in the COMS. The COMS study group appears to be quite proud of the fact that only 5 of 1,527 tumors (0.3%) in the medium and large choroidal melanoma subgroups treated by enucleation proved on histopathologic study to have a nonmelanoma lesion. On the other hand, given the fact that patients with atypical or unusual tumors were likely to be excluded from the trial (see published exclusion criteria) and recognizing that the enrolling ophthalmologist's clinical diagnosis needed to be confirmed by readers in the fundus photography and ultrasonography reading centers for the patient to be enrolled, the real surprise is that the diagnostic error rate was so HIGH! If all atypical and problematic cases are excluded, the diagnostic accuracy in the remaining typical and noncontroversial cases should be extraordinarily good. Because of this, the reported result should *not* be interpreted as a valid estimate of the overall diagnostic accuracy of the clinicians who participated in this study.

J.J. Augsburger, M.D.

Long-term Survival in Choroidal and Ciliary Body Melanoma After Enucleation Versus Plaque Radiation Therapy

Augsburger JJ, Corrêa ZM, Freire J, et al (Wills Eye Hosp, Philadelphia; Allegheny Univ of the Health Sciences, Philadelphia)

Ophthalmology 105:1670-1678, 1998 10–3

Background.—Patients with a primary choroidal or ciliary body melanoma are treated by plaque radiation therapy or enucleation. Although short-term results are similar with both techniques, there is concern that long-term results (>10 years) may be poorer with plaque treatment because many eyes that were treated with plaque show histologically intact residual melanoma cells. This study followed a previous group of patients treated more than 15 years previously to compare the long-term results of both methods.

Methods.—The original study group consisted of 237 patients with primary choroidal or ciliary body melanoma who were treated between

May 1976 and June 1980 by ^{60}Co plaque radiation therapy (n = 97) or enucleation (n = 140). All patients had 5 year or more of follow-up (median, 16.3 years). Patients were identified whose baseline clinical variables were substantially different than those of patients in the other subgroup, such as those who were significantly younger and those who had more extensive retinal detachment. To reduce baseline susceptibility bias, these patients were eliminated and the remaining 121 patients formed the residual group (51 treated by enucleation, 71 treated by ^{60}Co plaque). These patients had a median follow-up of 16.7 years (^{60}Co plaque group) or 17.7 years (enucleation group). Outcomes of interest were the mortality rate attributable to melanoma and survival.

Findings.—In the original group, throughout follow-up, survival was substantially better in the ^{60}Co plaque group, but the difference was not statistically significant. Cumulative survival rates of the original patients at 15 years in the ^{60}Co plaque and enucleation groups were 59% and 51%, respectively. In the residual group, survival was only slightly better in the ^{60}Co plaque group (again, not significantly so), which indicates that baseline differences between the patients in the original group likely explained the improved survival in the ^{60}Co plaque group. This conclusion is supported by the residual group's relative rate ratio for treatment effect of 0.97. Cumulative survival rates of the residual patients at 15 years in the ^{60}Co plaque and enucleation groups were 56% and 52%, respectively. In neither the original group nor the residual group did the patients who underwent ^{60}Co plaque treatment experience a late decline in survival or have survival worse than that of patients treated by enucleation.

Conclusion.—Survival after ^{60}Co plaque radiation therapy is not significantly worse than that after enucleation, and it is not associated with a late downturn in survival.

▶ This is potentially a very important article. It summarizes the results of a large, nonrandomized but well-controlled clinical trial of enucleation versus plaque radiation therapy for primary choroidal and ciliary body melanomas. As such, it anticipates the results of the Collaborative Ocular Melanoma Study's medium tumor trial by at least 5 years. The results of this study suggest that that study's expensive and prolonged medium tumor trial will show no clinically important or statistically significant difference in survival rates of patients assigned to enucleation versus plaque.

J.J. Augsburger, M.D.

Radiotherapy of Choroidal Metastases

Rosset A, Zografos L, Coucke P, et al (Centre Hospitalier Universitaire Vaudois, Lausanne, Switzerland; Univ of Lausanne, Switzerland)

Radiother Oncol 46:263-268, 1998 10–4

Background.—The most common malignant intraocular neoplasm is the choroidal metastasis. The role of high energy external beam radiation therapy in the treatment of choroidal metastases was investigated.

Methods.—The records of 58 consecutive patients undergoing external beam radiation therapy between 1970 and 1993 were reviewed. Patient ages ranged from 40 to 81 years. Sixty-two percent of the patients had unilateral disease. Patients had a mean of 2 lesions per eye. Sixty-five percent of cases had retinal detachment. The primary tumor was breast carcinoma in 75% of the patients, lung carcinoma in 17%, and gastrointestinal, genitourinary, or unknown in the remainder. The median interval between the primary tumor and metastases was 55 months. Treatment consisted of megavoltage irradiation, with a median prescribed dose of 35.5 Gy. Treatment was fractionated. The standard dose per fraction was 2 Gy.

Findings.—The complete response rate at 3 months or more after treatment was 53%. Results were significantly better after doses exceeding 35.5 Gy. In 62% of the patients, visual acuity was improved or stabilized, the results again being significantly better at doses exceeding 35.5 Gy. Metastasis in the opposite eye developed in 3 of 26 patients with unilateral CM who had no elective contralateral irradiation, but in none of the 10 patients undergoing bilateral irradiation. There were 5 complications: 3 cataracts, 1 retinopathy, and 1 glaucoma.

Conclusions.—Radiation therapy is efficient and safe in the palliative treatment of choroidal metastases. This treatment helps to preserve vision in many affected eyes. Doses greater than 35.5 Gy provide significantly better tumor response and visual acuity. A lens-sparing technique should be used when possible.

► This article is a useful source of current information about treatment techniques and results of conventional external beam radiation therapy for choroidal metastases from various primary tumor sources. I agree completely with the general principles of dosage, fractionation, and portals for radiation delivery recommended by the authors. However, I have 2 major reservations about this work. First, I disagree strongly with the authors' decision to irradiate both eyes of 10 patients with unilateral choroidal metastasis. Most patients with choroidal metastasis have monocular disease at presentation and do not develop metastatic lesions in the fellow eye during subsequent follow-up. Treating both eyes of patients with monocular choroidal metastasis may prevent clinical lesions from developing in a few patients, but would probably subject the majority to unnecessary and potentially detrimental effects of irradiation. Second, the authors did not report on prior, concurrent, or subsequent chemotherapy in these patients. Because many chemotherapy regimens enhance both the effectiveness of treatment and the likelihood of treatment-related complications, the guidelines on dosage provided by the authors may be inappropriately high for patients on concurrent chemotherapy.

J.J. Augsburger, M.D.

Second Nonocular Tumors in Survivors of Bilateral Retinoblastoma: A Possible Age Effect on Radiation-related Risk

Abramson DH, Frank CM (New York Hosp—Cornell Med Ctr)

Ophthalmology 105:573-580, 1998 10–5

Background.—External beam radiation therapy, often used to treat bilateral retinoblastoma, can increase the risk of second primary neoplasms. The relationship between the incidence of second tumors and the age at which external beam radiation (EBR) was delivered was investigated in survivors of bilateral retinoblastoma.

Methods.—Eight hundred sixteen patients with bilateral retinoblastoma were included in the retrospective analysis. All survived for at least 1 year after diagnosis.

Findings.—Patients treated with EBR before the age of 12 months had a significantly reduced tumor-free survival rate. No significant difference

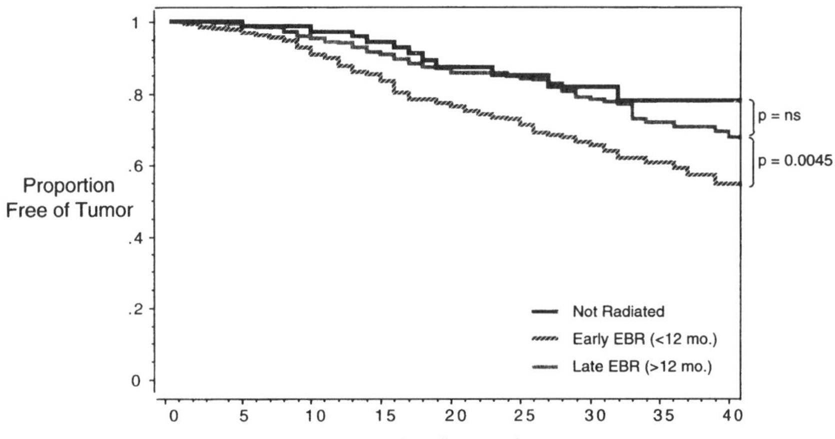

# no RT	78	68	43	22	12
# early RT	319	274	179	83	18
# late RT	320	273	211	130	43

FIGURE 2.—Effects of early, late, and no radiotherapy on tumor incidence. The subjects are divided into 3 groups: patients not treated with external beam radiation (EBR), patients treated with EBR before the age of 12 months, and patients treated with EBR after the age of 12 months, The end point of the Kaplan-Meier survival analysis is defined as the development of a second nonocular tumor. (Published courtesy of *Ophthalmology,* from Abramson DH, Frank CM: Second nonocular tumors in survivors of bilateral retinoblastoma: A possible age effect on radiation-related risk. *Ophthalmology* 105:573-580, 1998.)

was noted between EBR and non-EBR groups treated after 12 months of age. For tumors in the radiation field, tumor-free survival was significantly lower in the early EBR group than in the late EBR group, with no significant difference between the late EBR and no EBR groups. No significant differences occurred between groups for tumors outside the field of radiation. Significant differences that could be attributed to EBR use occurred only in tumors of the skull and face bones and in tumors of the soft tissue of the head (Fig 2).

Conclusions.—In the long term, radiotherapy increases the incidence and affects the distribution of second tumors in survivors of bilateral retinoblastoma. However, there is no increase in the risk of tumors outside the field of radiation among patients undergoing EBR. The risk of tumors in the field of radiation depends greatly on the age at which EBR is delivered and may be acceptably low in patients older than 12 months.

▶ The principal clinically recognized risk factor for development of nonretinoblastoma malignant tumors in the bones and soft tissues of the face and orbits in children with genetic retinoblastoma appears to be prior orbital EBR therapy for intraocular disease. This study revealed that the risk of nonretinoblastoma malignant tumors in the bones and soft tissues of the face and orbits was substantially higher in children who underwent EBR therapy for genetic retinoblastoma before the age of 12 months than in those who underwent such treatment after that age. A practical implication of this result is that clinicians should try to avoid EBR therapy (if it must be used at all) in children with genetic retinoblastoma until they reach the age of 12 months. Current treatment with chemotherapy followed by sequential aggressive local modalities makes this possible in the great majority of affected children.

J.J. Augsburger, M.D.

Management of Massive Orbital Involvement of Intraocular Retinoblastoma

Kiratli H, Bilgiç S, Özerdem U (Hacettepe Univ, Ankara, Turkey)
Ophthalmology 105:322-326, 1998 10–6

Background.—Retinoblastoma is the most common primary intraocular malignant tumor in children. Extraocular extension is the most significant risk factor predictive of death. One experience with the treatment of children with massive orbital involvement of intraocular retinoblastoma was presented.

Methods.—Sixteen patients seen between 1980 and 1995 were included in the retrospective review. Eight children had orbital involvement at the initial assessment, and 8 had orbital tumor after enucleation for intraocular retinoblastoma. Six children underwent orbital exenteration followed by external beam radiation therapy, 4,600 to 6,000 cGy in fractionated doses, and chemotherapy. Five were given chemotherapy alone. Three children were treated by exenteration and chemotherapy, and 2 underwent radiation therapy and chemotherapy.

Outcomes.—At a median 22-month follow-up, all treatments had produced satisfactory local and systemic tumor regression. Two children survived for more than 10 years. However, systemic metastases developed in 2 patients in the exenteration, chemotherapy, and radiotherapy group and in 1 patient in the chemotherapy group, all of whom died. One child was lost to follow up.

Conclusions.—The children in this series had highly individualized, aggressive therapy, including radical surgery, chemotherapy, and external beam radiotherapy. This approach enabled most patients to have longer survival and disease-free intervals than expected.

► Massive orbital involvement in retinoblastoma is, fortunately, rather rare today in most western ocular oncology centers. This report from Turkey on 16 patients with massive orbital retinoblastoma therefore represents a major experience. It is heartening to learn that a substantial proportion (81.3%) of these children were saved by a combination of chemotherapy and aggressive local treatment. All three of the children who died of retinoblastoma in this series succumbed within 9 months or less after diagnosis of massive orbital involvement and start of treatment. In contrast, all surviving patients had been observed for longer than 9 months, and 10 of the 13 surviving children had been followed up for more than 18 months. The results reported by Kiratli et al. are in marked contrast to the results presented by Ellsworth[1] in 1974; of 51 children with massive orbital retinoblastoma, only 5 (9.8%) survived.

J.J. Augsburger, M.D.

Reference

1. Ellsworth RM: Orbital retinoblastoma. *Trans Am Ophthalmol Soc* 72:79-86, 1974.

Cataract Surgery and Intraocular Lens Implantation in Patients With Retinoblastoma

Portellos M, Buckley EG (Duke Univ, Durham, NC)
Arch Ophthalmol 116:449-452, 1998 10–7

Background.—The authors' standard treatment for cataract removal in children consists of extracapsular cataract extraction, posterior chamber intraocular lens (IOL) implantation, pars plana posterior capsulotomy, and pars plana anterior vitrectomy. Their experience with IOL implantation in children with retinoblastoma and radiation-induced cataracts was presented.

Methods.—Eight patients with 11 affected eyes were treated. Patient age ranged from 1.5 to 8 years at the time of surgery for radiation-induced cataract. Follow-up ranged from 6 to 39 months. Nine eyes underwent extracapsular cataract extraction, posterior chamber IOL implantation, pars plana posterior capsulotomy, and pars plana anterior vitrectomy. Two eyes underwent secondary IOL placement.

Outcomes.—Visual acuities in all eyes treated with primary IOL implantation were equal to or better than the best ever recorded before development, of the cataract. No postoperative complications occurred. Postoperative inflammation was minimal in all eyes. Although the 2 eyes undergoing secondary IOL implantation achieved their best-corrected aphakic visual acuities, both had a prolonged course of postoperative inflammation.

Conclusions.—In the short term, IOL placement in eyes with regressed retinoblastoma appears to be a safe, acceptable method for rehabilitating vision. The long-term effects of such treatment have yet to be determined.

► The benefit-risk ratio of cataract surgery in typical survivors of retinoblastoma who were treated successfully with external beam radiation therapy (EBRT) in childhood is uncertain. In my opinion, the patients described in this report are not typical. Only 1 of the 11 affected eyes had advanced intraocular tumor (RE group IV or V) at the time of initial treatment. Only 6 of the 11 eyes contained macular tumors. Seven of the 8 described patients had unilateral retinoblastoma. Only 3 children (of the 4 with bilateral retinoblastoma) received EBRT to both eyes. The typical child treated with EBRT in the past was a child with bilateral retinoblastoma that was too advanced for local obliterative treatments. Most children of this type underwent either bilateral EBRT or enucleation of the worse eye and EBRT for the better one. Children with advanced monocular disease were usually treated with enucleation, and those with limited monocular disease were usually treated with local obliterative treatments that were unlikely to cause cataract. A large proportion of children with genetic retinoblastoma have macular involvement. Although the results reported in this article appear quite favorable, they should not be interpreted as representative of the anticipated outcome in typical survivors of retinoblastoma. Cataract surgery with IOL implantation in a child with only one remaining eye or with destroyed maculas poses special risks and concerns that the ophthalmic surgeon must take into account.

J.J. Augsburger, M.D.

Ruthenium-106 Brachytherapy for Peripheral Retinal Capillary Hemangioma

Kreusel KM, Bornfeld N, Lommatzsch A, et al (Freie Universität Berlin; Universitäts-Augenklinik, Essen, Germany)

Ophthalmology 105:1386-1392, 1998 10–8

Background.—Small peripheral retinal capillary hemangiomas are typically successfully managed by direct light or laser coagulation. For larger hemangiomas, the treatment is usually laser coagulation or cryocoagulation. However, neither treatment is completely effective in destroying large tumors, and both methods can cause retinal detachment. These authors evaluated the use of ^{106}Ru brachytherapy in patients with large peripheral retinal capillary hemangiomas.

Methods.—Between 1986 and 1996, 25 eyes in 24 patients (8 men and 16 women; mean age, 25 years) were treated by ^{106}Ru plaque brachytherapy because of a large peripheral retinal capillary hemangioma. Patients were evaluated at regular intervals to determine outcomes, including visual acuity, tumor regression after therapy, any retinal detachment, and retinal status.

Findings.—Preoperatively, mean visual acuity was 20/60. Mean hemangioma diameter was 3.8 mm (range, 1.5-7.8 mm), which corresponded to about 2 average disc diameters. In 14 eyes, the retina was attached, but 8 eyes had an exudative detachment and 3 had a traction detachment. Patients with exudative detachment had significantly worse visual acuity (mean, 20/200) and significantly larger hemangiomas (mean diameter, 5.2 mm), but otherwise there were no significant preoperative differences. A single brachytherapy treatment (over a period of 3 to 7 days) destroyed 23 to the 25 tumors by 5 to 14 months after therapy. Two patients required repeat brachytherapy, 1 with a very large tumor (7.8 mm) who was lost to follow-up and 1 whose tumor (4.5 mm) did not respond to an initial dose of 300 Gy. In the latter patient, a second dose of 500 Gy destroyed the hemangioma, but the patient experienced irradiation retinopathy.

Overall, 16 of 25 eyes (64%) had a favorable response to therapy. However, 9 eyes (36%) had an unfavorable outcome, including severe worsening of visual acuity, the development or persistence of an exudative retinal detachment, and the recurrence of a traction retinal detachment. Outcomes were significantly more likely to be favorable for patients whose preoperative hemangioma was smaller (2.8 vs 5.4 mm in patients with an unfavorable outcome) and whose retina was attached preoperatively (80% vs 22%). Brachytherapy was successful in destroying hemangiomas of up to 5.0 mm in patients who did not have exudative retinal detachment preoperatively.

Conclusion.—^{106}Ru brachytherapy can safely and effectively destroy large peripheral capillary retinal hemangiomas. Results are likely to be better for patients whose tumor is 5 mm or less in diameter (that is, less than 2.5 average diameter discs) and who have no preoperative exudative retinal detachment. Outcomes are worse for patients who have larger hemangiomas, primarily because these are associated with retinal detachment.

▶ The results of this descriptive analysis of a series of patients with a solitary peripheral retinal capillary hemangioma treated by ^{106}Ru plaque radiotherapy indicate that this treatment is frequently effective in destroying the hemangioma and preserving or preventing further tumor-related visual loss in the affected eye. Retinal surgeons should be aware of this alternative to intense, repeated transscleral cryotherapy (the most commonly used alternative treatment in recent years) and other less common therapeutic options for these retinal vascular tumors.

J.J. Augsburger, M.D.

11 Pathology

Recent Advances in the Corneal Dystrophies

by Ralph C. Eagle, Jr., M.D.

In classic ophthalmic usage, the term *dystrophy* usually denotes an inherited, relatively symmetric bilateral disease that is unassociated with vascularization or inflammation in its early stages. Dystrophies, usually not evident at birth, become clinically evident later in life. The etimological derivation of the word dystrophy is outdated because it refers to poor nutrition. The corneal dystrophies are now known to be caused by mutations in genes encoding enzymes or structural proteins. During the last decade, advances in molecular genetics have disclosed new important information about these rare, fascinating disorders. In some instances, the specific genetic mutations and biochemical abnormalities responsible for corneal opacification and visual loss have been identified.

The corneal dystrophies have been classified on the basis of their clinical manifestations and the results of routine light microscopic, histochemical, and electron microscopic studies. Clinically, they are grouped topographically according to the primary locus of involvement as epithelial, Bowman's layer, stromal, and endothelial dystrophies. The primary epithelial dystrophies include Meesman's dystrophy, the anterior basement membrane or map-dot and fingerprint dystrophy, and a heritable subepithelial form of amyloidosis called *gelatinous droplike dystrophy* or familial subepithelial corneal amyloidosis.

The dystrophies of Bowman's layer include Reis-Bückler's dystrophy (CDB-I) and the honeycomb dystrophy of Thiel-Behnke (CDB-II). Fuchs' dystrophy, congenital hereditary endothelial dystrophy, and the posterior polymorphous dystrophy of Schlichting are the major dystrophies that affect the posterior cornea.

The classic stromal dystrophies include autosomal dominantly inherited granular dystrophy and lattice dystrophy type I and macular dystrophy, which is autosomal recessively inherited.

Macular corneal dystrophy usually necessitates early penetrating keratoplasty because it is marked by diffuse stromal haze that involves the entire cornea and extends peripherally to the limbus. The term *macular* refers to denser grayish opacities with indistinct borders that are found in the superficial stroma and begin axially. Histochemical stains disclose positive staining for acid mucopolysaccharide within keratocytes and endothelial cells. The macules correspond to larger extracellular deposits.

In granular dystrophy, slit lamp examination shows multiple white crumb- or ring-shaped opacities in the central cornea. Visual acuity often is excellent because clear corneal stroma separates the opacities. The granular deposits are more eosinophilic and less PAS-positive than the surrounding normal stroma, and they exhibit intense acid fuchsinophilia (red staining) with Masson trichrome.

Lattice corneal dystrophy type I is a localized corneal amyloidosis. The amyloid deposits form a characteristic lattice-work of branching relucent lines in the corneal stroma. Histopathology reveals smudgy round or oval deposits of eosinophilic material in the stroma, which stain positively with amyloid stains such as Congo red and have a characteristic apple-green birefringence and dichroism with polarization microscopy.

A dystrophy that combines features of both lattice and granular dystrophies was described in 1988. The dystrophy was called *Avellino dystrophy* because all of the initial discovered patients traced their ancestry to the Italian province of Avellino.[1,2] A German kindred subsequently was identified, and a review of six unrelated families disclosed that there was significant phenotypic variation between families.[3]

Genetic linkage studies reported in 1994 initially suggested that the genes for lattice corneal dystrophy type I, granular dystrophy, and Avellino dystrophy were linked to the long arm of chromosome 5.[4] Histopathologic studies disclosed significant histologic overlap between the three dystrophies, strongly suggesting that they might be caused by mutations within the same gene.[5]

In 1997, Munier and coworkers[6] reported that these three corneal dystrophies that had been linked to chromosome 5q, and Reis-Bückler's dystrophy as well, were caused by allelic mutations in a gene called the *βig-h3 gene*. The βig-h3 or *transforming growth factor beta induced gene-h3* was identified when a human lung adenocarcinoma cell line was treated with TGF-beta.[7] The protein product of the *βig-h3* gene has been called *kerato-epithelin* because the gene is normally expressed in the corneal epithelium. The latter name is somewhat inappropriate, however, because the *βig-h3* gene is expressed in other tissues such as the kidney[8] and arteries.[9] The function of βig-h3 protein currently is uncertain, although it is known to bind to integrins and may be linked to type VI collagen.[7,10] Munier's findings have been confirmed by other workers, and additional mutations have been identified.[11-13] Increased amounts of βig-h3 protein have been demonstrated by electrophoresis and immunoelectron microscopy in dystrophic corneas.[14-16]

The dystrophies that are linked to *βig-h3* appear to be associated with specific missense mutations in the gene. Missense mutations cause a single amino acid substitution in the gene's protein product. All of the mutations that Munier reported affect codons that normally code for arginine. In granular and Reis-Bückler's dystrophies, the normal arginine at position 555 in the protein was replaced by tryptophan and glutamine, respectively. In lattice dystrophy type I and Avellino dystrophy the arginine normally found at position 124 was replaced by cysteine and histidine, respectively. Affected patients usually are heterozygous for the *βig-h3* mutations. However, a homozygous patient who has particular severe granular corneal dystrophy has been reported.[17]

These amino acid substitutions presumably affect the conformation and physicochemical properties of the βig-h3 protein, which leads to different patterns of aggregation or precipitation in the stroma. The mutations at position 124 in lattice type I and Avellino dystrophies presumably allow parts of the molecule that have a pleated sheat configuration to aggregate as filaments of amyloid. In contrast, the mutations at position 555 in patients who have granular and Reis-Bückler's dystrophy lead to the formation of osmiophilic protein crystalloids. The source of the mutant kerato-epithelin is probably the corneal epithelium, but *βig-h3* also is found in the serum, and that source cannot be totally excluded.

Both Thiel-Behnke (CDB II) and Reis-Bückler's (CDB I) dystrophies share many clinical and histopathologic features. Osmiophilic crystalloids that resemble those found in granular corneal dystrophy tinctorially (though smaller,) accumulate beneath the epithelium in cases of Reis-Bückler's dystrophy. The deposits are thought to interfere with epithelial adhesion and initiate recurrent episodes of desquamation and scarring that result in a thick multilaminar pannus composed of alternating layers of mutant keratoepithelin and collagen. The process destroys Bowman's layer and causes a characteristic irregular saw-toothed configuration of the epithelium. Although Thiel-Behnke dystrophy has linked to chromosome 10, an immunoelectron microscopic study by Streeten et al., has shown that the deposits in both Thiel-Behnke (CDB II) and Reis-Bückler's (CDB I) are immunoreactive for βig-h3 protein.[16,18] The mutant keratoepithelin in Thiel-Behnke forms "curly filaments" instead of crystalloids. The reader should note that it is now believed that patients previously identified as having Reis-Bückler's dystrophy in the United States actually had Thiel-Behnke dystrophy. The patients reported by Reis and Bückler have a superficial variant of granular dystrophy.[19] Another *βig-h3* mutation (Pro501Thr) has been found in patients with lattice corneal dystrophy type III A.[11] It is possible that other allelic mutations in *βig-h3* might be found in other dystrophies.

Important new information about several other dystrophies has been reported recently. Meesman's epithelial dystrophy has been shown to be related to mutations in types of cytokeratins that are expressed only in the cornea (cornea-specific keratin K3 or K12).[20] These mutations occur in the highly conserved helix boundary motifs of the keratin molecule and severely compromise cytoskeletal function, causing fragility of the epithelium. Meesman's dystrophy is nearly a medical curiosity because it has relatively little effect on vision. Both the epithelium and its basement membrane are thickened. The epithelium contains small microcystoid spaces that migrate towards the surface and pool fluorescein dye. The cytoplasm of some of the epithelial cells has a smudgy hyalinized appearance when viewed with light microscopy and contains what has been termed *peculiar substance* when viewed with electron microscopy. Recent studies suggest that the latter is comprised of abnormal extracellular matrix material.[21]

Amyloid deposits composed of proteins totally unrelated to *βig-h3* occur in other corneal dystrophies. Patients with lattice dystrophy type II (Meretoja's syndrome) have nonocular findings such as cranial nerve palsies, dry itchy skin, blepharochalasis and typical mask-like "hound dog" facies with protruding lips, as well as lattice-like deposits in the stroma.[22-24] The deposits of corneal amyloid occur later but are indistinguishable from those found in lattice dystrophy type I. They are composed of a mutant form of gelsolin, an enzyme that cleaves actin filaments and is involved in the isolation of actin gels.[25,26] Most cases are caused by a single amino acid substitution, asparagine for aspartic acid at position 15.[27]

Gelatinous droplike dystrophy (familial subepithelial corneal amyloidosis) is a rare autosomal recessively inherited dystrophy marked by the deposition of globular mounds of amyloid beneath the corneal epithelium. Although it has been reported that the amyloid deposits are composed of the antimicrobial protein lactoferrin, abnormalities in the lactoferrin gene are not present affected kindreds, and the disease has been linked to the short arm of chromosome 1.[28] The lactoferrin gene is located on chromosome 3.[29]

Macular corneal dystrophy is not as well characterized, but appears to be caused by the faulty sulfation of keratan sulfate, an important proteoglycan in the corneal stroma. Although the disorder has been termed a *localized corneal mucopolysaccharidosis*, the corneal stroma in macular dystrophy is not massively thickened as it is in the systemic mucopolysaccharidoses such as Hurler's, Scheie's, and Maroteaux-Lamy syndromes, which have corneal clouding. Defects in catabolic enzymes lead to the massive storage of normal mucopolysaccharides in the latter disorders. The material disclosed by the mucin stains alcian blue and colloidal iron in patients with macular corneal dystrophy is an abnormal nonsulfated form of keratan sulfate. The absence of sulfation interferes with stromal hydration and the proper spacing of collagen fibers, which degrades the optical properties of the cornea. The poorly hydrated stroma in macular corneal dystrophy is typically thinner than normal.[30]

Some patients who have macular corneal dystrophy (type I) have undetectable levels of keratan sulfate in their serum and cartilage.[31,32] Macular corneal dystrophy type I therefore appears to be the corneal manifestation of a systemic disease that presumably is innocuous elsewhere.[33] Macular dystrophy type I and II can coexist in the same family and both appear to be caused by allelic mutations in a single gene on chromosome 16.[34,35]

In summary, recent advances in molecular biology and genetics have increased our understanding of the corneal dystrophies. It now has been established that a variety of dystrophies that have dissimilar clinical and pathologic findings are actually caused by allelic mutations in a single gene. Furthermore, mutations in totally separate genes can cause dystrophies with similar phenotypes. Some dystrophies (e.g., Meesman's) are caused by mutations in genes that are expressed solely in the cornea. Other dystrophies (e.g., macular type I) appear to be the corneal manifestation of an otherwise innocuous systemic disease.

The *βig-h3* gene is expressed elsewhere in the body. It is unclear whether the osmiophilic crystalloids of granular dystrophy or the foci of amyloid found in lattice dystrophy can or do occur elsewhere in the body in patients with these dystrophies. To my knowledge, no one has ever specifically sought such deposits in extraocular tissues, and they could be readily overlooked. The availability of postmortem tissue from a patient with one of the *βig-h3* dystrophies could answer this interesting question.

References

1. Folberg R, Alfonso E, Croxatto JO, et al: Clinically atypical granular corneal dystrophy with pathologic features of lattice-like amyloid deposits: A study of these families. *Ophthalmology* 95:46-51, 1988.
2. Holland EJ, Daya SM, Stone EM, et al: Avellino corneal dystrophy: Clinical manifestations and natural history. *Ophthalmology* 99:1564-1568, 1992.
3. Rosenwasser GO, Sucheski BM, Rosa N, et al: Phenotypic variation in combined granular-lattice (Avellino) corneal dystrophy [see comments]. *Arch Ophthalmol* 111:1546-1552, 1993.
4. Stone EM, Mathers WD, Rosenwasser GO, et al: Three autosomal dominant corneal dystrophies map to chromosome 5q. *Nat Genet* 6:47-51, 1994.
5. Folberg R, Stone EM, Sheffield VC, et al: The relationship between granular, lattice type 1, and Avellino corneal dystrophies: A histopathologic study. *Arch Ophthalmol* 112:1080-1085, 1994.
6. Munier FL, Korvatska E, Djemai A, et al: Kerato-epithelin mutations in four 5q31-linked corneal dystrophies [see comments]. *Nat Genet* 15:247-251, 1997.
7. Skonier J, Neubauer M, Madisen L, et al: cDNA cloning and sequence analysis of beta ig-h3, a novel gene induced in a human adenocarcinoma cell line after treatment with transforming growth factor-beta. *DNA Cell Biol* 11:511-522, 1992.
8. Gilbert RE, Wilkinson-Berka JL, Johnson DW, et al: Renal expression of transforming growth factor-beta inducible gene-h3 (beta ig-h3) in normal and diabetic rats [see comments]. *Kidney Int* 54:1052-1062, 1998.
9. O'Brien ER, Bennett KL, Garvin MR, et al: Beta ig-h3, a transforming growth factor-beta-inducible gene, is overexpressed in atherosclerotic and restenotic human vascular lesions. *Arterioscler Thromb Vasc Biol* 16:576-584, 1996.
10. Hirano K, Klintworth GK, Zhan Q, et al: Beta ig-h3 is synthesized by corneal epithelium and perhaps endothelium in Fuchs' dystrophic corneas. *Curr Eye Res* 15:965-972, 1996.
11. Fujiki K, Hotta Y, Nakayasu K, et al: A new L527R mutation of the betaIGH3 gene in patients with lattice corneal dystrophy with deep stromal opacities. *Hum Genet* 103:286-289, 1998.
12. Korvatska E, Munier FL, Djemai A, et al: Mutation hot spots in 5q31-linked corneal dystrophies. *Am J Hum Genet* 62:320-324, 1998.
13. Meins M, Kohlhaas M, Richard G, et al: Type I lattice corneal dystrophy: Clinical and molecular genetic study of a large family [German]. *Klin Monatsbl Augenheilkd* 212:154-158, 1998.
14. Takacs L, Boross P, Tozser J, et al: Transforming growth factor-beta induced protein, betaIG-H3, is present in degraded form and altered localization in lattice corneal dystrophy type I. *Exp Eye Res* 66:739-745, 1998.
15. Klintworth GK, Valnickova Z, Enghild JJ: Accumulation of beta ig-h3 gene product in corneas with granular dystrophy. *Am J Pathol* 152:743-748, 1998.
16. Streeten BW YQ, Klintworth GK, Eagle RC Jr, et al: Immunolocalization of big-h3 Protein in 5q31-Linked Corneal Dystrophies and Normal Corneas. *Arch Ophthalmol* 117:67-75, 1999.

17. Fujiki K, Hotta Y, Nakayasu K, et al: Homozygotic patient with beta ig-h3 gene mutation in granular dystrophy. *Cornea* 17:288-292, 1998.
18. Yee RW, Sullivan LS, Lai HT, et al: Linkage mapping of Thiel-Behnke corneal dystrophy (CDB2) to chromosome 10q23-q24. *Genomics* 46:152-154, 1997.
19. Moller HU: Granular corneal dystrophy Groenouw type I (GrI) and Reis-Bucklers' corneal dystrophy (R-B): One entity? *Acta Ophthalmol (Scand)* 67:678-684, 1989.
20. Irvine AD, Corden LD, Swensson O, et al: Mutations in cornea-specific keratin K3 or K12 genes cause Meesmann's corneal dystrophy. *Nat Genet* 16:184-187, 1997.
21. Tremblay M, Dube I: Meesmann's corneal dystrophy: Ultrastructural features. *Can J Ophthalmol* 17:24-28, 1982.
22. Meretoja J: Familial systemic paramyloidosis with lattice dystrophy of the cornea, progressive cranial neuropathy, skin changes and various internal symptoms: A previously unrecognized heritable syndrome. *Ann Clin Res* 1:314-324, 1969.
23. Purcell JJ Jr, Rodrigues M, Chishti MI, et al: Lattice corneal dystrophy associated with familial systemic amyloidosis (Meretoja's syndrome). *Ophthalmology* 90:1512-1517, 1983.
24. Starck T, Kenyon KR, Hanninen LA, et al: Clinical and histopathologic studies of two families with lattice corneal dystrophy and familial systemic amyloidosis (Meretoja syndrome). *Ophthalmology* 98:1197-1206, 1991.
25. Gorevic PD, Munoz PC, Gorgone G, et al: Amyloidosis due to a mutation of the gelsolin gene in an American family with lattice corneal dystrophy type II [see comments]. *N Engl J Med* 325:1780-1785, 1991.
26. Kivela T, Tarkkanen A, Frangione B, et al: Ocular amyloid deposition in familial amyloidosis, Finnish: An analysis of native and variant gelsolin in Meretoja's syndrome. *Invest Ophthalmol Vis Sci* 35:3759-3769, 1994.
27. Haltia M, Levy E, Meretoja J, et al: Gelsolin gene mutation—at codon 187—in familial amyloidosis, Finnish: DNA-diagnostic assay. *Am J Med Genet* 42:357-359, 1992.
28. Tsujikawa M, Kurahashi H, Tanaka T, et al: Homozygosity mapping of a gene responsible for gelatinous drop-like corneal dystrophy to chromosome 1p. *Am J Hum Genet* 63:1073-1077, 1998.
29. Klintworth GK, Sommer JR, Obrian G, et al: Familial subepithelial corneal amyloidosis (gelatinous drop-like corneal dystrophy): Exclusion of linkage to lactoferrin gene. *Mol Vis* 4:31, 1998.
30. Donnenfeld ED, Cohen EJ, Ingraham HJ, et al: Corneal thinning in macular corneal dystrophy. *Am J Ophthalmol* 101:112-113, 1986.
31. Klintworth GK, Meyer R, Dennis R, et al: Macular corneal dystrophy: Lack of keratan sulfate in serum and cornea. *Ophthalmic Paediatr Genet* 7:139-143, 1986.
32. Thonar EJ, Meyer RF, Dennis RF, et al: Absence of normal keratan sulfate in the blood of patients with macular corneal dystrophy. *Am J Ophthalmol* 102:561-569, 1986.
33. Edward DP, Thonar EJ, Srinivasan M, et al: Macular dystrophy of the cornea: A systemic disorder of keratan sulfate metabolism. *Ophthalmology* 97:1194-1200, 1990.
34. Vance JM, Jonasson F, Lennon F, et al: Linkage of a gene for macular corneal dystrophy to chromosome 16. *Am J Hum Genet* 58:757-762, 1996.
35. Jonasson F, Oshima E, Thonar EJ, et al: Macular corneal dystrophy in Iceland: A clinical, genealogic, and immunohistochemical study of 28 patients. *Ophthalmology* 103:1111-1117, 1996.

Therapy With a Purified Plasminogen Concentrate in an Infant With Ligneous Conjunctivitis and Homozygous Plasminogen Deficiency

Schott D, Dempfle C-E, Beck P, et al (Univ of Heidelberg, Mannheim, Germany; Hyland-Immuno Division of Baxter Healthcare, Heidelberg, Germany; Hyland-Immuno Division of Baxter Healthcare, Vienna; et al)

N Engl J Med 339:1679-1686, 1998 11–1

Introduction.—Ligneous conjunctivitis is a rare acute or chronic recurrent conjunctivitis characterized by conjunctival membranes that acquire a woodlike consistency from deposits of fibrin. It has been linked to severe plasminogen deficiency. This disease may be caused by a genetic defect with an autosomal recessive pattern of inheritance. Described is a patient with homozygous plasminogen deficiency in whom ligneous conjunctivitis developed soon after birth.

Case Report.—Newborn, second son of parents who were first cousins, had bilateral inflammation of the palpebral portion of the conjunctiva, with hypersecretion and formation of pseudomembranes detected 3 days after birth. At 2 weeks, a thick, yellowish white, fibrous, woody pseudomembranous layer of conjunctival proliferation developed and spread from the inner side of the upper and lower eyelids and completely closed both eyes (Fig 1). The pseudomembranes were removed several times and regrew rapidly each time. Family studies revealed that the patient's parents and older brother had diminished levels of plasminogen antigen and activity, indicating heterozygous plasminogen deficiency. When the patient was 6 months old, a diagnosis of homozygous plasminogen deficiency was proposed. He was treated with continuous intravenous infusion of 1,000 caseinolytic units of lys-plasminogen per 24 hours. The patient's plasminogen level rose within 3 hours after treatment, and the level approached normal values within 24 hours. Within 3 days of the start of therapy, the patient's symptoms were markedly improved and he subsequently became normal. At around 2 weeks, the conjunctival pseudomembranes softened and were easily removed. Specimens were subjected to histologic and genetic examination. Hematoxylin-eosin staining of parts of the conjunctival pseudomembranes showed fibrin-rich granulation tissue with a mixed neutrophil-rich perivascular infiltrate. Staining with an antibody specific for fibrin and fibrinogen showed diffuse fibrin deposits. Direct sequencing of fragments of exon 11 revealed a homozygous point mutation at position 1511 (G→T), leading to a stop codon (TAA) at position 460 (Glu460Stop). The catalytic domain of plasmin is eradicated by this mutation. The healthy brother and the healthy parents of this patient were heterozygous for this mutation.

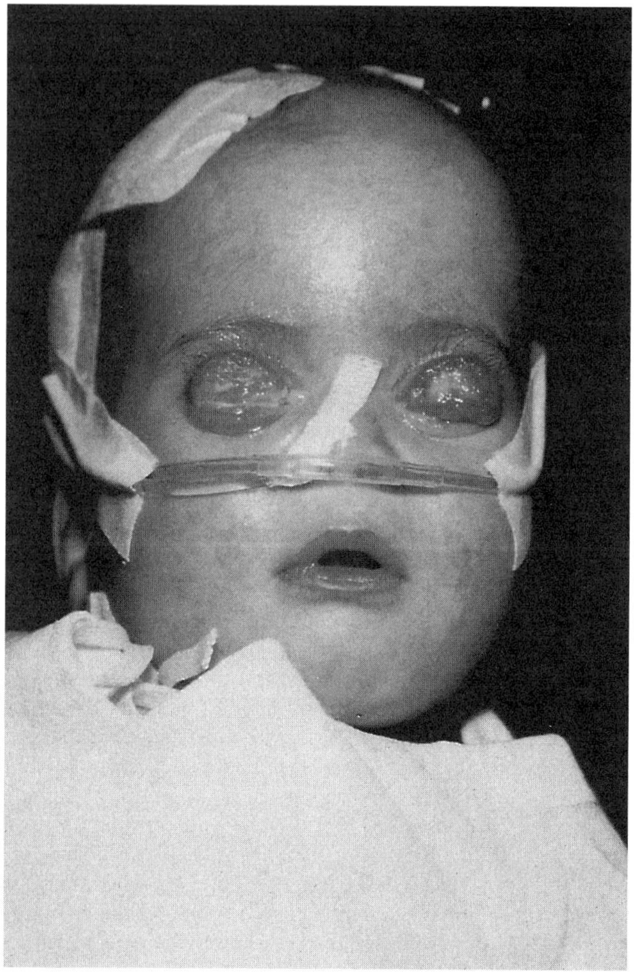

FIGURE 1.—Initial appearance of a child with homozygous plasminogen deficiency, showing the typical features of ligneous conjunctivitis. (Reprinted by permission of *The New England Journal of Medicine*, from Schott D, Dempfle C-E, Beck P: Therapy with a purified plasminogen concentrate in an infant with ligneous plasminogen deficiency. *N Engl J Med* 339:1679-1686. Copyright 1998, Massachusetts Medical Society. All rights reserved.)

Conclusion.—Absence of plasmin activity caused formation of the fibrin-rich viscous or membranous material usually seen in patients with ligneous conjunctivitis. It is notable that no intravascular thromboembolic episodes occur in patients with ligneous conjunctivitis.

▶ The treatment of ligneous conjunctivitis generally has been unsatisfactory. In the past, recommended therapy has included surgery, antivirals, anti-inflammatory agents such as steroids and cyclosporine, and hyaluronidase eye drops. The latter were recommended in the mistaken belief that mucopolysaccharides such as hyaluronic acid were a major constituent of the dense woody pseudomembranes that characterize the disease. In 1986, I reported that fibrin actually was the major constituent of ligneous conjunctivitis.

This study provides additional evidence that ligneous conjunctivitis is an autosomal recessively inherited disease caused by homozygous mutations in the gene for plasminogen, the precursor of the enzyme plasmin that breaks down fibrin. The child reported here presented shortly after birth with extensive bilateral involvement. His ocular disease responded remarkably to periodic intravenous infusions of purified plasminogen concentrate.

R.C. Eagle, Jr., M.D.

Histopathologic Characteristics of Uveal Melanomas in Eyes Enucleated From the Collaborative Ocular Melanoma Study: COMS Report No. 6

Albert DM, for the Collaborative Ocular Melanoma Study Group (Univ of Wisconsin, Madison; et al)

Am J Ophthalmol 125:745-766, 1998 11–2

Introduction.—The Collaborative Ocular Melanoma Study, is made up of 2 multicenter, randomized, controlled clinical trials for determining the efficacy of radiotherapy in prolonging the survival of patients with choroidal melanoma. In a series of enucleated globes from the Collaborative Ocular Melanoma Study (COMS), the principal histologic findings of patients with choroidal melanoma were described.

Methods.—Three ophthalmic pathologists independently examined 1,532 eyes enucleated in the COMS. The findings were recorded. After adjudication, a composite of findings was obtained.

Results.—In 99.7% of 1,532 eyes examined, the diagnosis was choroidal melanoma. Hemangioma (1) and metastatic adenocarcinoma (4) were the misdiagnoses. There were mixed cell (86%), spindle cell (9%), and epithelioid cell (5%) types seen (Table 1). Large tumors were located less posteriorly than medium tumors. Considerable local invasion was seen, with 87.7% having rupture of Bruch's membrane, 49.1% having invasion of the retina, 25.2% having tumor cells in the vitreous, 8.9% having

TABLE 1.—Cell Type by Tumor Size Group

Tumor Size	Spindle	No. (%) Cell Type Mixed	Epithelioid	Total No.
Medium	66 (12.3)	454 (84.7)	16 (3.0)	536
Large*	71 (7.2)	858 (86.7)	61 (6.1)	990
Total	137 (9.0)	1,312 (86.0)	77 (5.0)	1,526

*One tumor in the large group was completely necrotic and could not be graded.

vortex vein invasion, 13.8% having invasion of tumor vessels by tumor cells, and 55% having invasion into emissary canals. Local invasion was found in 81.1% of eyes, excluding rupture of Bruch's membrane. In 55.7% of eyes, scleral invasion was seen, and in 8.2% of eyes, extrascleral extension was observed. In eyes that had received pre-enucleation radiation treatment, mitotic activity was significantly reduced. With increased pigmentation and increased necrosis, the number of macrophages in the tumor increased.

Conclusions.—With the histopathologic confirmation of the diagnosis at 99.7%, there is a high accuracy of diagnosis in the COMS. There was extensive local invasion of the tumor. The number of mitotic figures was significantly reduced by pre-enucleation irradiation. The presence of macrophages, the level of pigmentation, and the degree of necrosis were found to have an association.

▶ There are few surprises in this histopathologic review of than 1,500 medium and large uveal melanomas enucleated from patients enrolled in the COMS. This paper suggests that there will be little new prognostic information from the pathology section of the COMS study. The COMS study was designed more than a decade ago and relies on standard techniques of histopathologic assessment. Many newly reported techniques that might predict patient outcome are based on molecular biology and require fresh tissue, which was not archived by the COMS study, or specially prepared slides. Even Callender cell type, which is a well-established prognostic standard, will be of limited benefit in this study, because the great majority (86%) of cases fall in the single category of mixed cell melanoma.

This is unfortunate because there currently is a need for new prognostic indicators that can identify patients at greater risk for metastatic melanoma who might benefit from new therapies, such as aggressive chemotherapy or immunotherapy.

R.C. Eagle, Jr., M.D.

Biologic Determinants of Uveal Melanoma Metastatic Phenotype: Role of Intermediate Filaments as Predictive Markers

Hendrix MJC, Seftor EA, Seftor REB, et al (Univ of Iowa, Iowa City; Hadassah Univ, Jerusalem, Israel)

Lab Invest 78:153-163, 1998 11–3

Background.—Although earlier research emphasized the use of vimentin and keratin intermediate filaments (IFs) as cell type-specific markers in differentiation and pathology, recent studies have included many demonstrations of their co-expression in epithelial and nonepithelial neoplasms. The co-expression of vimentin and keratins 8 and 18 in cutaneous melanoma has been associated with recurrent and metastatic disease. Cells co-expressing these IFs are considered "interconverted," as they display both mesenchymal and epithelial phenotypes. The current study focused on the biologic significance and prognostic importance of the interconverted phenotype in primary uveal melanoma and metastatic uveal melanoma in the liver.

Methods and Findings.—The IF phenotype and morphologic characterization in human uveal melanoma tissues and derivative cell cultures from primary choroidal or ciliary body melanomas and from foci of metastatic uveal melanoma to the liver were compared with those of normal uveal tissue and cultured uveal melanocytes. Cell cultures from primary choroidal or ciliary body melanomas expressed only vimentin IFs, had a spindle cell morphology or co-expressed vimentin and mainly keratins 8,18 IFs, and had a mixed population of spindle, intermediate, and epithelioid cells. The relationship between cell morphology and IF expression extended to biologic differences in invasive ability in vitro. Interconverted cells, expressing both vimentin and keratin 8,18 IFs, were significantly more capable of invading a collagenous matrix compared with cells expressing only vimentin. Keratins 8,18 in the M619 cells were transiently suppressed using antisense oligonucleotides, resulting in a marked decline in the migratory ability of these cells in vitro. Abrogation of keratin expression in the M619 cells induced a migratory response similar to that noted in the OCM-1 cell line, positive only for vimentin.

Conclusions.—Human uveal melanoma cells, which primarily co-express vimentin and keratin IFs, have an interconverted phenotype. Compared with cells expressing vimentin only, they are 6-fold more invasive through extracellular matrices. These interconverted cells are located specifically in highly invasive uveal melanoma cells and liver metastases in patients with uveal melanoma.

► Vimentin is the IF normally found in uveal malignant melanoma. This study shows that "interconverted" uveal melanoma cells that express keratins 8 and 18 as well as vimentin have increased invasive properties in vitro. The keratin, normally found in epithelial cells, may contribute to the morphology and behavior of epithelioid melanoma cells.

In 1992, Fuchs and colleagues first reported about one-half of posterior uveal melanomas are immunoreactive for these keratins.[1] The melanomas in that small series that expressed keratin seemed to have a worse prognosis, but the results were not statistically significant.

Further studies are necessary to determine if cytokeratin expression is a valid prognostic indicator. If it is, it could be used to identify patients who are candidates for prophylactic chemo- or immunotherapy. Unlike some of the newer techniques that have been touted to assess metastatic risk, which are labor-intensive or subjective, immunohistochemistry is widely available and can be performed using automated processors. In addition, one of the best antibodies for detecting cytokeratins 8 and 18 is CAM 5.2, which is used routinely as an epithelial marker in many labs.

R.C. Eagle, Jr., M.D.

Reference

1. Fuchs U, Kivela T, Summanen P, et al: An immunohistochemical and prognostic analysis of cytokeratin expression in malignant uveal melanoma. *Am J Pathol* 141:169-181, 1992.

Regulation of Uveal Melanoma Interconverted Phenotype by Hepatocyte Growth Factor/Scatter Factor (HGF/SF)

Hendrix MJC, Seftor EA, Seftor REB, et al (Univ of Iowa, Iowa City; Hadassah Univ, Jerusalem)

Am J Pathol 152:855-863, 1998 11–4

Background.—Uveal melanoma is the most common primary intraocular malignancy in adults. It spreads first and preferentially to the liver. Studies have shown that the interconverted phenotype of uveal melanoma (ie, expressing both mesenchymal [vimentin] and epithelial [keratin] intermediate filaments) is 6 times more invasive than phenotypes expressing the mesenchymal marker only. Hepatocyte growth factor/scatter factor (HGF/SF) stimulates motility of these interconverted cells, presumably via its ligand, the c-met proto-oncogene. These authors investigated the expression of c-met in interconverted uveal melanoma cells and their motogenic response to HGF/SF.

Methods.—Cell lines were derived from primary choroidal or ciliary body melanomas, from foci of uveal melanoma metastatic to the liver, and from normal uveal melanocytes. Immunofluorescence was used to label keratins 8 and 18, vimentin, c-met, and HGF/SF. RNA was extracted for the analysis of c-met and HGF/SF expression. Tumor cell invasion and motility were also assessed in vitro.

Findings.—Uveal melanoma cell lines that expressed c-met correlated with the expression of both keratin and vimentin and with invasive ability. Expression of c-met was highest in interconverted, highly invasive primary and metastatic uveal melanoma cell lines. Immunoperoxidase staining revealed no c-met in uveal melanoma cells that were not interconverted, but intense staining for c-met in uveal melanoma cells that contained both vimentin and keratin. Both primary and metastatic uveal melanomas contained HGF/SF. Invasive, interconverted, c-met–positive primary and metastatic uveal melanoma cell lines had the greatest motogenic/migratory response to HGF/SF. Cells that were poorly invasive, not interconverted, and c-met–negative barely had a response to HGF/SF.

Conclusion.—These data strongly suggest a link between the expression of c-met, the expression of both vimentin and keratin, and in vitro invasive ability. HGF/SF staining was most intense at the level of the choriocapillaris, which suggests that the endothelial cells in that layer may be an important alternate source for HGF/SF. Furthermore, tumors that are likely to disseminate have highly remodeled networks that connect to the choriocapillaris and the vortex veins. Thus, HGF/SF regulation of the interconverted phenotype of uveal melanoma appears to be important in the dissemination of metastases.

▶ Uveal malignant melanoma preferentially metastasizes to the liver. Hepatic metastases occur in more than 90% of patients with metastatic melanoma and are the first metastases detected in 80%. Why this occurs has been unclear. This study from the University of Iowa suggests that a multifaceted growth factor made in the liver called HGF/SF may play a major role in the orchestration of this hepatic honing. The authors have identified receptors for HGS/SF on certain uveal melanoma cells that contain cytokeratin intermediate filaments in addition to the normal complement of vimentin. The authors have previously shown that these so-called interconverted cells are more invasive. The liver is a major source of HGF/SF.

R.C. Eagle, Jr., M.D.

Accumulation of Tissue Inhibitor of Metalloproteinases-3 in Human Eyes With Sorsby's Fundus Dystrophy or Retinitis Pigmentosa

Fariss RN, Apte SS, Luthert PJ, et al (Univ of Washington, Seattle; Cleveland Clinic Found/Wb3, Ohio; Inst of Ophthalmology, London; et al)

Br J Ophthalmol 82:1329-1334, 1998 11–5

Introduction.—Sorsby's fundus dystrophy (SFD) is an autosomal dominant retinal degeneration characterized by accumulation of extracellular deposits in Bruch's membrane. Invasion of the thickened Bruch's membrane by newly formed, thin-walled vessels acquired from the choriocapillaris is a serious complication of SFD. Mutations in exon 5 of the gene for tissue inhibitor of metalloproteinases-3 (TIMP-3), a member of a family of matrix metalloproteinase (MMP) inhibitors, is observed in patients with SFD. The TIMP-3 in Bruch's membrane may be synthesized and secreted by the retinal pigment epithelium (RPE). The role of TIMP-3 in human retinal degenerative diseases was examined to determine whether TIMP-3 localization in SFD is unique or might also be present in a dominant form of retinitis pigmentosa (RP) not caused by TIMP-3 mutation but having sub-RPE deposits resembling those seen in SFD.

Methods.—The eyes of a 77-year-old woman with SFD caused by the *Ser-181-Cys* mutation in the TIMP-3 gene were obtained post mortem. This donor had poor night vision, which developed in her early 30s. By her early 40s, she had distorted vision in her left eye. Her visual acuities diminished to hand movements after choroidal neovascularization and development of disciform scars in both maculae. Samples from 3 patient donors with RP and from 2 normal donors with no history of ophthalmic disease were examined. A mouse monoclonal antibody to human TIMP-3 was used for immunocytochemistry.

Results.—Bruch's membrane and occasional drusen that demonstrated strong, specific TIMP-3 labeling were seen in normal eyes. Eyes with SFD had advanced disease, including loss of nearly all retinal photoreceptors

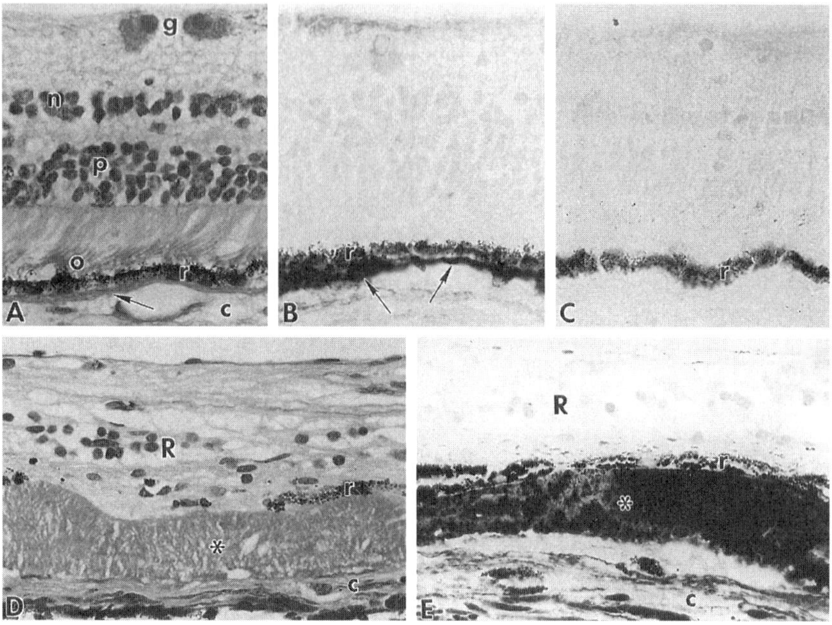

FIGURE 1.—Paraffin sections of normal human eyes (**A**, **B**, and **C**) and of eyes with Sorsby's fundus dystrophy (SFD; **D** and **E**). Magnification, ×625. **A**, Normal retina stained by PAS and hematoxylin: Bruch's membrane (*arrow*) is PAS-positive. **B**, Normal retina immunolabeled with anti-TIMP-3. Note strong reactivity (purple reaction product) of Bruch's membrane (*arrow*), which is somewhat thickened on the left side of the figure. **C**, Normal retina processed for immunocytochemistry with secondary antibody alone. Only weak, nonspecific labeling of scattered nuclei in the retina is observed. **D**, SFD retina stained with PAS and hematoxylin. Note thick layer of PAS-positive deposits (*) between the RPE (*r*) and choroid (*c*). The retina (*R*) is severely degenerate. **E**, SFD retina immunolabeled with anti-TIMP-3. Note strong reactivity of the sub-RPE deposits (*). *Abbreviations: o*, PAS-positive photoreceptor outer segments; *r*, retinal pigment epithelium (RPE); *c*, choroid; *p*, photoreceptor nuclei; *n*, inner nuclear layer; *g*, ganglion cell layer. *R*, retina. (Courtesy of Fariss RN, Apte SS, Luthert PJ, et al: Accumulation of tissue inhibitor of metalloproteinase-3 in human eyes with Sorsby's fundus dystrophy or retinitis pigmentosa. *Br J Ophthalmol* 82:1329-1334, 1998. By permission of the B.J. Publishing Group.)

and gliosis of the remaining retinal layers. Bruch's membrane was notably thickened with extracellular PAS-positive deposits ranging in thickness from 15 to 60 μm (Fig 1). The deposits were located between the RPE and the elastin sublayer of Bruch's membrane and were strongly positive for TIMP-3 throughout their thickness. Adjacent Bruch's membrane deposits were PAS positive and had no TIMP-3 immunoreactivity in occasional areas where RPE cells were lost. Eyes from an 80-year-old donor with RP of unknown genotype and no TIMP-3 gene mutation had thick deposits of about 50 μm internal to the elastin sublayer of Bruch's membrane. These deposits were PAS positive throughout and were strongly positive for TIMP-3. These were adjacent to surviving RPE cells and were less reactive to TIMP-3 where RPE cells had degenerated. Bruch's membrane was PAS positive and well labeled with anti–TIMP-3 where RPE cells were present in the remaining RP retinas. The inner retinal vessels, which were surrounded by migrated RPE cells, had pronounced accumulations of PAS-positive extracellular matrix (ECM) between the RPE and the endothelial cells. Perivascular deposits of ECM associated with the RPE cells were strongly positive for TIMP-3, as were those in normal eyes. The thick deposits of TIMP-3–reactive ECM occluded the lumina in some vessels.

Conclusion.—The TIMP-3 is an element of the increased ECM sequestered in Bruch's membrane in SFD. The fact that TIMP-3 accumulations in retinas with RP were not caused by TIMP-3 mutations highlights the importance of ECM remodeling in normal and diseased human eyes.

▶ The histopathologic findings in SFD are striking; massive deposits of ECM material accumulate on the inner surface of Bruch's membrane in affected patients. SFD has been shown to be associated with heritable mutations in the gene for tissue inhibitor of TIMP-3, which normally inhibits the actions of enzymes that are involved in the degradation of the ECM. There has been speculation that the massive subretinal deposits in SFD could result from abnormal matrix degradation or might even represent massive quantities of mutant TIMP-3 protein, which is made by the RPE. This immunohistochemical study confirms that the subretinal deposits are intensely immunoreactive for TIMP-3. However, the authors also examined several cases of RP, including tissue from one unusual patient who had somewhat similar subretinal deposits and a normal TIMP-3 gene. Surprisingly, the deposits in that case and the matrix material surrounding intraretinal "bone spicule" pigmentation in other cases of RP also were immunoreactive for TIMP-3. The latter observations indicate that the deposits are not composed of mutant TIMP-3 protein.

The sub-RPE deposits in SFD are somewhat reminiscent of the basal laminar or basement membrane deposits that are found in most eyes with exudative age-related maculopathy. The deposits in both diseases are subject to invasion by choroidal neovascularization and contribute to disciform scar formation.

R.C. Eagle, Jr., M.D.

Sebaceous Carcinoma: Tumor Progression Through Mutational Inactivation of p53

Gonzalez-Fernandez F, Kaltreider SA, Patnaik BD, et al (Univ of Virginia, Charlottesville)

Ophthalmology 105:497-506, 1998 11–6

Background.—Sebaceous carcinoma can mimic an inflammatory condition for years. Some authorities believe that human papilloma virus (HPV) plays a role in the development of sebaceous carcinoma by inactivating tumor suppressor gene p53. The current study investigated the molecular basis of the progression of ocular sebaceous carcinoma.

Methods.—Seven patients with sebaceous carcinoma were seen at 1 center between 1989 and 1996. In situ hybridization and polymerase chain

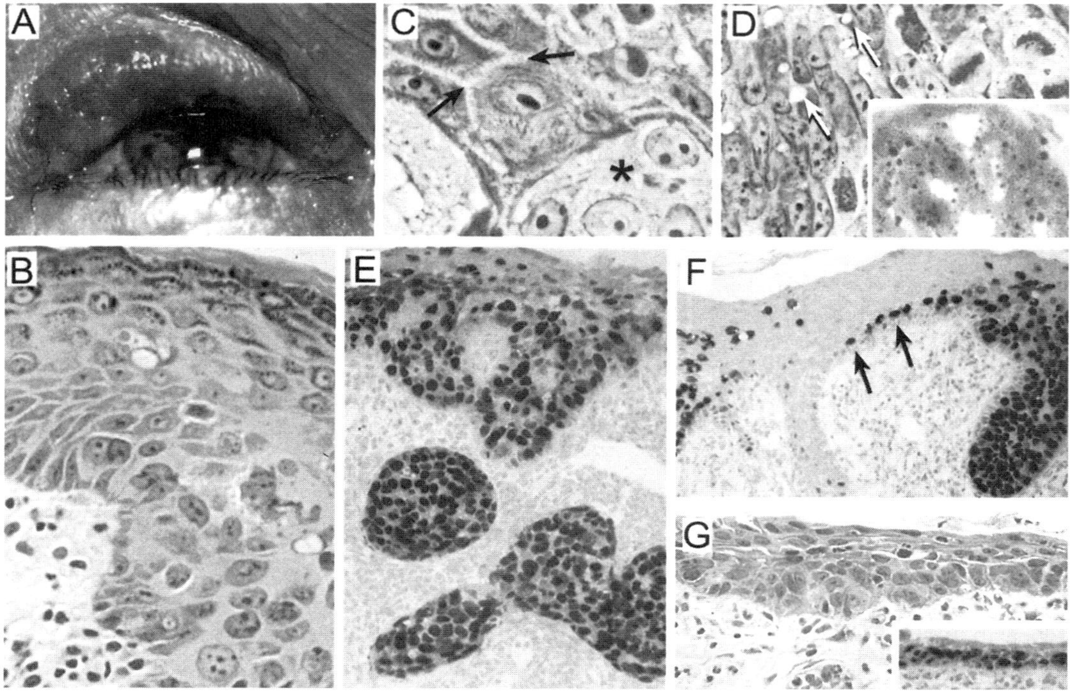

FIGURE 3.—Patient EF had a moderately differentiated sebaceous carcinoma with stromal invasion and intraepithelial pagetoid spread. She was treated for 2.5 years for apparent chronic blepharoconjunctivitis. **A**, destruction of the eyelashes in the erythematous and eczematous upper lid. **B**, sebaceous carcinoma extending into the dermal epithelium (stain, hematoxylin-eosin). **C** and **D**, higher magnification photomicrographs (stain, hematoxylin–eosin) taken under phase contrast. **C**, lack of intercellular desmosomal bridges (black arrows) between the malignant cells (*asterisk*). **D**, cytoplasmic vacuoles within the neoplastic cells (*arrows*) and several mitotic figures (*upper right*). **D** (**insert**), low-magnification photomicrograph of an Oil-red-O preparation showing numerous red cytoplasmic vacuoles indicative of fat. **E** and **F**, anti–p53 immunohistochemical preparations. **E**, lobules of tumor cells are invading the underlying stroma. **F** (*arrows*), the neoplastic cells also are extending within the dermal epithelium by pagetoid spread. **G** (**insert**), a sheet of malignant cells replacing the base of the conjunctival epithelium where they continued to overexpress p53. (Published courtesy of *Ophthalmology*, from Gonzalez-Fernandez F, Kaltreider SA, Patnaik BD, et al: Sebaceous carcinoma: Tumor progression through mutational inactivation of p53. *Ophthalmology* 195:497-506, 1998.)

reaction were done to determine the presence of HPV infection. Immunohistochemistry established the expression of p53, p21^{WAF-1}, Bcl-2, and epithelial membrane antigen. Frozen tumor was available from 1 patient, allowing sequencing of exons 5 through 9 of the p53 gene.

Findings.—All findings were negative for HPV. In patients with disease limited to dysplasia, p53 was negative but not p21^{WAF-1}. Patients with a component of invasive or metastatic carcinoma displayed a striking hyperexpression of nuclear p53 in all malignant cells (Fig 3).

Conclusions.—Mutational inactivation of p53 may play a role in the progression of sebaceous carcinoma. As well as being the most common genetic alteration in human cancer, p53 mutation corresponds to one of the most frequent mutations possible in a single gene.

▶ This study confirms that patients who do not have a distinct eyelid mass may have extensive involvement by in situ or intraepithelial sebaceous carcinoma. This is the basis for a classic ocular masquerade syndrome; affected patients are misdiagnosed as having chronic blepharoconjunctivitis. Conjunctival biopsy to rule out intraepithelial sebaceous carcinoma should be considered strongly in any patient who has chronic blepharoconjunctivitis that does not respond to therapy. The biopsy specimen should be handled carefully, because tumor infiltration predisposes to epithelial sloughing and loss. If the epithelium is lost, the biopsy is worthless.

This research provides a glimpse into the complex array of interrelated mediators and mechanisms involved in the pathogenesis and progression of cancer. Not unexpectedly, mutations in the p53 oncogene were found in sebaceous carcinoma. The role of these mutations remains unclear, however.

R.C. Eagle, Jr., M.D.

MIB-1 and PC-10 Immunostaining for the Assessment of Proliferative Activity in Primary Acquired Melanosis Without and With Atypia

Chowers I, Livni N, Solomon A, et al (Hebrew Univ–Hadassah Med School, Jerusalem, Israel; Univ of Iowa, Iowa City)

Br J Ophthalmol 82:1316-1319, 1998 11–7

Introduction.—Primary acquired melanosis (PAM) is a flat, superficial, and variably brown lesion that is typically unilateral and is usually seen in individuals who have fair complexions. On histologic examination, the presence of intraepithelial melanin deposition alone or with melanocytic hyperplasia without cytologic atypia is specified as PAM without atypia. These lesions have a negligible association with the subsequent development of malignant melanoma. Clinical appearance of a unilateral flat brown patch in the conjunctiva may be caused by intraepithelial melanocytic hyperplasia with melanocytic atypia, or PAM with atypia. This is associated with progression to melanoma in about 50% of patients. Findings of proliferating cell nuclear antigen (PCNA) and Ki-67 antigen with PC-10 and MIB-1 monoclonal antibodies are correlated with proliferating activity, histopathologic classification, and prognosis in many benign and malignant tumors. The correlation between degree of cellular proliferative activity and of intraepithelial melanocytes in PAM without atypia and PAM with atypia was compared by means of immunohistochemical staining for the Ki-67 antigen and the PCNA.

Methods.—Tissue blocks from 35 patients with conjunctival PAM were examined. Lesions were classified by experienced ophthalmic pathologists as PAM without atypia or PAM with atypia (19 and 16 patients, respectively). All PAM without atypia was required to include a histologic component of melanocytic hyperplasia. Slides were placed in citrate buffer and treated in a microwave oven to reveal masked antigen. With immunostaining, all melanocytic cells composing the PAM lesion that contained a distinct positive nuclear staining were considered positive.

Results.—Both pathologist examiners determined that PAM with atypia had a significantly higher MIB-1– and PC-10–positive cell count than PAM without atypia. Findings of positive cell counts were reproducible.

Conclusion.—It is possible to stain proliferating cells in formalin-fixed, paraffin-embedded sections with MIB-1. Antigen retrieval by microwave irradiation is required before staining with MIB-1 and PC-10. Both observers detected significantly higher proliferative activity in lesions with atypia with the use of both PC-10 and MIB-1 monoclonal antibodies. In earlier trials, staining of the Ki-67 antigen was a more accurate estimator of the proliferative activity and was more commonly found to correlate with histopathologic grading and prognosis than PC-10, which recognizes PCNA.

► Cases of severe PAM with atypia are relatively easy to diagnose. It is the lower-grade lesions that are problematic, even for experienced pathologists. It is often difficult to determine whether acquired conjunctival pigmentation merely reflects the accumulation of melanin in the basal cell layer of the epithelium or actually signifies melanocytic hyperplasia. This study suggests that immunohistochemical markers for proliferative activity may help the pathologist determine which lesions are more likely to progress to invasive melanoma.

R.C. Eagle, Jr., M.D.

Suggested Reading

Carden SM, Boissy RE, Schoettker PJ, et al: Albinism: Modern molecular diagnosis. *Br J Ophthalmol* 82:189-195, 1998.

► Pediatric ophthalmologists, retinal specialists, and interested ophthalmologists who have or may have albinos as patients should carefully read this excellent review article. Recent advances in molecular biology have led to a greater understanding and a reclassification of the variety of diseases that comprise albinism. The old "tyrosinase-positive" and "tyrosinase-negative" classification has largely been supplanted by new data. After reading this article, I had to update and revise the outlines and slides I use for teaching. The review also includes excellent guidelines for the clinical evaluation of the patient with albinism.

R.C. Eagle, Jr., M.D.

12 Social Economics

Role Models in the Age of Managed Care

by Elisabeth J. Cohen, M.D.

When it comes to role models in medicine, one is reminded of de Toqueville's view of America, "The more things change, the more they remain the same." In 1998, house officers considered as excellent role model doctors who spend a lot of time teaching and who stress the importance of the doctor-patient relationship and psychosocial aspects of care.[1] These are qualities many mature physicians agree their own role models possessed when they were in training years ago. Medicine is unique in regard to the central place role models have in teaching the essence of patient care at the bedside—or, nowadays, often in the office. Law and business focus on case studies, but in medicine the practitioner teaches by example. There is almost a parental quality to the relationship between attending and student, resident, or fellow. Actions speak louder than words.

Excellent role models take excellent care of patients and are genuinely committed to their residents and fellows. When we think of doctors who positively influenced our career paths, we recognize that their enthusiasm for their fields was contagious. I started out without any interest in surgery, but during the course of a intense required rotation under the direction of a meticulous attending I was won over by the excitement of the operating room. Positive relationships in medicine, and teaching in general, generate interest often more than the subject of study itself. Choice of a field within medicine is often determined by intangible aspects of a great learning experience, and the ability of the student to identify with the teacher.

How do changes in the health care environment affect the issue of role models in medicine? Ideally, the answer is, as little as possible. The crux of the doctor-patient relationship remains the same. However, the context of care has changed considerably. In the past, the financing of medical care was not a major, or even minor, issue in training. Cost-effective medicine was not taught to students, and physicians were not under pressure to control costs. In recent years, not only has reimbursement to many physicians been repeatedly reduced but, the level of hassles regarding insurance issues has increased dramatically. Every day there are problems related to referrals for care and approval for tests, admissions, and procedures that come between the patient and doctor as a result, the patient's insurer's efforts to control costs by limiting care. Managed care requires doctors to see more patients, which harms the doctor-patient relationship and makes it more difficult to teach. Training and time for teaching are ignored by managed care. It is not surprising these issues have a negative influence on morale and enthusiasm among attending physicians and threaten medical education.

It is critically important that attending physicians remember their importance as role models during these challenging times. To be a physician remains a sacred profession. We must pass this on intact to future physicians by the examples we set in the way we care for patients and how we interact with doctors in training. By focusing on the specific doctor-patient and attending-house officer interaction, we can maintain or restore the heart of our profession and be less distracted and discouraged by the larger environment in which we practice. The business of medicine has changed and will continue to change (hopefully, for the better in the not too distant future), but the essence of medicine, caring for the sick, will remain the same. Putting the patient first is here to stay. We must continue to set this example daily for the next generation of doctors.

Reference

1. Wright SM, Kern DE, Kolodner K, et al: Attributes of excellent attending-physician role models. *N Engl J Med* 339:1986-1993, 1998.

A National Bill of Patients' Rights

Annas GJ

N Engl J Med 338:695-699, 1998 12–1

Background.—In January 1998, President Clinton called for a national bill of rights in health care. Basic tenets are that patients have the right to know their treatment options, to choose their doctors, to have access to emergency room care, and to have their medical records kept confidential. This article discusses how the concept of patients' rights has evolved in the United States and how its realization could make the health care delivery system both more responsive and more responsible.

Early Advances in Patients' Rights.—In 1972 the courts established a patient's right to informed consent; the patient decides whether to move forward with treatment after he or she has been provided the basic information. The 1976 case of Karen Ann Quinlan prompted the courts to decree that a patient could refuse any treatment, even if it were life-sustaining treatment. Other rights recognized during the 1970s were patients' rights to medical privacy and confidentiality, access to their medical records, and access to basic emergency care. Although patients' rights advocates or ombudsmen were proposed, they never came into use.

The Managed Care Era.—Managed care has tried to make the patient a consumer. Consumers can choose the plan they want on the basis of cost, coverage, and quality. However, a problem with this belief is that employers—not the employees/patients—decide which health care plans to offer, and they typically select the plan based on cost considerations. Thus, efforts toward assuring patients' rights in managed care are directed at moving the power from managed care companies, health insurance companies, and health care facilities back into the hands of patients and their physicians. Health care delivery is not a business transaction, it is a relationship in which the patient must trust the physician to be working in the patient's best interests. Various responses to tipping the balance of power toward physicians and patients have included legislation (e.g., to allow physicians and patients to determine the length of hospital stay after childbirth); the "Putting Patients First" plan of the American Association of Health Plans (which, among other things, requests removal of "gag rules" regarding what physicians can say to their patients about treatment options); and others.

Steps Toward a National Bill of Patients' Rights.—In November 1997 a Presidential Advisory Commission provided the outline of a national bill of rights for patients. This proposal has at its core the patients' rights to complete treatment information, access to emergency care, confidentiality in medical records, and nondiscriminating and respectful treatment. Also advocated is an external, independent method to resolve grievances—an independent patients' rights advocate or ombudsman. This patients' rights advocate would, among other things, help patients navigate the grievance and appeals procedures with managed care and insurance companies. Ensuring patients' rights in health care is critical because, without these rights, Americans may see a health care system that is indifferent to their needs.

▶ President Clinton has called for federal legislation of patients' rights, including information on treatment options, choice of doctor, emergency care and confidential medical records. This represents a major change from the health plan proposed early in his first term, which promised to limit choice of doctors and emphasized cost control by competition among plans rather than information on treatment options.

This article makes clear the important distinction between patients who are sick and must be able to trust their doctors and consumers involved in business transactions. The vulnerability of sick patients can easily be forgotten by healthy businessmen and lawmakers, but illness is a humbling experience.

The right to an advocate to help patients assert their rights is an interesting concept. Physicians should be patient advocates, but with current health plans designed to reduce costs by limiting access to care, patients could well benefit from professional advocates who could help guide them through the current health care maze. Given the alleged excess of doctors, perhaps retired physicians will be able to enhance access to quality care by becoming professional patient advocates in the future!

E.J. Cohen, M.D.

Effect of Compensation Method on the Behavior of Primary Care Physicians in Managed Care Organizations: Evidence From Interviews With Physicians and Medical Leaders in Washington State

Zierler BK, Marcus-Smith MS, Cheadle A, et al (Univ of Washington, Seattle; Univ of Wisconsin, Madison)

Am J Managed Care 4:209-220, 1998 12–2

Background.—With managed care, the need to balance quality of care with cost-effectiveness is of paramount importance to physicians. Different managed care plans have different compensation arrangements, and this study examined these arrangements in 6 managed care plans to determine common principles and to see how physician behavior is influenced.

Methods.—Members of 67 physician groups affiliated with 1 of 6 managed care programs representing more than 1,500 physicians were surveyed. Goals of the survey were to determine the organizational arrangements that influenced how physicians practice and to understand how the groups transferred health plan payments into individual physician compensation. From the survey group, 72 key informants (33 primary care physicians and 39 medical or administrative leaders) were selected for open-ended interviews.

Findings.—Three broad categories emerged from the interviews. First, the method of compensation was a key factor that physicians considered when choosing a practice area. They selected a group whose compensation plan fit their lifestyles, and this led to high satisfaction with their compensation method (only 3% of physicians said they were dissatisfied). Second, compensation impacted production; the number of patients seen was influenced by the type of compensation. Eighty percent of respondents whose salary was based on some production measure said that production incentives increase physician production. Third, the participants expected future changes to plans, with more reliance on incentive-based methods. Almost three quarters of physicians expected their compensation plan to change in the near future.

Conclusions.—Compensation arrangements are critical in influencing physician satisfaction and behavior. Physician behaviors have a direct impact on quantitative outcome indicators, such as utilization and medical outcomes. Thus, future research is needed to determine how quantitative outcome indicators are affected by physician compensation arrangements.

▶ The results of this study ring true. Just as patients in the United States are more satisfied with their physicians when they have a choice, physicians are more satisfied when they choose their compensation method. The high priority Americans place on choice is linked to the U.S. ideal of liberty, a value that is by no means universal and may be unique to Americans. The observation that people work harder when they are rewarded for it reflects human nature. The success of capitalism as compared with socialism exemplifies this. Ophthalmologists are similar to primary physicians in this regard. Compensation models need to provide incentives for hard work without encouraging overutilization to try to both maintain quality and control costs.

E.J. Cohen, M.D.

Physicians' Perceptions of Managed Care

Levine RA, Lieberson A (Yale Univ, New Haven, Conn; Norwalk Hosp, Conn; Westport, Conn)

Am J Managed Care 4:171-180, 1998 12–3

Background.—Managed care plans are becoming more common, and more physicians are signing managed care contracts. This study evaluated physicians' opinions about and knowledge of legal and ethical issues involved with such contracts.

Methods.—All 315 medical staff of a community hospital in southwestern Connecticut were mailed a questionnaire. The questionnaire consisted of 9 questions addressing how knowledgeable physicians were about their managed care contracts and whether certain provisions were legal/illegal or ethical/unethical.

Findings.—Of the 315 physicians queried, 66 responded (20.9%). The respondents (more than 90% male) had an average age of 50 years and an average of 19.1 years in practice. Only 41 respondents indicated whether they participated in a managed care plan; 39 of these (95%) did so. In general, the legality of specific provisions was poorly understood. Most respondents did not understand the concept of "any willing provider"; only 69.6% knew this term means that any provider willing to join a managed care plan must be accepted. Furthermore, of 11 contract provisions addressed, only 1 was actually illegal, but most respondents believed that 7 of the 11 were illegal. Half the physicians thought any given provision was illegal, and from 53% to 95.4% thought it was unethical. The areas physicians thought most unethical were the requirement for a physician to perform procedures beyond his training, and the requirement to use specific laboratories and other diagnostic services even if their services are inferior. Another area of contention regarded nondisclosure provisions, which more than 85% of respondents said were unethical. Most physicians (97%) believed that managed care interferes with the patient's quality of care. Finally, while 92.4% of physicians believed themselves to be ethically responsible for providing quality care, 72.7% felt that the managed care industry should be legally responsible for ensuring such care.

Conclusions.—In general, physicians had a poor understanding of the legality of provisions in managed care contracts. Most respondents felt that the majority of the provisions were unethical. Further physician education is needed if physicians are to understand the legal and ethical aspects of managed care plan contracts.

▶ This article shows that physicians think many controversial managed care contract provisions are illegal, when in fact the provisions are legal (but perhaps should be illegal). The article also reveals that a large majority of physicians find managed care provisions unethical, and at the same time feel ethically responsible for quality patient care. Unfortunately, only a small percentage of physicians responded to the questionnaire. Assuming the respondents were not more ignorant or more ethical than the nonrespondents, it is not surprising that physicians are in a no-win situation when they sign managed care contracts. Physicians have a very legitimate concern that they will lose access to patients if they do not participate in managed care. Very few patients are able or willing to pay for their medical care, and many have little choice in their medical insurance. A large discrepancy between legal and ethical standards is to be expected. Managed care businesses must meet legal standards, but physicians and patients require ethical medical care.

E.J. Cohen, M.D.

How Large Employers Are Shaping the Health Care Marketplace: First of Two Parts

Bodenheimer T, Sullivan K (Univ of California, San Francisco; Minnesota Citizens Organized Acting Together, St Paul)

N Engl J Med 338:1003-1007, 1998 12–4

Introduction.—The managed care revolution of the 1980s and 1990s was set off by the largest U.S. corporations, in response to rising health insurance premiums. These employers began directing their employees into managed care insurance plans, particularly HMOs; new strategies for controlling health costs have since emerged. These strategies were reviewed in context of the growing impact of large employers on the health care marketplace.

Health Care Cost Control.—Employers began providing health insurance to employees in the years after World War II. Health care costs began to rise as corporate profits decreased during the 1970s. Still, by the early 1980s, few companies saw health costs as a major problem, and few Americans were enrolled in HMOs. As health care costs continued to rise, employers shifted the burden to employees by increasing premiums, deductibles, and copayments. Some small companies stopped offering insurance, while many large companies initiated self-insurance plans. By the late 1980s, health care costs were increasing by 17% to 19% per year; health costs now accounted for about 9% of wages and salaries, compared with 2% in 1965. These accelerating costs spelled the end of fee-for-service indemnity insurance, and the first response of big business was to direct employees into HMOs.

Channeling Employees into Managed Care.—In 1988, Allied-Signal became the first major employer to switch their employees to HMO plans. The number of Americans enrolled in HMO jumped from 15 million in 1985 to 50 million in 1996. Employees often have no choice in these arrangements, particularly at smaller companies. Larger companies generally offer a choice, but employees will pay more for the more expensive health plan. Experience has shown that employees are highly sensitive to increases in premiums, to the benefit of HMOs and PPOs.

Regional Purchasing Coalitions.—As HMO premiums continued to rise, often just behind the premiums of indemnity plans, employers began forming coalitions to purchase health plans collectively. A growing number of employers are joining these coalitions, such as California's Pacific Business Group on Health (PBGH), which represents 33 companies and 3 million consumers. Although such joint purchasing is not easy, it can have a major impact on costs; PBGH reduced HMO rates by 14% from 1995 through 1997. This coalition negotiates rates with HMOs, then decides which HMOs will be offered to employees, with the option to drop higher-priced HMOs. It also seeks to improve quality by tying part of the premium to quality of care and publishing consumer report cards on HMOs.

Direct Contracting.—One Minnesota coalition, called the Buyers Health Care Action Group, found that competition had faded in the face of mergers among health plans. In response, the coalition began contracting directly with integrated "care systems." Rates averaged about $100 per member per month, considerably less than HMOs. So far, however, the reduction has not increased the dollars allotted for actual medical services. Employers pay the care system a discounted fee for service under a "claim target," which averages $86 per member per month. If claims exceed the target, fees are discounted further; employer risk is limited. Employees have a choice of low-, middle-, and high-cost plans, thus producing price competition in favor of low-cost systems. Only the employee can make the decision to change plans, and thus change family physicians.

Discussion.—The impact of big business on the health care marketplace was reviewed, focusing on the forces leading to the rise of managed care and large employers' responses to changes in health care costs. A second part of this article discusses whether employers should have so much influence over health services.

► This article gives a nice historical perspective to the approaches large employers have used since the late 1980s to reduce health care costs, including use of managed care, purchasing coalitions, and direct contracting with health providers.

It is interesting how sensitive employees are to small differences in health premiums. In one study, an increase of $10 per month caused a quarter of employees to switch to cheaper plans. Increasing employee contributions rapidly causes large shifts toward cheaper options.

The employers have the power, and the employees appear to be very cost sensitive. The progressive lowering of prices is unrelated to the true costs of providing care. Quality does not appear to be anyone's priority, although patients tend to choose a plan that allows them to keep their current physician. With all the emphasis on cost, it's not surprising that hospitals are going bankrupt and physicians are earning less and less. Where will all this end?

E.J. Cohen, M.D.

Must Good HMOs Go Bad? First of Two Parts: The Commercialization of Prepaid Group Health Care

Kuttner R (Cambridge, Mass)

N Engl J Med 338:1558-1563, 1998 12–5

Objective.—Prepaid group health care—much later called HMOs—has grown from a radical form of medicine to the centerpiece of entrepreneurial health care in the United States. Driven by the need to cut health costs, HMOs have caught physicians between patients anxious about coverage on the one hand and demands by payers for further cost control on the other. The increasing trend toward commercialization of HMOs was reviewed.

Social Versus Commercial HMOs.—Socially oriented managed care plans emphasize prevention, pursue cost-effective care, and monitor care provided so as to reduce deviations from "best practice." Marketed-oriented HMOs additionally require that physicians assume financial risks, setting up an ethical conflict of interest. Physicians may be paid on the basis of capitation or otherwise put at financial risk. They must also serve as gatekeepers, in the face of large financial incentives to keep patients from seeing specialists. Commercial HMOs are also careful to select healthy, young patients while shifting the costs of sicker patients to other care plans. The emphasis on reducing variation in care may shift to simply reducing care, thus setting up a conflict between the desire to save money and the need for good care. In some cases, these HMOs stop "managing care" and start simply "managing costs."

Nonprofit plans vary in the extent to which they have adopted the characteristics of commercial HMOs, from Group Health Cooperative of Puget Sound, which remains largely faithful to the traditional model; to Kaiser Permanente, which has made more compromises; to Harvard Pilgrim Health Care, which uses many of the same cost-containment measures as for-profit HMOs. The entrepreneurial, commercial HMOs use more aggressive risk selection, follow more stringent care approval programs, and place a greater proportion of physician income at risk. Roughly half of gross income may be at risk, but this may amount to 100% of take-home income. Some plans even encourage physician groups to accept full risk, in return for which they offer a wide range of incentive payment plans. At the same time, some nonprofit HMOs use market-like disciplines while retaining a strong social conscience.

Convergence of For-Profit and Nonprofit HMOs.—Today, many so-called HMOs are actually distant groups of doctors with nothing in common except utilization controls or financial incentives. In response to utilization controls, patients demand more choice; the more choice that is offered by plans, the more they stray from the systemwide integration that is the advantage of HMOs. This shift away from staff-model HMOs also reduces organized resistance to clinical intrusions by doctors. Still, nonprofit HMOs continue to score better on objective indicators and consumer surveys. Nonprofit plans have lower disenrollment rates, higher quality scores, and spend more of the premium cost on health care.

Summary.—The differences between social (nonprofit) and commercial (for-profit) HMOs were highlighted. Although nonprofit HMOs appear to offer a more acceptable form of managed care, the pressure to cut costs will continue to increase. It remains to be seen whether counterpressures can provide adequate checks and balances.

Must Good HMOs Go Bad? Second of Two Parts: The Search for Checks and Balances

Kuttner R (Cambridge, Mass)

N Engl J Med 338:1635-1639, 1998 12–6

Purpose.—Unless a set of effective checks and balances emerges, an increasing number of HMOs may adopt policies that compromise medical ethics and patient care. Some of these forces rely on market discipline, whereas others are external. Potential checks and balances on HMOs were reviewed.

Checks and Balances.—Consumer choice of physicians is a potentially important source of market discipline. However, in contrast to almost all other countries, American employers increasingly limit the consumer's choice of plans. Even if there is a choice, it may be between only 2 or 3 plans, and it is difficult to switch plans under certain circumstances. The "quality" movement offers an approach to reducing negative outcomes, promoting more efficient use of scarce resources, and keeping the opportunistic tendencies of managed care in check. Various quality-monitoring approaches have been developed; however, most of these systems monitor overuse rather than underuse, and are relevant mainly to healthy populations. They also do not address the conflict of interest between the plan's desire to reduce costs and the patient's desire for access to care if they become seriously ill.

With the perceived failure of quality measures to protect consumers, state and federal regulatory measures have been considered. Competing "patient bill of rights" proposals are currently being considered by the U.S. Congress. However, the movement toward regulation has bipartisan support. In response, commercial HMOs urge competition and self-regulation as alternatives to federal regulation. The HMO industry blames the media for sensationalizing a few negative cases to illustrate HMO abuses. A government investigation found little evidence of such abuses, largely because they had been eliminated by media and regulatory pressures.

An alliance between physicians and health care consumers may be the best counter to claims of self-regulation by HMOs. Capitation has important ethical implications, in that it gives physicians an incentive to limit medical care. Yet the American Medical Association's code of ethics has been prohibited as an impermissible restraint of trade. Thus a measure to protect patients from financial arrangements that reward doctors for denying care has been thrown out in the name of consumer protection. Furthermore, physicians themselves are responsible for creating many of the systems that restrict their clinical autonomy.

Finally, although other approaches to health care reform may be possible, the United States now seems committed to cost control through managed care, with an emphasis on shareholder-owned HMOs and financial incentives for physicians. This ignores the fact that other countries use other approaches which rely less on bureaucracy and clinical intrusion. Commitment to the current approach raises difficult issues related to risk adjustment.

Discussion.—A number of types of checks and balances are potentially useful in protecting consumers against unscrupulous practices by HMOs. It remains to be seen, however, whether these approaches can provide adequate controls without placing too much of a drain on physicians and the premium dollar.

► This is an interesting 2-part report (Abstracts 12–5 and 12–6) comparing the older, socially oriented, staff-model, nonprofit HMOs and the newer, market-oriented, for-profit HMOs. Major differences between them are that physicians in the market-oriented HMOs are much more financially at risk for the care they provide, and there are various financial incentives to reduce referrals to specialists and hospitalization. U.S. Healthcare and Oxford are sobering examples of commercial HMOs that are close to home. In the U.S. Healthcare contract described in this article, 50% of a physician's pay is at risk, but given a 50% overhead, this translates into 100% of take-home pay! Oxford Health Plan offered liberal benefits and payments. Their advertising targeted young and affluent individuals, but when patients with chronic disease enrolled, severe financial troubles followed—well known to readers of the business section of newspapers.

Market forces to reduce care need somehow to be opposed effectively. Part 2 of this article outlines the limited nature of existing checks and balances to prevent market-oriented HMOs from leading a competitive "race to the bottom."

What can physicians do? As a minimum, we should not participate in contracts with excessive financial incentives to limit care. We should be very careful if and when we help in designing utilization management systems that restrict physician autonomy. Physicians should align themselves with patients rather than insurers and remain patient advocates.

E.J. Cohen, M.D.

Carve Outs: Definition, Experience, and Choice Among Candidate Conditions

Blumenthal D, Buntin MB (Harvard Med School, Boston; Massachusetts Gen Hosp, Boston)

Am J Managed Care 4:SP45-SP57, 1998 12–7

Background.—The increase of "carve-out" contracts—in which separate, specialized organizations provide health care services for particular conditions, procedures, diseases, or patient groups—is an interesting development in managed care. However, few systematic data are available on the effects of carve outs on cost, quality, and access to health care services. In the absence of this information, a conceptual framework is useful for deciding which conditions and populations may benefit from carve-out strategies. Carve-out contracts were discussed.

Discussion.—Carve-out contracts vary in scope or type of services, patients or conditions covered, the extent of financial risk, degree of integration between carve out and other care providers, and organizational characteristics. Carve outs may help improve functioning of the health care market as well as the quality and cost effectiveness of service delivery. The potential pitfalls of carve outs include administrative costs, which may negate expected benefits; interference with quality of primary care; and the possibility that the risk selection problem will merely be transferred from the general health insurance market to the new carve-out market. At least 5 characteristics increase the likelihood that the benefits of a carve out will outweigh its drawbacks:

1. The condition, disease, or procedure specified is likely to induce risk selection by insurers, plans, providers, or patients.
2. The condition minimizes the likely administrative complexity and cost of a carve out.
3. The condition is well suited to care in a separate, specialized system.
4. The condition tends to not be managed primarily or exclusively by primary care physicians.
5. The condition affects patients who are capable of and have the resources to assert their rights.

▶ Since the arrival of managed care, there has been a lot of talk about ophthalmology carve outs, but payers have not been as interested in implementing them as expected. This holds true not just for ophthalmology.

This article provides background information on the pros and cons of carve outs. Ophthalmology would be a specialty carve out, not a population carve out of patients with a specific condition such as HIV/AIDS. Ophthalmology could also be handled as a "carve in" if organized within a specific health plan. It is clear that eye care is better provided by ophthalmologists than by primary care doctors. Administering an ophthalmology carve out should be relatively straightforward because the boundary between eye care and other medical care is clear.

It is interesting that some programs intended as carve outs, i.e., those involving care of diabetics and cancer patients, have evolved into disease management programs instead. Apparently, this has happened because health plans are not interested in carve outs that limit patients' choice of physicians. Procedure-oriented carve outs have been more successful than disease-oriented ones. Procedures in which high volume has been associated with high quality are suited for carve outs.

Taken together, it would seem that many factors favor the development of ophthalmology carve outs if the patient's right to choose the ophthalmologist is preserved. Participation by ophthalmologists in potentially competing health systems actually enhances patient choice. Given the recent climate in health care, the development of ophthalmology carve outs will probably not be associated with exclusivity and closed panels of doctors.

E.J. Cohen, M.D.

Ethical Guidelines for Physician Compensation Based on Capitation

Pearson SD, Sabin JE, Emanuel EJ (Harvard Med School, Boston; Harvard Pilgrim Health Care, Boston; NIH, Bethesda, Md)

N Engl J Med 339:689-693, 1998 12–8

Introduction.—With managed care, there is a crisis of confidence. Fears are triggered that necessary health services are withheld and that health care decisions are driven by the financial bottom line. There are public fears about the effects of capitation and other financial incentives to physicians. Nevertheless, with limited health care resources, capitation cannot be dismissed as a method of compensating physicians, and it will not go away soon. The ethical dimensions of compensations systems based on capitation must be better understood. An analytic framework for considering how capitation agreements can be designed to achieve more cost-conscious and effective care without jeopardizing the integrity of physicians' decisions was described.

Design Principles.—Safeguards to minimize potential conflicts must be integrated into the design of compensation systems. The extent of physicians' conflict of interest is affected by the intensity of incentives, which is determined by the scope of services included, amount of financial loss or gain, timing and structure of bonuses or deductions, and provision of a limit on the financial risk faced by physicians. Primary physicians are at greater risk when the costs of referral services are covered directly out of the risk pool in which the referring physician participates. Capitation compensation systems should not present an intensity of financial gain or risk for physicians that would lead reasonable individuals to question whether the judgments of the physicians are influenced improperly.

Incentives.—The immediacy of incentives is also important, and this depends on the number of physicians and patients covered by a capitated payment or other financial incentives. When there are more patients, the potential for risk is spread out. The targeting of incentives involves using

TABLE 2.—Specific Design Features of Compensation Systems Based on Capitation and Their Effects on the Degree of Conflict of Interest Faced by Physicians

More Conflict of Interest	Less Conflict of Interest
>20% of income at risk	<10% of income at risk
No per-patient stop-loss insurance	Per-patient stop-loss insurance provided
Primary care physicians bear risk alone for services outside the scope of their practice	Primary care physicians at risk only for services they control
Bonuses and "withholds" calculated frequently and paid as distinct, lump sums	Bonuses and "withholds" calculated infrequently and paid according to a sliding scale
Individual physicians at risk	Larger groups of physicians at risk (>15)
Small groups of enrollees in risk pool (≤250)	Larger groups of enrollees in risk pool (>250)
Narrowly targeted incentives to reduce specific services, implemented without guidelines or monitoring for underuse	No incentives targeted to reduce costs of specific services such as radiology or drugs
Pure capitated payments with incentives linked only to use of services	Incentives for improved access to care, prevention, patient satisfaction, and clinical outcomes
No risk adjustment	Risk adjustment of capitation rates

(Reprinted by permission of *The New England Journal of Medicine*, from Pearson SD, Sabin JE, Emanuel EJ: Ethical guidelines for physician compensation based on capitation. *N Engl J Med* 339:689-693.)

deductions or bonuses to target specific costs for reduction. Narrowly targeted incentives, such as controlling the costs of radiology or decreasing the number of cesarean sections performed, can increase potential conflict of interest for physicians. Incentives must be balanced and must address high enrollee turnover. A system of incentives must not discourage physicians from caring for the patients who are most in need (Table 2).

Conclusions.—Research is vitally needed to clarify how capitation truly affects physician-patient relationships, decision making by physicians, and clinical outcomes.

► Capitation is an obvious threat to the ethical practice of medicine, which requires that the interests of the patient are placed first. Standard ethics have focused on the individual patient, but this discussion of ethics and capitation starts by shifting the focus from the individual patient to patients and the public. The public has good reason to think that capitation is a threat to the trust that is at the heart of the doctor-patient relationship.

The authors admit that research is needed to determine the level of financial risk needed to make physicians cost conscious without causing them to withhold necessary care. I have been told by high-ranking officials of a major insurer that in the end, physicians do the right thing for their patients (even if it means they will lose money). It is interesting that given experiments in capitation that have taken place in the United States there are not better data available. However, the authors proceed to make recommendations without any information, when it would be more appropriate to design research studies to obtain this information. There is no basis to suggest that 20% is the upper limit of acceptable financial risk or that capitation contracts should cover at least 250 patients and 15 doctors. Intuitively, the financial risk sounds high and the number of physicians and patients sounds very low. Because there are no valid methods to adjust for severity of patients' conditions, and it is ethically unacceptable to discourage physicians from caring for the sickest patients, capitation is not ethically viable.

E.J. Cohen, M.D.

The Urgent Need to Improve Health Care Quality: Institute of Medicine National Roundtable on Health Care Quality

Chassin MR, and the National Roundtable on Health Care Quality (Mount Sinai School of Medicine, New York; et al)

JAMA 280:1000-1005, 1998 12–9

Introduction.—Quality of care is central to the ongoing debate about health care in the United States. A series of discussions took place to identify issues related to health care quality including its measurement, assessment, and improvement, that require action by health care professionals and other constituencies in the private or public sector.

Methods.—The Institute of Medicine convened the National Roundtable on Health Care Quality. There were 20 individuals from the public and private sectors including representatives from medicine, nursing, academia, business, consumer advocacy groups, and the health media, as well as heads of federal health programs. During a 2-year period the group met 6 times to explore the changes.

Process.—The group held discussions with many experts, read commissioned papers, and drew on their own professional experiences. The members reached a consensus on the state of the quality of health care in the United States. They defined quality of care as "the degree to which health services for individuals and populations increase the likelihood of desired health outcomes and are consistent with current professional knowledge." Problems identified were underuse, or failure to provide a health care services when it would have produced a favorable outcome; overuse, when a health care service is provided under circumstances in which its potential for harm exceeds the possible benefit; and misuse, when an appropriate service has been selected but a preventable complication occurs and the patient does not receive the full potential benefit of the service.

Conclusions.—A national focus on improving the quality of health care is imperative. There can be a precise definition of the quality of health care. Quality can be measured just as accurately as the majority of clinical problems. All delivery systems and financing mechanisms have problems with health care quality. Only a few health care groups have made impressive efforts to improve their quality of care. The delivery of health care services must be reengineered to improve quality.

► This article presents the conclusions from a series of meetings sponsored by the National Academy of Sciences regarding quality of care, but does not report results of research. Fortunately, the experts concluded that the focus should shift from concern over health care costs to quality. Quality is defined and quality issues are categorized as underuse, overuse and misuse. Improvement in the areas of overuse and misuse can reduce costs, but addressing problems of underuse (which capitation encourages) usually increases costs. Randomized controlled studies of efficacy are the gold standard, but they are limited in scope and costly. The lack of an information infrastructure is considered critical because with it, computer-assisted guidelines for care can be used to try to improve quality. Developing this infrastructure is a major, expensive undertaking that is worthwhile. The article describes quality issues more than solutions. It is harder to measure quality than the article suggests.

E.J. Cohen, M.D.

A New Method of Developing Expert Consensus Practice Guidelines

Frances A, Kahn D, Carpenter D, et al (Duke Univ, Durham, NC; Columbia Univ, New York; Cornell Univ, New York; et al)

Am J Managed Care 4:1023-1029, 1998 12–10

Introduction.—The only enduring way of improving the quality of health care while simultaneously reducing the cost of medical care is to standardize "best practice" treatment delivery. When developing practice guidelines, the strategy is to identify expensive illnesses treated with highly variable and less-than-optimal interventions. The Institute of Medicine's definition of practice guidelines is "systematically developed statements to assist practitioner and patient decisions about appropriate health care for specific clinical circumstances." Research is not always available to answer problems encountered in everyday practice. A valuable bridge between clinical research and clinical practice is expert consensus. A new method of gathering expert consensus guidelines was described.

Survey method.—Limitations of previous methods to develop expert consensus included lack of quantification, specificity, representativeness, and implementation. The new method of developing, documenting, and disseminating expert consensus guidelines addresses these limitations. The method involves a survey of leading clinical researchers studying a given disorder. Their opinion is solicited on the most important disease management questions that are not covered well by definitive research.

Method Applied.—This method has already been applied to 4 disorders in psychiatry, and other medical conditions could equally benefit from this method. There was an 85% response among the experts for the 4 different psychiatric disorders. By surveying separately a large group of practicing clinicians, the views of the clinician researchers were validated. This ensured that the guideline recommendations were widely generalizable. Using criteria that were established a priori for defining first-, second-, and third-line choices, all the suggestions made in the guidelines were derived from and referenced to the experts' survey responses.

Conclusions.—A high level of reliability and reproducibility was achieved with this method of quantifying expert responses. For standardizing practice for decision points not well covered by research, this survey method is probably the best available means.

▶ This is a very nice article describing a new approach to develop valid, useful, and up-to-date practice guidelines, which are central to the practice of quality medicine under managed care. The authors point out that current guidelines are inadequate because they are vague and difficult to apply to specific clinical situations. To be useful, guidelines must go beyond what is known from valid scientific research because research is limited in scope and complexity. The approach advocated includes identifying what is known and key decisions that are not covered by the scientific literature. A questionnaire regarding many clinical situations and possible options is then sent to a large number of clinical researchers and validated by responses of practicing clinicians. Results are presented so they can be quickly used for specific clinical situations.

This approach should be applied to ophthalmology, but who can accomplish this major undertaking? Having the experience with the difficulty of developing technology assessments by the Academy of Ophthalmology, it is unlikely this organization can do it. Alternatives include the U.S. government through research or funding agencies, insurance/managed care companies, private corporations, or a combination, with the Academy offering guidance.

E.J. Cohen, M.D.

The Risk-Adjustment Debate
Kuttner R
N Engl J Med 339:1952-1956, 1998 12–11

Background.—Risk adjustment is an insurance reimbursement process that takes into account the actual health status or recent medical experience of patients in a particular health plan. This author examined risk adjustment while keeping in mind the idea behind insurance: that, in a large population, people at high risk are balanced by people at low risk.

The Physician's Perspective.—Under the fee-for-service system, risk adjustment was not needed; physicians spent as much time with a patient as they thought appropriate and charged accordingly. The capitation system, however, carries an inherent bias toward selecting low-risk patients. Furthermore, a physician group that accepts high-risk patients and provides them with good care runs the risk of attracting more such patients, which in a capitation system can actually reduce income.

Adjusted payments to reflect the actual risks of a practice have typically been based on age and sex (which predict 20% or less of the variation in medical costs). Other adjustment plans also take into consideration diagnosis (with the risk of exaggerating diagnoses for reimbursement purposes) or base outpatient costs on inpatient experience (which accounts for about 75% of the variation in medical costs). There is no clear consensus as to which risk adjustment program is best, and accordingly, most medical groups do not have a risk adjustment mechanism in place with insurers. Typically, only the large provider organizations have the clout to bargain with insurance companies about risk adjustment.

The New "Fourth Party."—Risk management efforts today are directed toward paying adjustments to a plan or "fourth party" rather than directly to physicians or groups. The fourth party collects premiums and redistributes payments from third parties (such as insurance plans) according to the calculated adjustment. However, most Americans do not receive their health insurance through a plan that can assume the role of a fourth party. Are "health alliances" or multivendor health plans for state employees the answer? Whatever the answer, it must be found soon, as the Health Care Financing Administration must have a risk-adjustment mechanism in place by January 1, 2000.

The United States Experience.—Currently only a few purchasers are pursuing systematic risk adjustment; one is Colorado's Medicaid plan, which takes into account the patient's diagnosis. Risk adjustment is particularly thorny for our Medicaid program, because the most needy populations have a disproportionate number of health problems. Whether risk adjustment is the best solution remains to be seen; after all, in any capitated system, physicians make more money by not seeing their patients. Risk management can help plans with sicker populations of patients to avoid unfair losses, but it will not solve all our problems.

▶ This is a nice review of the issues involved in risk adjustment, or methods to have payments appropriate for patients' health care needs so that managed care organizations do not avoid sick patients and physicians who care for sick patients are not punished financially. Although there are ways to adjust for risk—to some extent—on the basis of diagnosis, hospital records, and disease severity, most managed care organizations use only age and sex. Given the aim of maximizing profits by health care plans, it is not surprising that many have withdrawn from Medicare since the Health Care Financing Administration has mandated the introduction of diagnosis-based risk adjustment by the year 2000.

I think the authors vastly overestimate the ability of physician hospital organizations to develop risk adjustment systems and influence payments—at least in a market such as Philadelphia where 2 larger insurers dominate and determine reimbursement. There is a fundamental inconsistency, which risk adjustment cannot fix between the purpose of health insurance to provide care for the sick and the aim of managed health care plans to maximize profits by denying care. Americans deserve better and will not tolerate this.

E.J. Cohen, M.D.

Attributes of Excellent Attending-Physician Role Models

Wright SM, Kern DE, Kolodner K, et al (Johns Hopkins Univ, Baltimore, Md)
N Engl J Med 339:1986-1993, 1998 12–12

Background.—An integral part of medical education is role modeling. But what attributes make an attending physician a good role model? These authors performed a case-control study to identify the distinguishing characteristics of excellent role models.

Methods.—All internal medicine house staff at 4 large teaching hospitals was surveyed, and staff members were asked to identify the colleague(s) they thought was "a standard of excellence to be imitated." The case physicians were the 165 role models named; the control physicians were the 246 attending physicians who were not identified by at least 1 respondent as being an excellent role model. These 411 attending physicians were asked to complete a 55-item questionnaire regarding their career-related characteristics and achievements, attitudes toward teaching, and other aspects of their career. Of the total sample of 411, 341 (83%) completed the questionnaire (144 cases [42%] and 197 controls [58%]).

Findings.—The cases and controls did not differ in demographics, number of degrees, academic rank, or employment status (full-time vs. part-time). Significantly more of the cases were generalists (odds ratio [OR], 3.37) rather than subspecialists. Cases had significantly greater assigned teaching responsibilities than controls; thus, data were adjusted to take into consideration the respondent's assigned teaching responsibilities. Even after this adjustment, the cases and controls differed substantially in many aspects (Table 3). In general, cases spent more time with house staff, had a teaching style that stressed the importance of the doctor-patient relationship, and built more relationships with house officers; they were also more likely to have received training in teaching and to enjoy teaching. Multivariate analysis identified 5 attributes that were independently associated with case status. First, attending physicians who spent more than 25% of their time teaching were more likely to be considered an excellent role model (OR, 5.12). Spending 25 or more hours/week teaching or conducting rounds while attending was also associated with the cases (OR, 2.48). Teaching styles that stressed the importance of the doctor-patient relationship (OR, 2.58) and the psychosocial aspects of medicine (OR, 2.31) were also associated with the excellent role models. Finally, many of the cases had served as a chief resident (OR, 2.07).

Conclusion.—Excellent role models share many common characteristics. They spend a lot of time with trainees, they build positive relationships with their patients, and they take a comprehensive approach to patient care. Many of these attributes can be acquired, and doing so might create more excellent role models for our trainees.

► This is a well-designed case-control study of attributes associated with excellent role models by internal medicine house officers. It is not surprising that attending physicians who spent a lot of time teaching were identified as

TABLE 3.—Association of Selected Characteristics of Attending Physicians With Identification as an Excellent Role Model

Characteristic	Physicians Named as Excellent Role Models (N = 144)	Control Physicians (N = 197)	Adjusted Odds Ratio (95% CI)*
	no. (%)		
Additional time spent with house staff			
Time spent with house staff when not attending			
≤2 hr/wk	37 (26.4)	94 (49.7)	1.00
3-5 hr/wk	58 (41.4)	64 (33.9)	2.02 (1.18-3.46)
≥6 hr/wk	45 (32.1)	31 (16.4)	3.13 (1.67-5.84)
Time spent with team when attending			
<10 hr/wk	29 (20.6)	67 (35.4)	1.00
11-24 hr/wk	57 (40.4)	72 (38.1)	1.79 (1.00-3.20)
≥25 hr/wk	55 (39.0)	50 (26.5)	2.49 (1.35-4.56)
Training in teaching			
Attended teaching workshops	53 (38.1)	43 (22.1)	2.06 (1.25-3.39)
Served as chief resident	52 (36.4)	42 (21.6)	2.00 (1.20-3.30)
Had any formal training in teaching	67 (48.2)	63 (32.3)	1.89 (1.18-3.01)
Attended faculty-development programs	43 (30.9)	38 (19.5)	1.75 (1.03-2.98)
Received feedback on teaching from colleagues†	51 (35.7)	60 (30.5)	1.14 (0.71-1.84)
Teaching style and methods			
Stresses importance of the doctor-patient relationship†	29 (20.6)	17 (8.9)	2.68 (1.40-5.20)
Teaches psychosocial aspects of medicine†	85 (59.0)	82 (42.5)	2.00 (1.30-3.00)
Gives in-depth feedback†	51 (35.4)	45 (23.9)	1.74 (1.08-2.81)
Prepares for teaching sessions†	54 (38.0)	57 (30.2)	1.35 (0.84-2.17)
Directs teaching according to needs of learners†	55 (38.2)	62 (33.0)	1.29 (0.81-2.06)
Attitudes toward teaching			
Enjoys teaching house staff†	121 (84.0)	128 (66.3)	2.70 (1.60-4.60)
Rates self highly as a role model for house staff†	68 (48.2)	59 (31.1)	2.12 (1.32-3.39)
Enjoys teaching medical students†	47 (32.6)	46 (23.8)	1.80 (1.09-2.98)
Perceives role models to be important in medical education†	44 (31.0)	47 (24.4)	1.54 (0.93-2.54)
Believes role models influence trainee's career†	37 (25.7)	46 (23.4)	1.27 (0.75-2.14)
Notes strong influence of role models on own career†	63 (44.4)	79 (41.6)	1.26 (0.80-1.99)
Building relationships with house officers			
Organizes end-of-month dinner	121 (84.6)	143 (76.1)	1.90 (1.10-3.50)
Shares professional experiences with house staff†	58 (40.3)	54 (27.5)	1.73 (1.07-2.78)
Shares personal life with house staff†	68 (47.3)	67 (34.0)	1.70 (1.10-2.70)
Learns about the lives of house staff†	71 (49.3)	71 (36.0)	1.69 (1.07-2.67)
Brings doughnuts to house-staff team	92 (64.3)	112 (59.9)	0.76 (0.47-1.21)

Note: Characteristics were assessed after adjustment for assigned teaching responsibilities. Adjustment for assigned teaching responsibilities included both months spent as an inpatient attending physician (on the wards, in the coronary care unit, or in the ICU) and number of sessions per week as a preceptor in an outpatient clinic. Because of rounding, percentages do not always total 100. All percentages have been calculated on the basis of the number of physicians with valid data available. For each variable, physicians with missing data were omitted from the calculation of odds ratio.

*For characteristics related to the amount of time spent in teaching, odds ratios are expressed in relation to a reference category (odds ratio, 1.00). For other characteristics, odds ratios show the likelihood of identification as an excellent role model among physicians with the characteristic as compared with those without it, unless otherwise specified.

†For this variable, the "high" group is compared with the combined "low" and "medium" groups.

Abbreviation: CI, confidence interval.

(Reprinted by permission of *The New England Journal of Medicine*, from Wright SM, Kern DE, Kolodner K, et al: Attributes of excellent attending-physician role models. *N Engl J Med* 339:1986-1993.)

excellent role models, probably because they were interested in teaching and were well known to house officers. However, it is interesting that generalists were considered better role models than subspecialists, including those who spent a lot of time on a consulting service. This would suggest that the desired shift in favor of primary care over subspecialty care has been achieved among house officers.

It is reassuring that physicians who stress the importance of the doctor-patient relationship are recognized as excellent role models, as this is at the heart of the issue of teaching in clinical medicine and may be jeopardized by managed care priorities of cost control and care of populations rather than individual patients. Recognition of the importance of psychosocial aspects of patient care is appropriate and not surprising.

Physicians involved with research were less likely to be recognized as role models because they spent less time teaching. There are only so many hours in a day, so this is to be expected. However, it is of concern if we hope to train physicians for academic medicine. Physicians who were satisfied with their positions were identified as excellent role models most frequently. Discontent among current physicians threatens the successful training of future physicians.

E.J. Cohen, M.D.

13 Office Management

Practice Management

by Patricia M. Salmon

Much of the discussion in practice management this past year has focused on two "hot" areas: Y2K and billing and coding compliance.

By now, you have heard endless stories about the problems that may happen with computers and computer-dependent equipment at the stroke of midnight 2000. Hopefully, you have already ensured that your computer and computer-related equipment are compliant, and you have back-up plans developed in case they are not.

No doubt, you have also read equally as many articles about the government's commitment to crack down on fraud and abuse and the importance of a compliance plan to help you avoid the risk associated with coding and billing.

Both of these topics are critical to practice operation and future success. They do, however, represent only two areas where practices are at risk or potentially noncompliant.

Compliance, translated into business terms, is an effort to avoid allegations of illegal business procedures. Is the potential for allegation in your practice—is the *risk* for your practice—limited to billing and coding or your computer's ability to operate on January 2, 2000? Certainly not.

To demonstrate the fact that risk is everywhere in a practice, consider the following:

1. Does your practice have written triage procols for screening phone calls?
2. Does non-clinical staff give instructions over the phone?
3. Is patient information discussed casually either within the practice or outside of the office?
4. Are the practice's problems discussed casually either within the practice or outside of the office?
5. Does your practice keep a log of tests ordered to ensure that results are received and reviewed?
6. Are patient-related phone calls documented?
7. Is your Occupational Safety and Health Administration (OSHA) Manual up to date?

8. Do you have a standard methodology for screening and hiring new employees?
9. What is your policy on checking references?
10. Do you ask for a release before checking references?

If the answer to any of these questions is "no," the practice is non-compliant. It is at risk for some type of allegation.

Take the concept of risk one step further:

1. *Do your office policies create risk*? Does your office have a Policy and Procedure Manual which governs office operations—both in terms of office operations and personnel? Where is that manual? Collecting dust on a shelf? Is every employee required to review it as part of their introductory period? Do employees indicate their understanding of the policies in writing? Is that attestation statement in the employee personnel file?

   When was your manual last updated? Practices that do have manuals create risk by failing to live up to stated policies and to keep existing policies current in all respects.
2. *Does your corporate culture create risk*? The creation of a written policy and procedure manual is often viewed as a luxury—particularly in smaller practices.

This is true for many reasons:

a. No one has time to develop formal policies. "There are more important things to do."
b. No one has time to update policies annually.
c. "Everyone knows what they are supposed to do." "We are small, we talk every day." "We are trying to keep expenses down." "It takes time to do policy manuals." "We don't want to spend the money."

While there is no doubt that it takes time to develop effective policies and procedures and to keep those policies up-to-date, the above-mentioned mindset implies that it is okay to "fly by the seat of your pants." Flying carries some risk: It takes only one "oops" to cause a great deal of damage.

As we enter a new millennium, it is critical to address Y2K and billing and coding compliance issues. It is, however, also critical to recognize that compliance and risk management are one and the same. They are not just a "gimmick" used to promote discounts on malpractice insurance or to drum up work helping you keep the "Feds" out of your practice. Compliance and risk management are synonymous with good-quality patient care and overall business success.

Building a Compliance Program: Guidelines for Physician Practices
Hart R, Sheidy D (Coopers & Lybrand, Harrisburg and Pittsburgh, Pa)
Med Group Manage J 45:17-22, 1998 13–1

Background.—Physician practices are now being closely monitored for compliance with federal legislation. Submitting a claim based on incorrect coding can result in a civil monetary penalty or a criminal penalty if willful misrepresentation is detected. Aberrant billing practices may trigger a review that is costly in time and legal fees and can even affect reputations. Many physicians remain unsure of Medicare's documentation requirements and rely on "default coding," which can trigger audits. The government uses software programs to detect aberrant billing patterns and also relies on *qui tam*, or "whistle blower" lawsuits.

Compliance Programs.—To avoid suits and investigations, many health care organizations are establishing an effective compliance program. Responsibility for this program must rest with a compliance officer, who should develop the program, establish policies, oversee monitoring, train staff, report findings, and initiate corrective action as necessary. Physician practices can consult the U.S. Sentencing Commissions Guidelines for Organizations on voluntary disclosure. These guidelines include establishment of standards and procedures; designation of a compliance officer; establishment of procedures; training and monitoring; and disciplinary and corrective action plans as necessary. The Health Care Financing Administration's documentation guidelines should be used to review evaluation and management codes for office and hospital visits. The current procedural terminology coding system changes annually, so CPT coding courses are important to stay current. Continuous audits and physician profiles are necessary to detect problems, and feedback must occur to correct these problems. A formal disciplinary process must be in place. Because most "whistle blower" suits are brought by disgruntled employees, a compliance program should provide a method for resolution of employee concerns. It should be emphasized that the use of billing companies does not resolve physician responsibility for accurate coding and claims submission. The billing company should be audited as part of the compliance program.

Conclusions.—The fraud provisions of the Health Insurance Portability and Accountability Act should encourage physicians to ensure that coding procedures are accurate and internal monitoring procedures are in place. Compliance programs are an important step in ensuring compliance with federal regulation to reduce liability and avoid government audit.

▶ Early 1998 was surrounded by much controversy over the 1997 multi- and single-organ system Evaluation and Management Guidelines slated for implementation by the Health Care Financial Administration on July 1, 1998. The complexity of those guidelines generated more physician involvement in this aspect of practice management than I had seen in a long time.

The indefinite delay in the implementation of these guidelines raises concern as to whether physicians will continue to recognize the importance of their role in proper code selection and documentation. This article reinforces a practice's vulnerability to third-party audits and government sanctions.

The 1995 evaluation and management documentation guidelines are in effect. Practices can, and will, be audited based on existing criteria. In my experience, the area of documentation that is most vulnerable during an audit is the area of medical decision making. Practices must take a proactive approach to ensuring the accuracy of current procedural terminology and ICD-9-CM coding and the documentation of service provided. Even the smallest practice should have an internal process in place to monitor compliance in that area. This article provides practical suggestions for how to accomplish that goal.

P.M. Salmon

HIPAA Hits the Group Practice Radar Screen: Administrative Simplification Provisions and Issues

Tennant RM (MGMA Government Affairs Dept, Washington, DC)

Med Group Manage J 45:9-14, 1998 13–2

Background.—Part of the Health Insurance Portability and Accountability Act (HIPAA) is intended to simplify the administrative burden of providing and paying for health care. Once the regulations are finalized, the health care industry must be able to send and receive electronic transactions in a standard format within 2 years (3 years for small health plans). In 1998, the Health Care Financing Administration (HCFA) released 4 Notices of Proposed Rule Making (NPRMs). This article reviews these NPRMs and discusses the issues that remain.

National Provider Identifier.—Each health care provider will be issued an 8-digit alphanumeric National Provider Identifier. Part of the data in this National Provider System will include demographics of the physician's practice and business information. Providers, health plans, and clearinghouses will have restricted access to selected data. Each National Provider Identifier entry into the National Provider System is expected to cost the HCFA $60. Costs to providers during implementation (through 2004) will be $200 million, and health plans are expected to see a net gain of $1.7 billion over this time.

Standards for Electronic Transactions.—A standard form will be created for the electronic transmission of 9 administrative and financial transactions: health claims, health claims attachments, health plan eligibility, health plan enrollment, health plan disenrollment, health plan payment premiums, health care payment and remittance advice, health claim status, and certification and authorization of referral.

National Employer Identifier.—For conducting electronic health care transactions, each employer will be assigned a National Employer Identifier. This will be the current Employer Identification Number assigned by the Internal Revenue Service, although the HCFA admits that it has not yet decided how to handle National Employer Identifiers for employers with 1 or more Employer Identification Numbers. Note that employers will not be required to use the National Employer Identification. The costs for implementing this NPRM is estimated to be $1.5 billion over 5 years.

Security Standards and Electronic Signatures.—This NPRM was created to ensure the safety of transmitted data. Security standards fall into 4 categories: administrative procedures, physical safeguards, technical security services, and technical security mechanisms. Although physicians would not be required to use electronic signatures, those who did would have to follow certain regulations, such as the requirement that such signatures be cryptographically based.

Unresolved Issues.—Who will pay for implementing the HIPAA regulations, Congress or the health care industry through enumeration tariffs, user fees, and noncompliance fines? Also, which Federal agency will be in charge of ensuring HIPAA compliance? Finally, can group practice managers realistically be expected to comply with the HIPAA regulations given the projected year 2000 computer problems? Although the administrative simplification process is in its infancy, group practice managers must begin to prepare for standardized electronic transmission of health care data.

▶ Practices familiar with the HIPAA (and it is still surprising how many are not) have, most likely, heard about it through the fraud and abuse implications associated with it. This article discusses the far reaching implications of the HIPAA—and it is a bit unsettling,

Many small-to-medium–size groups are struggling with the financial implications of bringing their computers into Y2K compliance. The HIPAA introduces carrier-wide standards for electronic transmission as well as the probability of a national provider number and the ever controversial unique patient identification number. Any one of these items spells an outlay of time and money for the average practice.

Although none of these potential changes have been put into effect as of yet, the article reinforces the ever-increasing complexities associated with running a medical practice. The average practice may not have the administrative depth needed to tackle the complexity of some of these issues while still "making things happen" in the practice on a day-to-day basis. Although the article is not written to emphasize the need for professional management support; that is a lesson that should not be ignored as you read through it.

P.M. Salmon

Y2K a Serious Business Risk Management Issue

Lazarus SS (MSA Corp and Boundary Information Group, Denver)
Med Group Manage J 45:88-90, 1998 13–3

Background.—Has your practice addressed the Year 2000 computer problem? This article offers sound advice to make sure you are ready for business in the new millennium.

Managing the Y2K Problem.—Create a risk management team to identify and address the Y2K issues in your practice. The team will need to perform the following steps: First, inventory the information system and any devices that have a microcomputer chip (such as electrocardiography machines) to determine whether they are Y2K-compliant. Second, inventory all the infrastructure components of your facility that depend on computer chips, such as burglar alarms, elevators, and so forth, and determine whether they are Y2K-compliant. Third, rank all of the identified potential problem elements as to their importance in the maintenance of your basic business practices, and also as to their potential risk to patient care.

Fourth, estimate the costs to test and fix or replace each of the items, putting the highest priority items first. Then calculate the capital required and the operating costs, and allocate the funds so the work can be completed by the end of 1999. Note that if budget constraints are an issue, other capital improvements may need to be deferred in favor of making sure your practice is Y2K compliant. To keep on track, prepare a written document that specifies the action item, the budget, the time frame, and the person(s) responsible for making sure it gets done. Fifth, start correcting the problems. This step can take considerable time and resources, not only to replace equipment but to ensure that the upgraded equipment is Y2K compliant. In many cases, this will require upgrading current financial and clinical systems to the most current version to ensure that these systems are compliant with the vendors' Y2K upgrade fix.

Sixth, you have enough work to do to ensure your current systems are Y2K-compliant; so plan not to incorporate new software or computer devices until at least the second quarter of 2000. Seventh, identify key strategic business partners (major payers, hospitals, your bank) and identify and document contingency plans for continuing your business operations and patient care. Remember that the practice that is well prepared for Y2K has a competitive edge and may well be inundated with patient requests for care that its less-prepared competitors cannot provide. Eighth, test all interfaces (internal and external) thoroughly, testing them with business partners as necessary. Finally, create a validation protocol to evaluate every corrected system and device to ensure that it will work properly on January 1, 2000.

Sources of Information About the Y2K Problem in Health Care.—The RX2000 Solutions Institute sponsors a website devoted to health care; its Internet address is: http://www.rx2000.org.

▶ Much of the focus in the average practice in respect to Y2K has been geared toward billing and scheduling routines. Millennium readiness seems to vary significantly in medical practices. Many practices have discussed system considerations with their computer vendors and are moving toward necessary changes. Others have not yet gotten to that part of their "to do" list. That is particularly true of smaller practices which have bought low-end systems and do not have the support they need to consider their options. Not enough practices have gone further than their billing and scheduling routines, however. Very few have formal contingency plans.

This article provides an excellent checklist for practices in accessing their overall Y2K risk—- beyond the obvious areas. In addition, it includes several resources to help practices keep abreast of this critical area. On the downside, the article does assume a level of computer knowledge that does not exist in the average small practice.

P.M. Salmon

Making a Difference: What Staff Needs to Know About Service
Bradford V (The Bradford Company, Denver)
Med Group Manage J 45:55-62, 1998 13–4

Background.—Your office staff plays an integral role in patient satisfaction. This article describes tips for helping staff members realize that what they do *does* make an important difference in the lives of your patients.

Let Staff Know That Their Contributions Are Important.—Staff members have a direct impact on how patients perceive the practice. In fact, patients often say that staff members contribute in a significant way to their improved health. Conversely, patients also say that negative perceptions about staff contribute to their decisions to seek another physician. Therefore, make sure your staff knows that they make a real contribution to your patients' care. Even a quick note left on their desk can let staff know that you appreciate what they do.

Help Your Staff Build Relationships With Patients.—Despite the popular misconception, people really don't "just know" what it takes to provide good service. To build positive relationships with patients, staff members need information, feedback, coaching, and reinforcement. How to provide satisfying service to patients must be a part of staff training, and there are numerous keys to creating positive patient interactions. First, staff members should treat patients with respect and be friendly. They should offer patients encouragement, which also does wonders for patient compliance. Another key point is that staff should be aware of what is important to the patient and tailor messages accordingly. In a related manner, staff should realize that too much socializing or disagreement between staff members is not something patients want to see; it can make them feel ignored or unimportant.

Staff members should help educate patients; many patients are reluctant to ask their physicians for clarification, but they will ask a nurse or other staff member. Staff members must also truly listen to the patient and show an interest in what the patient is saying. Staff members should dress and carry themselves like professionals and should maintain a positive attitude, even when dealing with difficult patient situations. Difficult patient situations can be handled more easily if the staff member has empathy for the patient and truly listens to what the patient has to say.

Help Your Staff Build Relationships With Physicians.—Staff members should make an effort to know the individual physician's preferences, communication style, and personality and to be interested in the physician as a person. The best way for a staff member to earn the physician's respect is to be professional and competent, to use concise communications, and to have a positive attitude. Also, staff members should not be afraid of the physicians, even though some can be intimidating.

Help Your Staff Build Relationships With Co-workers.—The quality of the service that staff members provide to patients is directly related to how well staff members get along in the workplace. Staff should realize that conflicts are going to occur and that they should be handled in a problem-solving manner.

▶ Compliance, risk management, HMO quality indicators are all critical buzz words essential to the success of a practice. Although there are many facets to each of those items, they share a common bond: staff impact. Your staff is your most valuable asset. A good staff can make the worst systems work. You can spend all the money you want on computers, etc., and a poor staff will still struggle. This is not news to anyone. Unfortunately, however, staff training and development is an "under served" area in many medical practices.

This article reminds us that training and development go beyond teaching someone how to schedule an appointment or fill out a 1500 form. Practice success is aided by making Mrs. Jones feel as though she is the most important person who ever walked in the door when she arrives at the desk for her appointment—by having the resources available to answer questions or call for that taxi if needed; by remembering to smile even if you've had a bad day. Although much of what is discussed seems like common sense, this should be a must read article for every practice.

P.M. Salmon

---

10 Keys to Running a Good Meeting

Lowes RL (St Louis)

Med Economics 75:73-82, 1998 13–5

Background.—Although physicians have traditionally considered meetings to be distractions from the work of patient care, they are attending more meetings than ever. Many resent time spent in this seemingly non-productive way. The answer: make meetings effective and productive.

Strategies for Effective Meetings.—Only meet when it is necessary, not just to disseminate information that could be delivered by other means. Only meet with a specific agenda and planned speakers with specific time limits. Assign meeting-oriented roles, such as time keeper, facilitator, and secretary. Schedule realistically and start and stop on time. Encourage promptness by putting important things near the top of the agenda. Meetings that end early encourage attendance. Announce ground rules for meetings and stick to them. Avoid traditional meeting formats to encourage creativity. Don't let trouble makers hijack the meeting. Assign committees to carry out the meeting's agenda and trust their findings. Assign follow-up action so implementation occurs. Inviting a meeting expert to attend and offer suggestions can help to break a group out of a nonproductive rut.

Conclusions.—Physicians may resent the increasing number of meetings they must attend but also understand that these meetings are an essential part of their work. With good planning, meetings can be both effective and brief.

▶ Many of the groups with which I have worked express frustration with the lack of decision making within their group. One of the first things I do when I hear this concern is ask to sit in on their next group meeting. Contributing factors to this dilemma become apparent as such meetings proceed. Meetings are conducted without a formal agenda. The meeting, therefore, lacks structure from the start. Meeting participants often drift in at different times throughout the meeting. Because they were late, these members often then sidetrack discussions, revisiting issues that have already been addressed and, occasionally, resolved. And, too much time is often spent on topics that should be referred to a committee.

No one likes to spend their early mornings or evenings in meetings less than I. They are, unfortunately, essential to the success of any entity. The points raised in this article are key to increasing meeting productivity and business profitability and to making them much less tedious for everyone.

P.M. Salmon

The Seven Deadly Sins of Physician Practice Management: How to Stop Committing Them to Gain a Competitive Edge

Sterling J (Smock Management Consultants, Lake Forest, Ill)

Med Group Manage J 45:17-22, 1998 13–6

Background.—Today's physicians and practice managers face unprecedented challenges in the health care marketplace. This article describes the type of internal, self-imposed challenges many practices create and how to avoid these mistakes.

The "Seven Deadly Sins" of Physician Practice Management.—First, practices often fail to make management decisions with a sense of urgency. If part of this delayed response is caused by searching for universal consensus on big decisions, one must realize that this is rare and should act accordingly. Second, physicians often prefer to perform a procedure or prescribe a treatment only after they know that others have successfully done so before them. But rather than asking what other groups are doing (which may or may not work for your patient base), try solving the problem in such a way that you gain a competitive advantage. Third, practices often chase the latest management trend. Rather than chasing trends, implement management processes and structures that will more definitely make a difference.

Fourth, practices often fail to accept management concepts that have proven successful in other industries, such as creating strategic plans, marketing, and taking a total quality management approach to patient care. Try them, they work! Fifth, practices often create meaningless networks. Rather than spending energy and money on networks to which no one is truly committed, spend those resources in alliances that will actually strengthen the practice. Sixth, practices often resist change; this resistance, and the denial that anything needs to change, prevent progress. Seventh, practices often adopt the "hamster wheel" strategy: running harder and harder to maintain the same income. Physicians should develop a strategy that focuses on our control of a greater share of health care dollars.

How to Avoid These Pitfalls.—The first step is to recognize these pitfalls in your practice and decide to do something about them. Make decisions and take action to remove these obstacles. Develop strategies that help you build revenue in ways other than seeing more patients or performing more procedures. Create alliances that can truly benefit your practice, and commit to making them work. Make sure your partners and staff are also avoiding these pitfalls, and be ready to deal effectively with those who are not. Apply proven management techniques such as developing a strategic plan and marketing your services; these techniques really do work for medicine as well as for other industries. Focus on making your patients satisfied and on providing measurable outcomes (both clinical and financial). Finally, focus on what *you* need to do, not what others are doing. Certainly, be aware of what the competition is doing, but use that information to create other approaches that give you a competitive edge.

► The first half of this article paints a rather dismal, but all too true, picture of how many practices are run. The 7 deadly sins, as described in the article, are, in fact, alive and thriving in many medical practices. There is a lesson to be learned from the discussion of these sins. All too many practices waste time and dollars responding to the latest trend when those dollars might have been better spent in a better management information system or effective staff development. Other practices have taken a more conservative "wait and see" approach changing little and assuming that patients will still come because they always have. Although there are certainly examples of how each approach has worked for a practice, they are even more examples of how it has not.

The real lesson of this article comes in the last quarter: Stop spending all of your time looking over your shoulder and focus on the things about the practice that inhibit progress. Correcting the "sins" and playing to your strengths as they apply to the market is probably the best recipe for a successful practice.

P.M. Salmon

Train Your Newly Hired Physician the Right Way
Beck LC (Advisory Publications, Conshohocken, Pa)
Physician's Advisory May:1-2, 1998 13–7

Background.—Most newly recruited physicians to your practice are well prepared clinically. However, the recruit will not be prepared for how your practice operates. Setting aside the time for a couple of meetings each month can orient new colleagues to their role in your practice and help improve their efficiency. This article offers a 4-part plan for ensuring that your new colleague is happy and productive in the new role.

Teach.—Each new colleague must "learn the ropes" of your practice. As the employer, you have the right and the obligation to ensure that the new physician is indoctrinated into your systems. Items to teach your new colleague include making chart entries. Although this might be considered too basic to teach to an accredited professional, nonetheless chart entries must be consistent in style with those of the other physician(s) in the practice. Another important area for education is selecting the correct diagnostic and procedural codes, which is particularly difficult for newcomers. Other areas include the responsibilities of each office staff member, budgeting and a financial overview, restraints of managed care contracts and other managed care protocols, and ancillary operations such as laboratory and radiographic studies. Teaching sessions can also include more subjective issues, such as hospital demeanor and issues regarding referral.

Mentor.—One partner should serve as the new person's mentor. This role should be looked upon as a privilege and taken seriously.

Communicate.—The mentor should make sure the new physician knows what he or she is doing right—and just as importantly, what is being doing wrong. Constructive criticism and helpful hints help give your new colleague performance feedback. A lack of feedback is the number 1 complaint of new associates.

Evaluate.—In addition to daily comments, a structured process for evaluating the new associate should be instituted. For example, the mentor might give the other established physicians in the group a written evaluation form for assessing the new member. Then the mentor can cull these comments and provide the new member with both the good points and the areas needing improvement. An appropriate schedule for these formal evaluation meetings might be quarterly during the first year, then semi-annually.

▶ Established physicians reading this article may have a tendency to think "Great idea. Who has the time?" New physicians think "You have got to be kidding." Practices—particularly solos adding their first doctor—often experience unexpected delays in needed productivity once the new physician is on board. Simple things like finding supplies, filling out charge tickets, and interpreting "old" records takes a toll on the volume of patients a new provider can see on any given day. Practices would be wise to follow the advice presented in this article. Up front time with a new associate will result in a real return on your investment. Equally important, it will create a more collegiate atmosphere on all levels and help assure longevity.

A side that the article does not address, however, is the fact that the new physician probably comes to you with some valuable ideas and observations. Create an environment in which the new person feels comfortable sharing those ideas by designating a "feed back time" for them at each of your sessions.

P.M. Salmon

A Female Member Wants to Cut Back: Now What?

Beck LC (Conshohocken, Pa)

Physician's Advisory Feb:1-3, 1998 13–8

Background.—Practices nationwide face situations in which a female member wants to cut back her work level because of family responsibilities. The current article advises practitioners what to do in this situation.

Discussion.—Legally, female and male physicians must be treated equally. There is even a strong case for being more accommodating to female physicians who are of high value to the group. A member who is a valued practice "resource" should be employed for the sake of the practice's business interest. Female physicians can provide a "female perspective" that attracts new patients to the practice. Many women today seek female physicians. Female patients then bring other patients—husbands, siblings, etc.—into the practice. When a practice member wishes to cut back, compensation becomes an issue. A lighter work schedule merits less pay. However, many fixed costs, such as malpractice insurance, remain the same whether a clinician is working full- or part-time. Thus, a variety of expense factors must be considered. Another important issue is partner status. An excellent female physician may stay on the partner track or in the owner club, even if she cuts back her hours, just as a male senior member may remain a partner after "phasing down."

Conclusions.—Practices should be prepared for the possibility of full-time clinicians wishing to cut back. Policies can be established objectively to avoid subjective decision-making, which can lead to tensions among the practitioners, when the issue arises.

► For a long time, this question posed the greatest challenge to primary care practices. But more women have entered medicine, the issue has become pervasive. This article hits the nail on the head in respect to physician work schedules: don't wait until the first request for a leave of absence to develop a policy, and develop a policy that is gender neutral.

Many of today's physicians, male and female, have lifestyle issues that make it difficult for them to balance a full-time practice load and personal commitments. For some, those commitments are child related. For some, they may come in the form of an aging parent. Other physicians may take a different direction—for example, they may have political ambitions, whether on the local, state, or federal level or within their own medical society. Whatever the conflict, a balance benefits everyone—including the practice—if handled correctly.

This article offers a variety of perspectives on the topic, as well as an overview of a few practices' solutions. Equally as important, it points out that a successful group will not see this as a "woman's issue," but as a key ingredient in developing a successful and productive physician team.

P.M. Salmon

Ten Key Questions to Ask a PPMC Representative
Beck LC (Conshohocken, Pa)
Physician's Advisory Feb:5, 1998 13–9

Background.—Before entering a relationship with a physician practice management company (PPMC), it is important to investigate all aspects of the contract. There are 10 key questions to ask a PPMC representative.

Ten Key Questions.—First, clinicians should ask about the PPMC management: what restrictions apply to their PPMC? In other words, what keeps the management financially and emotionally committed to the company? Second, the clinician should ask about the PPMC's mission and goals. Third, what services does the PPMC provide, or what will the PPMC actually do in exchange for its management fee? The clinician should then read and re-read the proposed management services agreement carefully to determine to what extent and how the PPMC will control the practice. The fifth question concerns what the management services agreement provides if the PPMC does not deliver adequate services or breaches a material term of the contract. Sixth, what are the clinician's options if the PPMC is negligent, inefficient, or faulty in billing and collecting for the practice? Is there a restrictive covenant? If the clinician is to receive stock in the PPMC, when can he sell the shares? What are the clinician's options on a public offering? Last, the clinician needs to ask what other groups have signed on with the PPMC. These groups can be contacted to verify or obtain additional information.

Conclusions.—When asking these 10 questions, clinicians should be careful not to be sidetracked by incomplete answers. Clinicians must ensure that their interests will be well served by the PPMC and its proposed arrangements.

▶ Not a month goes by without our hearing of a group who has been contacted by a PPMC regarding a possible "relationship." At first blush, the idea of being relieved of day-to-day management frustrations, and being associated with an organization which can help you and your practice compete for that all-too-elusive contract, is more than appealing. The business of medicine has become overwhelming. The idea of selling your practice and going back to concentrating on patient care is a goal worthy of some sacrifice.

This article highlights critical points which should be considered during any serious discussions with a PPMC. Know the deal; don't get caught up in the glint and glitter of sales promotions and financial promises. Recognize that you are giving up a fair amount of control over many aspects of your practice. Over and above the effect the change may have on your day-to-day operations and staff, the loss of control may have an unexpected impact on your role in the practice as well.

Physician Practice Management Companies may be a viable option for some physicians, particularly those who are at the latter part of their career. There is, however, a lot more to the deal than you may realize. Proceed with caution.

P.M. Salmon

14 Medicolegal Issues in an Era of Health Care Reform

Legal Issues for Ophthalmologists: Choosing the Right Path

by Alice G. Gosfield, Esq.

In listing the legal issues challenging ophthalmologists and all other physicians, it would be impossible to overstate the rising importance of antifraud and antiabuse law enforcement efforts at federal and state levels. That the government has significantly intensified its focus in this regard can be seen in two policy documents through which they are trying to project a "kinder, gentler" fraud and abuse environment.

Ranging from a purportedly easier process to voluntarily disclose problems found to instructions from high levels in the Department of Justice to U.S. attorneys with respect to what types of false claims cases to pursue, the government is making efforts to indicate that it really is interested only in significant patterns of problems. The context is a confusing one to physicians and should be clearly understood and managed within the context of each physician's practice.

Against this background, two articles presented here describe in practical and realistic terms the risks physicians face and the methods by which they should be approached.

1. In "Physician compliance plans: Walking the walk—not just talking the talk," the real significance of efforts to prevent problems before they start and to correct those that may arise are discussed. The current landscape teems with consultants who claim to be in a position to develop compliance plans for all healthcare providers. This article makes the argument that the best plan is one that a physician will actually follow and therefore ought to be homegrown.

Similarly, in "Assessing the risks of physician false claims enforcement," the new false claims environment is explored. With recent announcements that pre-payment review is garnering far greater use by the carriers, it is clear that appropriate claims submission with the medical necessity clearly documented is the best safeguard against a cascade of events that can otherwise ensue.

Little appreciated in the world of fee-for-service false claims under Medicare is the developing interest of the government in fraud and abuse emanating out of managed care programs. From underservice as a quality-based false claims issue to physicians' claims submissions to a Medicare HMO, the fraud and abuse world is shifting its attention to managed care. Physicians who do not understand their risks in this setting remain ignorant at their own peril. "Fraud and abuse in managed care: The next wave" describes the new theories and initiatives at work.

Despite the significantly daunting implications of all of this fraud and abuse attention, there are positive steps that physicians can take to maximize their positions. Ophthalmologists, like all other physicians, are faced with a multitude of conflicting demands, from documenting their fee-for-service encounters, to becoming more efficient for managed care, to avoiding risk from malpractice liability, to focusing on disease specific behaviors. These pressures create significant challenges to most physicians who really would just like to practice medicine. In fact, the practice of medicine is conceptually expanded to include many of these business issues. At the same time, physicians and their business managers have not been very successful at finding a common language or common ground on which to accomplish multiple goals. In the last piece in this chapter, "Gosfield's unified field theory of health care management," a clinically based approach to managing administrative processes is offered as a potential solution to the fragmented nature of practice management. No one could deal with the multiplicity of forces at work on physicians today if these demands were managed as disconnected silos of activity. Using clinical practice guidelines as the basis for administrative systems seems to be an approach that offers physicians opportunities to build management systems from a foundation that reflects the way they actually think.

Over the last ten years, the legal issues faced by physicians have multiplied and crystallized. Throughout, however, common themes remain in play. Doing what is right for the patient in accordance with mainstream concepts of medical necessity, as appropriately documented, remains the bulwark against most forms of legal liability. Successful physicians will develop techniques to consolidate their positions even in light of these new challenges.

Physician Compliance Plans: Walking the Walk—Not Just Talking the Talk*

As health care enters an era of wary compliance with the federal fraud and abuse regulations, internists find themselves in an environment abounding with compliance warnings—and with compliance consultants. Many physicians are confused about the significance of compliance plans. This article describes the genesis of compliance plans, presents their essential features, debunks some common myths about them, and introduces specific compliance issues to which internists should devote attention.

Genesis and Revelations

The federal sentencing guidelines—which establish a rigid mathematical formula for imposing penalties on convicted criminals—have been the predicate for most compliance plans. Evidence that a defendant, even though convicted, had in place a systematic approach to prevent breaking the law can mitigate a federal judge's determination of the sentence.

The role of compliance plans in health care came about when the government settled its false claims case against National Medical Enterprises (NME) for $379 million. In that case, the Office of the Inspector General (OIG) of the Department of Health and Human Services also imposed a compliance plan on the company, requiring focused internal management of claims submissions, correction of the problems, and close monitoring by the government. Since then, all major settlements in the health care arena have required compliance plans; these include cases involving the University of Pennsylvania, the Tucker House nursing home, and SmithKline Beecham Clinical Laboratories.

Despite this historical link of the health care industry to the federal sentencing guidelines, internists ought to hope fervently that these guidelines never have any direct significance for them. However, there are two other reasons why internists should think about using a formal compliance program in their office:

1. The advent of *qui tam*, "whistleblower" lawsuits oriented around false claims liability; and
2. Evidence that proactive management of liability issues can forestall both the time and expense of a defensive position.

In 1996 and 1997, Congress increased and strengthened not only the penalties for false claims but also the avenues for enforcement. Even so, a major stimulant to false claims prosecutions is the reward: a whistleblower, or relator, stands to receive as much as 25 percent of any amount the government recovers in settlement or gains from a verdict in a case based on the whistleblower's information. The man who brought the National Health Laboratories case to the government's attention, for

*Permission granted to reprint from Gosfield AG: Physician compliance plans: Walking the walk—Not just talking the talk. *Today's Internist* 39:10-13, 1998. The American College of Physicians—American Society of Internal Medicine is not responsible for the accuracy of the translation.

example, gained more than $20 million. The three relators in the SmithKline Beecham Clinical Laboratories case will share $52 million.

Disgruntled ex-employees bring most of these false claims cases to the government's attention. The government is more likely to pursue a whistleblower case if the relator can show that the enterprise had ignored the problems brought to its attention. In addition, a separate provision in the law states that those who retain government money they know they are not entitled to—and do not take action to repay the sum—are criminally liable.

In this context, physicians should create an environment in which they work assiduously to comply with the law, assuring that their employees understand the practice's genuine commitment to do the right thing. Creating a culture of compliance requires the commitment and involvement of the physicians whose actions drive all other activities in the practice.

Approaching Compliance

After launching into the business of guiding compliance plans with its NME settlement, the government published its suggested "guidelines for compliance programs"—originally referred to as "model compliance plans"—for clinical laboratories, hospitals and others. Soon it intends to publish guidelines for physician practices, billing companies, managed care organizations and other enterprises. In the meantime, the American Medical Association has published its own compliance plan guidelines.*

It is a myth that an effective compliance program must follow a specific format. In addition, OIG's model plans are not a mandate. The law does not impose a specific way to adopt a compliance program.

Typical elements of an approach to compliance that will create a culture of doing it right include:

1. Documenting all processes and procedures in clear, usable and accessible formats to guide those in the office who can create or influence liability.
2. Creating a system to identify problems and bring them to the attention of those authorized to make changes.
3. Monitoring activities over time, to detect errors and demonstrate actions to solve problems.
4. Encouraging staff and physician continuing education and constantly refining plans to stay current.
5. Correcting errors by repaying amounts received improperly.

---

*For a copy of "Federal Fraud Enforcement and Physician Compliance," call the American Medical Association, 800/262-3211.

Homegrown Plans

Today there is a plethora of consultants who work with companies to develop compliance programs. Many of them have entered this burgeoning business in health care only recently. As a result, consultants vary in their knowledge of the technical content and the operational requirements of the closely watched Medicare and Medicaid programs.

It is not necessary to hire a lawyer to develop a compliance program. Lawyers, however, should play a significant role in establishing policies regarding the management of the information created by a compliance program, to take advantage of attorney-client privilege. Since there are so few health care fraud prosecutions, it is difficult to determine any consultant's track record of effectiveness. The proof comes when the physician practices that have hired the consultant survive overpayment audits or investigations—or better yet, prevent them.

A homegrown plan is far more viable for most physician practices. Depending on the size and complexity of the practice, with some outside assistance in using attorney-client confidentiality to protect information, many internal medicine practices can develop meaningful, functional compliance programs that both reflect their specific operating realities and foster a culture of doing it right.

It is extremely important that a compliance plan reflect the priorities and realities of the individual practice. In terms of liability, it is far worse to adopt a canned compliance plan that no one either adheres to or looks at than to have a simple, less grandiose system in place. Some practices, though, are large enough that undertaking a compliance plan that reaches throughout the organization would be daunting and time consuming; outside consultants are then necessary. However, it is essential to customize any process to reflect the day-to-day operation of the practice itself.

Problem Areas

For most physician practices, avoiding false claims liability is the compliance program's priority. Evaluation and management services documentation is a critical first step. Knowing when to bill for a consultation as opposed to a visit is another potential pitfall for most internal medicine practices. When the referral is for a specific evaluation of the patient with a written report back to the referring physician, who will use the findings in treating the patient, it is appropriate to bill for a consult. If the referral is to take over the management of a course of treatment for the patient, then bill all of the services as visits, not as consults.

Submitting claims for nonphysician practitioners is increasingly a challenge for internists. Medicare now pays for the services of nurse practitioners, physician assistants and clinical nurse specialists either as "incident to" physician services or as provided individually and paid at 85 percent of the physician fee schedule. For other ancillary personnel, the reimbursement options require strict adherence to the incident-to reimbursement rules.

Relationships with billing companies also merit attention in managing compliance issues.

Who is responsible for both procedural and diagnostic coding? Does the company have its own compliance program? What obligations are there to convey information received from payers? How knowledgeable is the billing company about differences in payer requirements? These are important questions to take into account.

Managed care fraud and abuse is now the focus of increased attention from the federal government. When physicians take on financial risk—via capitation or otherwise—working out the implications of the financial incentives as well as claims submission to the managed care program for fee-for-service payments becomes commensurately important.

High Level Commitment

It is beyond the scope of this article to identify all the issues to consider. It is undeniable, though, that avoiding false claims liability should command the attention of internal medicine practices. A compliance program approach also is applicable in other regulated areas, including those under the purview of the Occupational Safety and Health Administration, the Clinical Laboratory Improvement Amendments, the "Stark" and anti-kickback regulations, and—for some entities—antitrust laws.

The scope of a compliance program, the specifics of its implementation, and the cost of developing and operating one will vary from practice to practice. Nonetheless, physician practices should implement some type of systematic, organized approach to avoiding liability and encouraging employees to bring problems to the attention of those in a position to effect change.

As annoying as it may seem at first to establish a compliance program, its success requires commitment from the highest levels of the enterprise. The physicians whose liability is on the line must be involved intimately in the development, adoption and operation of a successful practice compliance program—they cannot delegate this undertaking.

Those who only talk the talk may well find themselves talking to enforcers they would rather not know.

Alice G. Gosfield, Esq.

Assessing the Risks of Physician False Claims Enforcement: Avoiding Pre- and Post-Payment Audit Should Be a Management Imperative*

In the wake of the now diminished PATH program and other initiatives scrutinized by Congress, the Department of Justice has issued guidelines professing a kinder-gentler approach to false claims enforcement.

The implementation of PATH and other efforts around nonprofit hospitals made fraud and abuse liability much more real to the bulk of the medical community. Congressional aggressiveness in the Health Insurance Portability and Accountability Act (HIPAA) and the Balanced Budget Act, providing major new weapons in the enforcers' armamentarium, did nothing to calm those fears (nor should it have).

It was not surprising then, that when HCFA launched new evaluation and management code documentation standards, many physicians for the first time began to understand the connection between documentation and fraud liability. Physicians hear that compliance plans are required by law—which is not true—and as a result, paralyzing paranoia and high anxiety characterize many of their reactions.

Still others do not believe the government can or will pay attention to them unless they have bad intent to defraud the government.

A realistic assessment of physician risk in the current environment lies somewhere in between. Staying out of trouble and deciding how to expend physician practice energies on these issues cannot be effective without a realistic understanding of the issues. This brief article looks at some of the issues related to a proper assessment of risk.

Intent

First of all, intent for fraud and abuse purposes is often not what physicians think. For criminal and civil false claims prosecutions, federal statutes provide that the standard is a knowing and willful submission of improper claims.

But caselaw has established that unartful coding, reckless disregard as to the accuracy of the claim, a pattern of improper claims, or even a decision to remain affirmatively ignorant of the appropriate rules can all be evidence of intent.

At the same time, the new Department of Justice position is that it will not pursue cases involving innocent mistakes. Whether physicians and the department have a shared perception of what qualifies as a mistake remains to be seen.

Apart from the cases that the U.S. attorneys will bring in court, though, HIPAA provided a very different standard for civil money penalties for false claims. Here, whoever submits claims they knew or should have

---

*Reprinted/adapted, with permission, from Gosfield AG: Assessing the risks of physician false claims enforcement: Avoiding pre- and post-payment audit should be a management imperative. *J Health Care Compliance* 1(1):52-53, 1999.

known demonstrate an improper pattern of services, including upcoding or ordering services which are not medically necessary, can lead to penalties of up to $10,000 per claim and triple the charges.

Significantly, the statute explicitly states that no proof of specific intent—"gee, I know, let's find a way to cheat the government"—is necessary to make these cases stick.

Most physicians do not knowingly submit claims for services they never provided. On the other hand, though, many physicians have been relatively recalcitrant in recognizing the need to learn and adhere to documentation standards relevant to their specialty.

Most physicians do not upcode, but they frequently under-document. Their anger at a generalized environment of less autonomy (in managed care and otherwise) and greater regulation interferes with effective compliance efforts. These are people, however, who got top marks in organic chemistry. Learning the documentation standards and making them work is indeed quite manageable.

As a practical matter, based on the new guidelines for prosecution, those physicians who have been reviewed in a post-payment audit who change their behaviors will likely not have difficulty when they are re-evaluated in the next subsequent time frame. (Once you have been tagged for repayment you are in the hopper for additional follow-up.) Those who do not change their practices will become fodder for the Department of Justice. Administrative processes, however, do feed the false claims pipeline.

Administrative Dilemmas

A new development, though, has the potential for more immediate and devastating effects for physicians. Where a carrier has reason to believe claims may not be proper or medically necessary the carrier may implement prepayment review, requiring additional documentation. In some cases this is done on every claim submitted and payment is held pending evaluation.

The dilemma here is that there are no procedural rules regarding this process. It can be imposed without appeal, evaluation, or challenge of the reason for the suspicions leading to it; and there is no limit on how long it may extend.

Some may recall statements made by OIG officials in the wake of the launch of the PATH program that the days of "pay and chase" were coming to an end. HCFA officials announced in 1996 to the Physician Payment Review Commission that they would place far more emphasis on prepayment review and they have been good to their word.

At the same time, post-payment audits, particularly of evaluation and management coding, remain a vital part of the government's initiatives as implemented by the carriers.

It is noteworthy that under HIPAA, carriers can lose the right to make fraud and abuse judgments if they are seen as too lenient. The post-payment process has been refined recently so it seriously limits approaches which had existed in the past. Equally troubling is the fact that the carriers have a certain degree of discretion in determining how to proceed.

Some carriers do an initial assessment of a number of cases, request repayment on those cases and do not proceed with any extrapolation of the results across a time frame. When they come to a determination that overpayments have been made, they offer three options:

- repay the entire amount within thirty days;
- repay the entire amount within thirty days and submit additional information for review but relinquish the right to a fair hearing to challenge any determination; or
- submit a much larger sample of cases but retain the right to go to a fair hearing.

Others do not use informal samples of review but move directly to stratified statistical sampling. The variability around the country is itself problematic.

What Does It Mean?

For most physician practices, avoiding pre- and post-payment audit should be a management imperative. Under the new guidelines, those who have been identified initially are at far greater risk for false claims liability than those who are being scrutinized for the first time.

Compliance plans are really not about the impact of the sentencing guidelines; they are about actually avoiding trouble and convincing the employees, by real behavior, that the practice is committed to doing the right thing. There is real risk in false claims liability. It is, however, mostly avoidable and worthy of concerted effort and attention to avoid the earliest steps that can lead to real trouble.

Alice G. Gosfield, Esq.

Fraud and Abuse in Managed Care: The Next Wave*

Many in the industry believe that the primary focus of fraud and abuse enforcement is fee for service false claims and anti-referral violations. In fact, managed care is a developing target of prosecutors and the Office of the Inspector General. Liabilities run both to the managed care entities (MCOs) and providers who do business with them. Quality is a specific focus of interest. This *AGG Note* (1) presents managed care fraud and abuse enforcement efforts to date; (2) discusses plan-based risks; (3) focuses on provider and physician based pitfalls; and, then (4) offers guidance for staying out of trouble.

Enforcement Efforts To Date

Enforcement against managed care based fraud is here today and will only increase in the future. At both state and federal levels initial skirmishes can be documented where managed care has provided a basis for penalties and prosecutions.

- A product manager at Blue Cross Blue Shield of Massachusetts senior division was convicted of making false statements to HCFA and intermediate sanctions were imposed on the plan.
- Blue Cross of Northeast Pennsylvania's Medicare HMO was assessed $700,000 in intermediate sanctions for failing to give enrollees the benefits packages the plan advertised.
- Medica and Pacificare were assessed overpayments of more than $600,000 each for claiming enhanced institutional payments for their Medicare HMO products.
- The California Department of Corporations in three waves assessed first 43 plans, then another 12 and later still another 25 plans for failing to comply with a 1995 law requiring them to notify enrollees of their right to complain to the Department of Corporations and of the Department's toll free number for complaints.
- In a Maryland state court, an HMO marketing executive was convicted of fraud for her role in supervising sales representatives that bribed state employees to get leads on Medicaid recipients.
- Texas slapped an $800,000 penalty on the Harris Methodist Health Plan for violating a state insurance regulation that prohibits health plans from using financial incentives to encourage doctors to withhold medically necessary care.
- Oregon fined Pacificare of Oregon for improper claims denial in a consistent pattern of denying payment of emergency services.
- In New York 18 MCOs were fined for non-compliance with the state's patients bill of rights.

*From *AGG Notes*, published by Alice G. Gosfield, Esq.

- The Texas Attorney General has just filed suit against 6 HMOs for improper physician incentive plans which motivate underservice.

New OIG Initiatives

In its Work Plan for 1999 alone, the OIG has identified fifteen separate managed care initiatives. Among them are for *plans*: (1) whether payments made to risk based Medicare HMOs are based on patients improperly classified; (2) payment for end-stage renal disease beneficiaries; (3) assessment of the usefulness of the national marketing guidelines for Medicare plans; (4) assessing HCFA's uses of and the quality of mandated HEDIS data submitted by plans; (5) under Medicaid, state uses of external quality review entities, and (6) how states detect and review for referral for investigation Medicaid managed care fraud. For *providers*, the OIG will, among other issues, focus on (1) physician incentive plans including contract language which may affect quality; (2) duplicate fee for service billing when capitation has been paid; and (3) enrollee access to emergency service.

New Theories Against MCOs

In addition, two novel theories of liability demonstrate the aggressiveness with which these issues are being addressed:

(1) In Florida, a US Attorney has filed kickback charges against providers and operators of an ERISA managed care program. ERISA as a federal employment benefit law has its own statutory and regulatory bases for false claims and kickback liabilities.

(2) In Pennsylvania, in the long term care arena, federal prosecutors have settled several cases where failure to provide appropriate services was the predicate for threatened false claims prosecutions. This approach has such significance for managed care that it merits review of the theory and the facts:

US v. Geri-Med and Tucker House was the first case. There, under the care of a now-defunct nursing home management company, patients were found to have serious decubitus ulcers. Rather than pursue the traditional remedy of closing the home to further admissions, the prosecutors investigated the cause for the decubiti. Geriatricians informed them that in addition to nursing care deficiencies such problems arise because of malnutrition. If the patients had been properly fed their conditions would not have deteriorated to such an extent. Their theory of the case then moved to one of threatening to charge the home and its managers with a false claim for every day of skilled nursing facility care for which they had received reimbursement since each claim inherently implied that the patients had been fed. When the home paid $565,000 to avoid the costs and risks of litigation, they entered into a settlement agreement that imposed a compliance plan which, in part, required them to adhere to the AHCPR clinical practice guidelines on treatment of decubitus ulcers.

Why discuss this case in the context of managed care fraud and abuse? Because the theory that claims for payment can be characterized as false when services impliedly part of the basis for payment are not provided is designed for managed care underservice cases. The US Attorney's Office in Philadelphia has distributed a managed care concern form which inquires of those who interact with managed care entities about the nature of the problems they have experienced when plans fail to deliver or authorize services. The Office is looking for the right fact pattern to use to either make new law or enter into a settlement which will have an intended chilling effect on problematic industry behavior.

The following actions of managed care entities have been identified by prosecutors as potential bases for these types of false claims cases:

- Denying treatment requests without legitimate medical evaluation;
- No standards for evaluation of claims;
- Assigning unreasonably high numbers of beneficiaries to providers making adequate service impossible;
- Specialist unavailability;
- Sending patients to skilled nursing care when they would benefit from rehabilitation services;
- Drug formulary issues which shift patients to preferred drugs and foreclose other options.

In addition to quality based fraud and abuse there are other business behaviors which can generate false claims liability: misrepresentations in sales regarding performance and outcomes, financial condition and history, provider and physician qualifications and availability; accreditation status; or even submitting selective or misleading data to obtain insurance department approval or HCFA approval could all be targeted as false claims in the publicly funded programs. And, of course, there are always mail fraud and conspiracy charges which federal prosecutors can use even where commercial plans are concerned. In addition, Congress has dealt with specific managed care fraud and abuse concerns.

Traditional Medicare Managed Care Fraud

Since the advent of Medicare and Medicaid managed care, Congress has provided weapons to address managed care problems.

Marketing issues are a major focus under §1876 of the Social Security Act dealing with Medicare risk programs. Not providing benefits advertised, expelling or refusing to reenroll expensive, sick beneficiaries and charging excessive premiums are all punishable by $25,000 civil money penalties (CMPs)—a program controlled by the Office of the Inspector General, and therefore not subject to ordinary judicial rules of civil procedure.

Other bases for penalties are even more ominous. Failure to provide medically necessary items and services that have adversely affected or have a substantial likelihood of adversely affecting an individual is punishable by a $25,000 CMP. Misrepresenting or falsifying information furnished to the Medicare program or "to other individuals and entities" is punishable by a whopping $100,000 CMP; and failure to comply with the rules governing physician incentive plans is punishable by a $25,000 fine.

Intermediate Sanctions

Where plans breach the imposed standards, Congress has provided a mechanism short of termination of their participation status. Where the Secretary of DHHS determines intermediate sanctions are appropriate, she may not only suspend enrollment of and payments for beneficiaries enrolled after a specific date, but also may suspend the plan's right to market to Medicare beneficiaries. The Secretary has imposed such sanctions even where plans have brought the precipitating problem to the attention of the government on their own initiative.

The Health Insurance Portability and Accountability Act of 1996 (HIPAA) extended intermediate sanction authorities to include situations whenever a plan is in violation of its contract with Medicare or is carrying out the contract in a manner "substantially inconsistent with efficient and effective administration." Civil money penalties are now up to $25,000 where the deficiency of the plan has a substantial likelihood of adversely affecting an individual and then up to $10,000 for each week the plan remains deficient. The plan is offered a chance to file a corrective action plan; and mitigating and aggravating factors are taken into account in determining the scope of the penalty to be imposed.

HIPAA and Managed Care

HIPAA has been the single most significant fraud and abuse enactment since 1977. In a major statement of its real commitment to the problem, Congress provided appropriations for enforcement and created a self-generating pool of money to feed prosecutors. Monies produced in recoveries, verdicts or settlements are retained in separate funds for prosecutors. As a result every state will have at least one Office of the Inspector General and some will have more by the year 2000. U.S. Attorneys have increased their ranks, and there are more investigators and FBI agents available to work on health care issues.

Reporting Requirements

In multiple sections of the Act, health plans including managed care plans—whether commercial or as part of the public programs—are now part of the army of fraud enforcers. HIPAA established a new clearinghouse for reporting of actions taken against providers (other than malpractice actions). "Health plans", for reporting purposes, include a policy of insurance, a contract of a service benefit organization (a Blues program) and a membership agreement with an HMO or other prepaid health plan. These entities must report final adverse actions which include civil judgments against a provider, supplier or practitioner. Proposed regulations were published in October, 1998.

Criminal Penalties

Since this statute extended fraud and abuse enforcement authorities in so many ways, it is not surprising that for the determination of what qualifies as a health care offense punishable by criminal penalties, the definition of the affected programs is extended to a "health care benefit program" which is defined to mean any public or private plan or contract affecting commerce under which a medical benefit is provided. This definition encompasses virtually every mechanism through which health care benefits are offered or paid, including ERISA plans and subcontracts under managed care contracts.

Penalties include fines plus up to ten years in jail for health care fraud, including theft or embezzlement. If the fraud results in bodily injury the violator can be sentenced to up to 20 years in jail. If death results from the scheme, life imprisonment may be imposed. Think of these penalties in light of the nursing home cases!

Fines and up to five years in jail may be imposed where false, fictitious or fraudulent statements are knowingly and willfully submitted "in any matter involving a health care benefit program." Under this extremely broad provision of the law, whoever is paid by a managed care program or submits claims to one is as liable for false claims as a plan, in relationship to government financing.

Enrollment Violations

HIPAA provided new civil money penalties for improper remuneration to induce individuals to enroll in specific plans. Improper remuneration includes waivers of co-insurance or deductibles, or transfer of free items or for other than fair market value, unless these are not offered routinely, are not advertised, or the waiver is offered only after a good faith investigation of financial need. Similarly, differentials in co-insurance or deductible amounts are permitted when they are part of health care benefit design, but only if such differentials have been disclosed to all beneficiaries, third parties and providers to whom claims are presented. Nor does remuneration include incentives given to an individual to promote preventive health, in accordance with regulations.

Physician Incentive Plans

Physician incentive plans and their capacity to stimulate underservice have been targeted in two separate congressional issuances: in the Medicare risk statute as well as in Stark II. Luckily, for once, a single set of regulations (March 27, 1995) addresses both programs. These rules impose obligations on plans but they, in turn impose administrative burdens on providers so the plans can comply with the law.

The fundamental principle of these provisions is that a Medicare or Medicaid plan, and those intermediate entities operating within such plans, must not make specific payment to physicians as an inducement to reduce or limit medically necessary services with respect to a specific individual. If the physician incentive plan places physicians at "substantial financial risk" for referral services, then plan must provide adequate stop loss protection and conduct periodic surveys of previous and current enrollees to determine enrollee access to and satisfaction with the HMO's services. In addition, the plan must furnish descriptive information to the Medicare program to permit a determination of whether the plan is in compliance with these requirements.

"Substantial financial risk" has been defined to focus on several aspects of the physician payment system: such risk exists only when a physician entity is given financial risk for more than its own services. Downstream risk for referrals is a necessary predicate to the application of the rules to an intermediate entity. Referral services means any specialty, inpatient, outpatient or laboratory services that a physician or a physician group orders or arranges for but does not furnish directly. In addition, risk only exists for these purposes when the physicians are at risk for more than 25% of the payment they could get as a maximum. Simple capitation for physician services is not substantial financial risk. Risk of no more than 20% is *not* substantial and therefore not regulated under these rules. Physician groups at risk for less than 25,000 covered lives are at risk unless that number is reached on the basis of establishing pools of physicians. The rules for establishing pools are also specified. Even where such risk exists, the rules do not prohibit the arrangements, but rather require the specified safeguards.

Safe Harbors

The federal anti-kickback statute, which now applies to all federal payors, has been interpreted in safe harbor regulations which have implications for managed care relationships. Violation of the statute has long been criminal, but the Balanced Budget Act of 1997 provided for a $50,000 CMP for each violation. Keep in mind that for CMPs, no proof of criminal intent is required.

The safe harbor regulations related to managed care programs have mostly focused on plans waiving co-insurance and deductibles or offering certain inducements for enrollment, issues which HIPAA has taken even further.

For physicians, the safe harbors offer some protections when they discount their fees in order to obtain business from a federally paid managed care entity. The Medicare+ Choice regulations (see below) will apply these provisions to those types of entities and their relationships with providers too.

Price reductions offered to health plans do not violate the anti-kickback statute if certain requirements are met. In the 1992 managed care safe harbors, price reduction discount issues are addressed in the context of Medicare or Medicaid cost contracts. The term must be one year, the services, items and methodology of payment must be specific and the plan must accurately report on cost reports the amounts paid to contract providers. And the provider may not seek additional payment for the discounted services. The 1996 safe harbors extended these protections to capitated arrangements too in accordance with similar criteria.

The dilemma for providers under these provisions is that they only protect for the amount of the discount in obtaining the business. There is a separate provision under the Social Security Act (§1128(b)(6)) which permits a provider to be excluded from the federal payment programs if the provider or practitioner charges Medicare substantially in excess of its usual charges. There have been no standards yet established as to what qualifies as the "usual charge".

Prior to the advent of RBRVS, physicians were paid on the basis of the lower of their usual charge or the reasonable charge. This provision created individual physician profiles. With RBRVS, payment is made on the lower of the actual charge or the fee schedule amount. There is no longer a usual charge calculated under Part B.

Last year, two proposed regulations would have initially addressed this provision. The proposals were so controversial they were ultimately dropped, but they offer some insight into the government's concerns over the relationship between discounted managed care and fee-for-service Medicare payments.

In one issuance HCFA would have taken the position that if a physician or provider bargains with a managed care plan for a discounted rate, and that rate is below Medicare rates, but Medicare is a secondary payor, Medicare would have no obligation to cover the difference. The second version was much more directly interpretive of the exclusionary authority. Here HCFA astoundingly took the position that the usual charge would be any charge made to any customer. Needless to say this would have disrupted virtually all managed care contracting arrangements. The proposals were withdrawn, but they do portend additional regulatory controls over charging practices.

Today, providers have no standard against which to measure their behavior under the statute. We do not know how much discounting by payor mix would trigger the exclusionary authority. We generally advise our clients that if the volume of discounted business of a physician group or physician approaches 40% it is time to keep tabs on what charges are being made fee for service to the Medicare program.

Medicare+ Choice Issues

The themes of anti-kickback, safe harbors, physician incentive plans and intermediate sanctions are all present in the Medicare+ Choice "mega-reg", which HCFA published on June 26, 1998 as an Interim Final Rule with comment period. Many of its provisions are so detailed and potentially unwieldy that as this *AGG Note* was being written, HCFA expected to revise some of its more onerous provisions. It is unlikely HCFA will back off much on the fraud and abuse sections. Although Congress may also intervene, fraud and abuse remains a major concern and its focus therefore unlikely to be watered down.

In addition to stating that the anti-referral and physician incentive plan provisions apply within Medicare+ Choice plans—which include HMOs, CMPs, medical savings accounts (MSAs) and PSOs—HCFA also stated that any grounds for termination of a Medicare+ Choice contract would also be grounds for intermediate sanctions including submission of false data to HCFA.

In a departure from other regulatory issuances though, HCFA also went further to require Medicare+ Choice plans to have a compliance program in effect which must include written policies, procedures and standards of conduct, the designation of a compliance officer accountable to the senior management of the organization, provisions for internal monitoring, auditing accountability, and an adhered to process for disclosing repeated violations of the law by the organization "or their subcontractors".

Not only is the regulatory imposition of a compliance plan dealing with fraud and abuse a major departure from the voluntary efforts of every other government effort to date, the last phrase puts these plans in the position of snitching on their providers. This approach means all providers doing business with Medicare+ Choice plans should expect to have these plans require *them* to have compliance plans in place and those plans will have to deal with quality concerns in addition to billing and other administrative issues. This emphasis only shines further light on developing concerns around provider behavior in managed care programs.

Provider Pitfalls

Similar to managed care entity concerns regarding underservice, prosecutors are also interested in the ways in which physicians respond to financial incentives. Examples of provider behaviors which prosecutors have cited as worthy of attention include:

- Inflating encounter data to get higher capitation rates and conceal underutilization;
- Submitting duplicate claims to the primary payor when the physician has already received capitated payments, which, actuarially, is intended to cover all financial risks for that patient (This type of behavior has been cited by plan attorneys in the commercial sector as a basis for their concerns about false claims.);
- Paying kickbacks to primary care physicians for referrals to fee for service specialists;
- Splitting fees with non-participating (out of network) physicians;
- Inconvenient office hours or locations to discourage visits by capitated patients;
- Making the patient come into the office for prior authorizations when he can't get around easily.

Practical Guidance

This brief survey of the context for managed care fraud and abuse makes it clear that providers and plans will have new pitfalls to consider in managing fraud and abuse risk.

1. Compliance plans for MCOs and provider entities should take managed care liabilities into account in design and implementation.

2. Providers should expect MCOs to require that they represent that they have a compliance plan in place, and providers dealing with Medicare+ Choice programs can be assured of such requirements. Some MCOs may even impose the terms of certain elements of compliance plans.
3. Those who advise MCOs suggest a range of fraud avoidance activities which extend from hiring investigators to pursue questionable provider behavior about providers to simply thinking about how the plan could be victimized. Some steps which are more mainstream include:
   - Develop fraud screens in computer software programs to detect billing problems.
   - Require compliance plans in provider agreements.
   - Contract to allow investigators to come into providers when a problem is suspected.
   - Develop model programs for contracting providers.
4. That blueprint for MCOs should motivate corollary activities from providers:
   - Ask what fraud and abuse avoidance programs the MCO has in place.
   - Ask for explicit rules regarding billing requirements of the plan.
   - Do not agree to allow plan investigators to come into the office unconditionally.
   - Develop your own compliance program which addresses the legitimate concerns of MCOs.
5. All managed care players—plans and providers—should pay attention to clinical behavior which results from financial incentives. Use of clinical practice guidelines as a safeguard against underservice and overservice will be important in defending any challenge from a government investigator. (A forthcoming *AGG Note* will elaborate further on how guidelines can serve multiple purposes.) Jim Sheehan, Chief of the Civil Division in the U.S. Attorney's office in the Eastern District of Pennsylvania has specifically cited the use of guidelines as a protection against fraud and abuse based on quality.
6. All public statements used in marketing, responding to RFPs, or reporting to state agencies which contain factual statements (e.g., qualifications of physicians, success rates on surgeries) should be reviewed carefully for accuracy.
7. All statements (including balance sheets, profit and loss statements, cost reports) made to federal payment sources (or those who get money from federal sources) to obtain managed care payments should be scrutinized carefully for accuracy.

8. Submission of claims to managed care payors should be incorporated as a matter of course into provider billing compliance programs.
9. Providers which accept financial risk—whether physician groups, IDSs or PHOs—should consider their activities equivalent to those of an MCO and reevaluate their fraud and abuse risk in that light.
10. Quality improvement activities and utilization management systems should be reviewed and evaluated in light of fraud and abuse exposure.

Conclusion

Better MCO internal information systems (by comparison with physician groups at least) will make it easier for prosecutors to show improper behavior. Invidious comparisons between care provided to MCO patients and care under programs without financial incentives to control services ought be considered by provider managers as an operational risk. Quality as a fraud and abuse issue will be targeted in the world of managed care. Like most fraud and abuse liability, these risks are manageable; but to avoid liability, managed care fraud and abuse risks first must be appreciated and addressed.

Alice G. Gosfield, Esq.

Gosfield's Unified Field Theory of Health Care Management*

Since failed Clinton health reform, physicians have been subjected to many multiple mixed messages on how to change their behavior to conform to new realities. From false claims liability to risk management and functioning efficiently for managed care, physicians are pummeled from all directions. At the same time, business managers struggle to communicate effectively with physicians around business issues. Within this context a new way of thinking about how to conduct health care businesses may be useful. This *AGG Note* elaborates a theory about how to integrate clinical predicates into administrative processes to achieve multiple goals. The theory is potentially applicable in physician practices, independent practice associations and similar MCOs physician practice management companies, hospitals and HMOs.

Conflicting Mixed Messages

From 1982 with the Tax Equity and Fiscal Responsibility Act through the Balanced Budget Act of 1997, in the last fifteen years each congressional iteration dealing with health care has meant new and heightened regulatory, compliance and administrative challenges for health care businesses. For physicians the regulatory environment has become virtually unmanageable. Concurrently, the industrial revolution around them has required physicians to be more responsive to new managed care demands for efficiency and cost containment. Meanwhile, they still must manage their malpractice liability risks as well as compliance and false claims liability risks. Still further, new health care management processes, particularly in the guise of disease management programs[1] offer them tantalizing possibilities if they could only concentrate their energies in a singular manner. The conflicts present major challenges for health care managers in a wide variety of organizations who are themselves struggling to survive much less succeed in a changing market.

In an era when the American public is extremely concerned about the business values which seem to propel the existing health care environment, efforts to safeguard clinical quality become extremely important. Some players are revaluing the vital role physicians can play in accountable health care organizations which chart new courses to success.[2] Six themes characterize the shifting tides and eddies.

Fraud and Abuse

False Claims

Although recent government pronouncements from the Department of Justice proclaim a kinder, gentler civil false claims world, pitfalls abound. In fee for service Medicare, "incident-to" billing rules versus billing for nurse practitioners, physician assistants, and clinical nurse specialists with-

*From *AGG Notes*, published by Alice G. Gosfield, Esq. Copyright 1997 Alice G. Gosfield, Esq.

out those restrictive requirements is a decision many physician-related practices must now make. Inadequate documentation to support the level of the code submitted is, under the Health Insurance Portability and Accountability Act (HIPAA), a basis for civil money penalty (CMP) false claims. This authority, which is managed by the Office of the Inspector General and not the U.S. Attorneys, does not require the rules of court procedure. Penalties can rise as high as $10,000 for each improper claim plus triple the charges.

In addition, the Medicare definition of a consultation still eludes many. A consultation is a request from another physician (even a physician within the same group) for an evaluation of the patient with a written report back to the requesting physician. If the referring physician transfers the responsibility for a segment of the patient's care with the consult request ("consult and treat") or simply hands off to the consultant, none of the visits qualifies as a consult.

Violations of the anti-kickback statute are now punishable by $50,000 CMPs. Going even further, a case in federal court in Texas, *U.S. ex rel Thompson vs. Columbia/HCA*, has taken the position that Stark statute violations can qualify as false claims. This makes these laws far more attractive to prosecutors.

Quality as Fraud and Abuse

In *U.S. vs. GeriMed and Tucker House* in 1997, the U.S. Attorney in Philadelphia dealt with a significant quality failure in the skilled nursing facility context by charging the home with false claims. (See *AGG Note*, "Fraud and Abuse in Managed Care: The Next Wave", December, 1998.) PRO penalties, exclusions from the federal payment programs for premature discharge or failing to provide medically necessary services are examples of a plethora of fraud and abuse penalties related to quality.

In addition, the U.S. Attorney in the Eastern District is aggressively pursuing managed care under-service as a potential false claim. His concerns include referrals related to financial incentives in managed care, under treatment, inadequate service and availability of care. "Promises made but not kept" are his focus.

Managed Care Demands

In a 1995 study for the Physician Payment Review Commission it was found that HMOs and PPOs do not rely on financial incentives alone to motivate physician behavior. Prior authorization of services, clinical practice guidelines, postservice review and profiling of physicians were all cited as techniques to change care.

Physicians find themselves attempting to comply with a myriad of utilization management initiatives which are variable from plan to plan. Often they cannot learn the guidelines that are used to judge them. Infuriating physicians, plans cite ERISA preemption as protecting them from liability for these practices which only increases the tensions. (See *AGG Note*, "Managed Care and Liability: As The World turns", October 1997.)

Physicians and physician entities that take financial risk find that they must change their previous fee for service behavior to survive. For many physicians this is difficult because they fear malpractice liability for not providing traditional services to their patients. In addition, they worry that their behavior will stint on quality by responding to financial incentives.

Fee for Service Medicare Controls

While managed care makes its demands known, the fee for service environment in Medicare has itself become more daunting. In the last year, using prepayment review the carriers now often demand medical record documentation on a claim by claim basis prior to payment. This process has no limits. Some physicians find themselves with vast chunks of their practice subject to this slowed payment mechanism.

Post-payment audits for conformity with the documentation and medical necessity standards continue. Large dollar amounts are recouped but in the current approach, carriers offer compromised settlements only if the physician will waive fair hearing and appeal rights. These rights are only available when the physician who has been assessed an extrapolated over-payment agrees to a statistical sampling which is almost always less favorable to the physician practice. Post-payment review is a precursor to false claims liabilities since failure to respond effectively to an overpayment situation can lead directly into a false claims charge.

Malpractice Liability in a Dynamic World[3]

Data show that the malpractice liability for primary care physicians is increasing as the gatekeeping function changes Dr. Welby into Dr. No. ("No, you don't need that study.") Since historically it has been demonstrated repeatedly that patients do not sue the physicians whom they love, gatekeeping may begin to undermine the patient's view that the physician is acting purely in the patient's interest. Failure to diagnose continues as a significant risk. Characterized in the health plan context, this often takes the form of a suit based on the failure to perform a service which would have led to the diagnosis. Although the ERISA laws have seriously undermined plan liability, developing caselaw is increasingly eroding that insulation. More and more, MCOs find themselves faced with liability for the outcomes of their management systems.

Even as that liability increases, more provider entities are taking on increased financial risk. This transforms them into the same liability target as an HMO. When a provider sponsored organization (PSO) or integrated delivery system (IDS) takes on global risk as a percent of premium, the financial incentives that drive liability concerns about managed care entities will devolve onto the new structures as well.

Performance Measurement

From articles in *USA Today* addressing the state of managed care as reported by NCQA based on HEDIS data, to new law in Texas requiring performance measurement reporting, the emphasis on comparative quality performance is unarguably increasing. As more public entities—including the Pennsylvania Cost Containment Council, the New York Department of Health, the Medicare program and HCFA—publish data, some players about whom observations have been made use their rankings in marketing. For others, anxiety over the market implications of not ranking well has led a number of managed care plans to choose not to publicly disclose HEDIS data which they otherwise report to NCQA.

While the locus of reporting has been primarily HMOs, hospitals and IDSs publish their own report cards. Business coalitions and even health plans are now publishing physician and practice group data.

As employers increasingly restrict the insurance offerings they make available to their employees, MCOs find themselves in more intense competition with each other. The determination as to which organization will be offered by the employer is increasingly made on the basis of data. NCQA's HEDIS measures have become more clinical over time. Use of beta blockers postmyocardial infarction, diabetic eye exams, lowering cholesterol and treatment of asthma are all addressed in HEDIS measures. Moreover, Accreditation '99 of NCQA will use HEDIS outcomes in the accreditation decision. Twenty-five percent (25%) of a plan score will turn on reported HEDIS data. NCQA accreditation standards themselves focus on the plan's use of clinical practice guidelines, preventive health measures, and appropriately documented medical records, among other issues. This in turn drives the way plans relate to providers and practitioners.

Quality Improvement Generally

Physicians have traditionally been interested in what works for their patients. Medicine has always been dynamic, adopting better techniques and discarding old. Principles of total quality management and continuous quality improvement have been introduced into health care generally. Quality improvement has made its way firmly into public policy if not into health care corporate boardrooms. Medicare's new Quality Improvement System for Managed Care (QISMC) quality improvement will be a major factor in the Medicare+ Choice program.

These six themes define a range of market and regulatory demands to which providers, payors and managed care entities will have to respond. Within this context, new models of managed care are also emerging and capturing the attention of the industry.

New Approaches to Care

As managed care has evolved in this country, it has become clear that approximately eighty percent (80%) of the costs of health care are generated by twenty percent (20%) of the population. Management by financial incentives has not accomplished the goals that the original concept of managed care would have claimed. Still, providers coalescing into IDSs find that without some new management technique, they have little infrastructure to justify their reorganization. Three new approaches to care delivery offer the potential to take delivery of care to a new level.

Case Management

In 1989, case management and out-of-contract benefits were the fastest growing benefits incorporated in employer health plans. Today, case management is often embedded in managed care programs. This technique utilizes specially trained personnel, usually nurses, to intervene in either high cost or high volume patient cases to work with the physician, the family, and the payor to develop an organized plan of treatment across a continuum. The case manager helps to develop the treatment plan and then monitors its implementation with the relevant parties thereby optimizing resource consumption. Case managers are no longer an insurance company phenomenon. Hospitals, IDSs and physician practices use them, too.

Demand Management

Even in an aggressive managed care environment, hospitals, physicians, and MCOs find that patients still present in the emergency department for relatively minor issues. Demand management is the new approach to decrease unnecessary emergency services by using call-in centers and other triage mechanisms, including better patient education and self care. Patients often end up more actively involved in their own care. Although physicians can be initially resistant to others entering into the doctor-patient relationship in this way, successful demand management programs find that physicians are eventually pleased when they find that this approach decreases the burden on their offices.

Disease Management

Disease management combines both case management and demand management into condition specific processes which emanate at their core from a clinical practice guideline. By focusing across the full continuum of delivery sites and using creative interventions for more proactive patient compliance, this approach to care delivery is increasingly practiced by MCOs, IDSs, and large physician groups. Services are provided either by disease specific outside vendors or are developed in house. One commentator has used the following description of disease management:

> "An integrated system of customized interventions, measurements and refinements to current processes of care designed to optimize clinical and economic outcomes within a specific disease state by facilitating proper diagnoses, maximizing clinical effectiveness, eliminating ineffective or unnecessary care, using only cost-effective diagnostics and therapeutics, maximizing the efficiency of care delivery and improving continuously."

Typical disease states targeted are diabetes, congestive heart failure, asthma, high risk pregnancy, kidney stones, breast cancer, HIV/AIDS, high cholesterol, high blood pressure, arthritis, peptic ulcer, and depression.

Some have stated that a sophisticated disease management program requires eight elements:

a. Disease mapping;
b. Analysis of the cost of treatment;
c. Health economics research;
d. Formulary integration;
e. Practice guidelines;
f. Patient education;
g. UR management; and
h. Outcomes measurement and management.

Since the comprehensiveness of traditional managed care approaches has been a barrier to effective management of chronic care, this new more focused technique may have the capacity to increase patient satisfaction, improve the quality of life for physicians, maximize efficiencies and save money while improving care.

CPGs at Work

Clinical practice guidelines are the foundation for disease management. But "systematically developed statements to assist practitioner and patient decisions about appropriate health care for specific clinical circumstances", good clinical practice guidelines can be used in many ways.

1. Fundamentally, they help the clinician and patient decide what to do in a specific situation.
2. They can provide a basis to profile practitioner behavior to benchmark stellar performance and identify those who need assistance.
3. CPGs can be used to negotiate payment rates since they provide the only legitimate basis on which to make a judgment about what it actually costs to treat a patient for a specific condition.
4. From a risk management perspective, they can be used to define a standard of care.

There are good practice guidelines and then there are others. Many specialty societies now develop evidence-based, scientifically valid CPGs. On the other hand, some guidelines are utterly self-serving and simply reflect local variation without a scientific basis for such variation. The Institute of Medicine in its guidance to the Agency for Health Care Policy and Research identified eight attributes of good clinical practice guidelines which have gradually emerged into the standard of care for guidelines development.

A guideline alone, however, does not create any activist management of care unless it is linked with administrative systems. Translating a guideline into medical review criteria—yes or no statements which can be gleaned from the guideline for purposes of evaluating conformity—provides a basis on which to measure behavior in relationship to the guideline. Performance measures can be calculated from the application of these medical review criteria to the care provided. In other words, by counting the presence or absence of relevant elements in the CPG, one can determine the extent to which any practitioner, group, division, department, or any other focus of inquiry has followed the guideline. Based on that ratio, a number of conclusions could be drawn. This data can be used to profile clinicians, increase or decrease payment rates, or take corrective action against those who cannot comply. Besides these uses, however, it is a different more pervasive application of guidelines which forms the core of the Unified Field Theory.

The Theory in Practical Steps

By basing essential administrative processes on the platform of a CPG, the next nine steps provide the basis for coordinating administrative processes with clinical thinking.

1. *Select a clinical practice guideline for the analysis.* A national guideline is better than a local guideline since the premise for CPGs is that much variation in care has no scientific basis and science itself ought not vary by geography. Still, local variation is sometimes legitimate. For example, in the evaluation of an upper respiratory infection in a northeastern state, it would not be typical to consider whether the patient has Valley Fever. However, in Scottsdale, Arizona this would be appropriate.
2. *Translate the guideline into applicable ICD-9 and CPT codes.* This step links the guideline to typical billing and claims systems. This connection can give physicians clear direction as to what level of code to bill for their services in a system which relies on CPT codes.
3. *Translate the CPT code analysis into documentation standards.* Documentation is vitally important for physician practices but also provides a rational medical records system for MCOs and IDSs seeking to actually draw conclusions based on medical records. By using consistent medical records documentation processes, analysis across a universe of actors can be accomplished.
4. *Articulate the full pathway (activities of others besides physicians).* Clinical practice guidelines often speak in relatively cursory terms. The actual implementation of a full pathway of care across the delivery sites (inpatient, SNF, outpatient) and practitioners (nurses, therapists, specialists) who interact with the patient is frequently missing from this type of analysis. Moreover, clear guidance about when referrals are appropriate can be offered through this kind of rigorous clinical analysis. Reference to the full continuum of care is important from a risk management perspective to address follow up and continuity of care.
5. *Accommodate deviations from the CPG.* Sometimes a patient will have a co-morbid condition that the guideline does not anticipate. Deviation from the guideline is then not only clinically appropriate but required. Protocols to accommodate such deviations should be articulated as well.

6. *Analyze the cost of treatment.* In order to engage in clinically relevant cost management, it is essential to determine literally what it costs to treat a patient for a specific condition. For example, in the AHCPR guideline on treatment of otitis media with effusion in primary care, there is a point in the algorithm when the guidelines suggest that if the patient returns with the third infection it would be appropriate to consider a bone conduction study. The costs associated with this service would include not only the fixed costs of the examining table and the otoscope but also the paper on the table, the patient's gown, the cover on the otoscope, the tongue depressor to look in the patient's mouth, and the inputs of the physician and any ancillary personnel. These are the actual costs for that patient visit. Many physician practices and provider systems still focus on charges which in no way reflect the actual cost of treating the patient. Consequently, assessment of reimbursement rates is often dissociated from the actual costs of providing care.
7. *Measure compliance and outcomes from applying the guideline.* This is a process that takes place over time. While a computerized process would make the technique more efficient, this approach need not be applied comprehensively in any clinical setting. Initial applications can be done without such technology although, obviously, some personnel to gather the data will be necessary.
8. *Analyze the data.* There is no point in engaging in this exercise unless there are conclusions to be drawn from the application of the guideline.
9. *Review and refine.* Based on data about outcomes to patients as well as cost of services, the algorithm itself should be changed to reflect both the dynamism of medicine and what is learned from implementation.

Advantages

This relatively straightforward approach can produce meaningful data with multiple uses. It is essential for all health care organizations to know what works clinically and what it costs to produce positive clinical results.

This technique has the capacity also to provide for unified clinical management of patients in a logically justifiable manner. By beginning the analysis with state of the art clinical practice guidelines, there is no reason to treat patients differently, for the most part, on account of insurance benefits packages. Moreover, the disputes that have emerged in managed care about necessary and appropriate services can be focused in a far more persuasive manner using this technique.

This process can provide a basis to measure clinical performance for the purpose of improving efficiency as well as patient outcomes. By referring back to the guidelines as implemented, appropriate changes in process can be developed.

Perhaps most critically, this methodology speaks to physicians the way they think. Throughout the health care system there have been culture clashes between the worlds of business and clinical care. Business managers have difficulty persuading physicians to change behavior. Moreover, they are often unsure as to what behavior needs to be changed. Physicians live in the world of practicing medicine. Consequently, if business processes are to be changed without improperly impacting on clinical service, some clinically relevant analysis is necessary. This theory can create a basis for common understandings by business managers and clinicians.

Potential results include the following:

1. The process can lower the fraud and abuse risk from overservice, failure to document effectively as well as from underservice by integrating clinical needs with documentation standards to support them.
2. The technique can maximize efficiency without sacrificing quality. Physicians are legitimately anxious about cutting back in a way that could harm patients. There is often little dialogue of a clinical nature about how to contain costs. This process provides the ability to have substantive dialogue on that subject.
3. The data which can emerge is useful both for internal management purposes as well as for use in external negotiations. The process embraces the capacity to involve physicians in actual business management decisions in a way that works for them, based on real data.
4. Over time, the application of these kinds of techniques may eliminate intrusive medical management by MCOs. To the extent that a provider organization can demonstrate the ability to perform in accordance with guidelines and can produce data showing their results, MCOs which are increasingly liable for their medical management decisions, may be more comfortable in delegating authority to physicians who use this approach to act with greater clinical autonomy.
5. With the rigorous cost analysis associated with this approach, payment negotiations can be shifted to something more meaningful for the delivery system. Case rates are a logical analogue to the theory, but other methodologies based on budgets and outcomes can result as well.
6. This explicitly articulated system can preempt the heart of a malpractice claim and lower liability risks.
7. Finally, in many IPAs and other provider entities that incorporate otherwise independently practicing physicians, this technique creates the kind of clinical integration that is explicitly recognized by the Department of Justice and the Federal Trade Commission as appropriate to avoid antitrust risk where physicians seek to negotiate fees for otherwise competing colleagues.

Disadvantages

Some respond to the theory with a variety of counter-arguments.

1. *There are not enough clinical practice guidelines for this to work.* But, this theory need not be applied for every clinical condition that may be treated. It has its greatest appeal for high volume and high cost services.

2. *Information systems are too cumbersome and expensive to implement the theory.* As indicated above, for initial exercises at least, this technique can be used in a low technology manner. Once it proves itself, the cost of the infrastructure to apply the system can be subjected to a cost-benefit analysis.
3. *Cookbook medicine doesn't work.* Of course cookbook medicine doesn't work. This is not a rigid one size fits all approach. Accommodation of deviations is necessary and appropriate. This system should be applied with a degree of flexibility.
4. *This system is a liability sword rather than a shield.* This argument may be true if the approach is adopted only in part. In most instances a clinical practice guideline merely states the standard of care that otherwise would pertain. So express recognition of the standard of care and then failure to meet it can increase liability but under the theory if a physician must deviate from an adopted guideline, as long as he justifies why he did so, the standard of care still is complied with. If CPGs are adopted, but then are not followed, this information could be used in a lawsuit over a bad outcome, but the system itself does not create liability. Improper care does that.

Conclusion

The demands imposed on physicians today from multiple regulatory and market forces are too often dealt with as if they are unrelated. Many of the forces at work today are ultimately directed toward assuring the value of healthcare services—appropriate quality at reasonable cost. To produce that value some technique which facilitates a unitary organizational approach would advance the state of the art. This Unified Field Theory may permit such efforts to proceed.

Alice G. Gosfield, Esq.

References

1. See, Gosfield, "Disease Management, Demand Management and Telemedicine: The Leading Edge of Managing Care", HEALTH LAW HANDBOOK 1998 Ed., The West Group, pp. 235-265.
2. For a formal consideration of the values physicians bring to bear in accountable health care organizations and the issues to which they ought direct their energies as well as how such organizations can more effectively utilize physicians to drive a clinical culture, see Gosfield, "Quality and Clinical Culture: The Critical Role of Physicians in Accountable Health Care Organizations", American Medical Association, 1998, omss@ama-assn.org.

Subject Index

A

B

D

E

I

K

L

M

O

Q

R

S

Author Index

A

B

C

D

E

F

G

H

I

J

K

L

M

N

O

P

R

S

T

U

V

W

Y

Z